Current Management of Diabetic Retinopathy

Current Management of Diabetic Retinopathy

CAROLINE R. BAUMAL, MD
New England Eye Center
Tufts University School of Medicine
Boston, MA, United States

JAY S. DUKER, MD
New England Eye Center
Tufts University School of Medicine
Boston, MA, United States

ELSEVIER

ELSEVIER

3251 Riverport Lane
St. Louis, Missouri 63043

Content Strategist: Kayla Wolfe
Content Development Manager: Taylor Ball
Content Development Specialist: Alison Swety
Publishing Services Manager: Deepthi Unni
Project Manager: Janish Ashwin Paul
Designer: Gopalakrishnan Venkatraman

Printed in United States of America

Last digit is the print number: 9 8 7 6 5 4 3 2 1

Working together
to grow libraries in
developing countries

www.elsevier.com • www.bookaid.org

List of Contributors

Alexandra Acabá
Bryn Mawr College
Bryn Mawr, PA, United States

Sophie Bakri, MD
Professor of Ophthalmology
Mayo Clinic
Rochester, MN, United States

Caroline R. Baumal, MD
Associate Professor of Ophthalmology
Tufts University School of Medicine
New England Eye Center
Vitreoretinal Service
Tufts Medical Center
Boston, MA, United States

María H. Berrocal, MD
Berrocal & Associates
San Juan, PR, United States

Xuejing Chen, MD
Vitreoretinal Fellow
Tufts Medical Center
Boston, MA, United States

David Eichenbaum, MD
Retina Vitreous Associates of Florida
Affiliate Assistant Professor
Department of Ophthalmology
Morsani College of Medicine
University of South Florida
Tampa, Florida, United States

Avni P. Finn, MD, MBA
Vitreoretinal Fellow
Duke University Eye Center
Durham, NC, United States

Karen Jeng-Miller, MD, MPH
Department of Ophthalmology
Massachusetts Eye and Ear Infirmary
Boston, MA, United States

Rahul N. Khurana, MD
Partner
Northern California Retina Vitreous Associates
Mountain View, CA, United States
Associate Clinical Professor of Ophthalmology
University of California, San Francisco
San Francisco, CA, United States

Kendra Klein, MD
Clinical Instructor
Vitreoretinal Service
New England Eye Center
Tufts University School of Medicine
Tufts Medical Center
Boston, MA, United States

Daniel Learned, MD
Vitreoretinal Fellow
Massachusetts Eye & Ear Infirmary
Boston, MA, United States

Yannek I. Leiderman, MD, PhD
University of Illinois at Chicago
Department of Ophthalmology and Visual Sciences
Department of Bioengineering
Illinois Eye and Ear Infirmary
Chicago, IL, United States

Michelle C. Liang, MD
Assistant Professor
Tufts University School of Medicine
New England Eye Center
Vitreoretinal Service
Tufts Medical Center
Boston, MA, United States

Anat Loewenstein, MD
Director, Department of Ophthalmology
Tel Aviv Medical Center
Vice Dean, Sackler Faculty of Medicine, Tel Aviv university
Sidney Fox Chair of Ophthalmology, Incumbent
Tel Aviv, Israel

Lindsay Machen, MD
University of Illinois at Chicago
Department of Ophthalmology and Visual Sciences
Illinois Eye and Ear Infirmary
Chicago, IL, United States

Elad Moisseiev, MD
Department of Ophthalmology
Tel Aviv Medical Center
Sackler Faculty of Medicine
Tel Aviv University
Israel

Dante J. Pieramici, MD
Partner, California Retina Consultants
Co-director, California Retina Research Foundation
Santa Barbara, California
CA, United States

Sean Platt, MD
Vitreoretinal Fellow
Mayo Clinic
Rochester, MN, United States

Geraldine Slean, MD
Department of Ophthalmology
California Pacific Medical Center
San Francisco, CA, United States

Michael D. Tibbetts, MD
Tyson Eye
Cape Coral, FL, United States

Lejla Vajzovic, MD
Assistant Professor of Ophthalmology
Adult and Pediatric Vitreoretinal Surgery and Disease
Duke University Eye Center
Durham, NC, United States

Randee Miller Watson, MD
Retina Consultants of Michigan
Southfield, MI, United States

Darin R. Goldman, MD
Retina Group of Florida
Affiliate Associate Professor
Charles E. Schmidt College of Medicine
Florida Atlantic University
Boca Raton, FL, USA

Charles C. Wykoff, MD, PhD
Retina Consultants of Houston
Associate Professor of Clinical Ophthalmology
Blanton Eye Institute
Weill Cornell Medical College
Houston Methodist Hospital
Houston, Texas

Preface

TARGETING DIABETIC RETINOPATHY

Diabetes is a major health problem that is increasing in epidemic proportions globally in both developed and developing countries. This appears to be in a large part driven by obesity, although genetics, diet, sedentary lifestyle, and coexisting medical and cardiovascular risk factors also play a role. Corresponding to the increasing incidence of diabetes, there has been an increase in secondary diabetic sequelae, including diabetic retinopathy. Projections from prevalence data show that the number of individuals in the United States with diabetic retinopathy will triple from 5.5 million in 2005 to 16 million by 2050, whereas vision-threatening diabetic retinopathy will increase from 1.2 million people in 2005 to 3.4 million in 2050.[1]

Over the last 50 years, diabetic retinopathy has changed from a blinding disease to one that is treatable, with maintenance of vision in most cases. For example, in the 1960s, invasive and minimally effective pituitary ablation was evaluated to treat proliferative diabetic retinopathy because of lack of other options at that time.[2] Fortunately, major advances in pharmacologic therapy (with intravitreal anti–vascular endothelial growth factor agents or corticosteroids), laser, and surgical vitrectomy have revolutionized the current treatment paradigm for diabetic retinopathy.

Despite progress in diabetic retinopathy management, there remain many hurdles, including prevention of diabetic retinopathy, identification and directing therapy to individuals at the highest risk for diabetic visual loss, and extending the treatment effect of current therapies to make them more permanent. This book serves to discuss the risk factors and classification of diabetic retinopathy, followed by a chapter on each treatment modality. Clinical cases are presented by the authors to demonstrate complicated diabetic retinopathy management issues. The editors hope that this book answers questions and stimulates new ones regarding this complex subject.

Caroline R. Baumal, MD
Jay S. Duker, MD

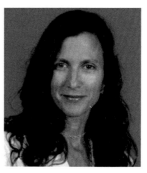

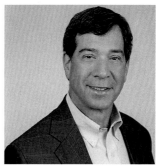

REFERENCES

1. Saaddine JB, Honeycutt AA, Narayan KM, Zhang X, Klein R, Boyle JP. Projection of diabetic retinopathy and other major eye diseases among people with diabetes mellitus: United States, 2005-2050. *Arch Ophthalmol*. 2008;126(12):1740–1747.
2. Speakman JS, Mortimer CB, Briant TDR, Exrin C, Lougheed WM, Clarke WTW. Pituitary ablation for diabetic retinopathy. *Can Med Assoc J*. 1966;94:627–635.

Acknowledgment

The editors would like to acknowledge all the contributors to this book and the team at Elsevier who worked on a timely schedule to ensure the material presented is current and concise. As well, thank you to the staff, residents, fellows, and our colleagues at New England Eye Center for being part of an amazing and thought-provoking team.

Contents

SECTION I
DIABETIC RETINOPATHY BACKGROUND

1 **Epidemiology and Natural History of Diabetic Retinopathy,** *1*
Dante J. Pieramici, MD and Daniel Learned, MD

2 **Clinical Diagnosis of Diabetic Retinopathy,** *7*
Randee M. Watson, MD, Lindsay Machen, MD and Yannek I. Leiderman, MD, PHD

3 **Classification of Diabetic Retinopathy,** *15*
Geraldine R. Slean, MS, MD and Rahul N. Khurana, MD

4 **Imaging in Diabetic Retinopathy,** *25*
Caroline R. Baumal, MD

5 **Genetics of Diabetic Retinopathy,** *37*
Karen Jeng-Miller, MD, MPH and Caroline R. Baumal, MD

SECTION II
TREATMENT OF DIABETIC RETINOPATHY

6 **Effect of Modifiable Risk Factors on the Incidence and Progression of Diabetic Retinopathy,** *41*
Michael D. Tibbetts, MD

7 **Anti–Vascular Endothelial Growth Factor Therapy for Diabetic Eye Disease,** *53*
Kendra Klein, MD and Michelle C. Liang, MD

8 **Corticosteroid Therapy for Diabetic Retinopathy,** *79*
Elad Moisseiev, MD and Anat Loewenstein, MD

9 **Laser Treatment of Diabetic Retinopathy,** *89*
Sean Platt, MD and Sophie Bakri, MD

10 **Surgical Treatment of Diabetic Retinopathy,** *101*
María H. Berrocal, MD and Alexandra Acabá

11 **Treatment of Diabetic Retinopathy in Pregnancy,** *115*
Avni P. Finn, MD, MBA and Lejla Vajzovic, MD

12 **Novel Treatments for Diabetic Retinopathy,** *123*
David Eichenbaum, MD

SECTION III
CLINICAL SCENARIOS

13 **Clinical Scenarios: Introduction,** *133*
Cases from David Eichenbaum, MD, Darin R. Goldman, MD, Charles C. Wykoff, MD, Caroline R. Baumal, MD

Clinical Scenarios: Case 1
Clinical Scenarios: Case 2
Clinical Scenarios: Case 3
Clinical Scenarios: Case 4

APPENDIX

A Summary of Diabetic Retinopathy Clinical Research Network (DRCR.net) Protocols, *149*
Caroline R. Baumal, MD and Xuejing Chen, MD

B Diabetic Terminology, *157*

INDEX, *159*

CHAPTER 1

Epidemiology and Natural History of Diabetic Retinopathy

DANIEL LEARNED, MD • DANTE J. PIERAMICI, MD

INTRODUCTION

Diabetes is an epidemic that takes a devastating toll on the body and strains healthcare systems worldwide. Although diabetes damages all organ systems, ocular complications can be particularly distressing to an otherwise functional individual. Diabetic retinopathy is currently recognized as the leading cause of vision loss in working-age adults (ages 20–65 years) and the most common cause of blindness in this population in the developed world.[1] The classic triad of clinical manifestations in diabetes includes retinopathy, nephropathy, and neuropathy. Of these, diabetic retinopathy is the most common cause of morbidity. The prevalence of diabetes mellitus (DM) continues to increase in both developed and developing countries, and thus the prevalence of diabetic retinopathy and associated vision problems is expected to grow as well. It has been shown that after 20 years, virtually all patients with type 1 diabetes and the majority of patients with type 2 diabetes have some degree of diabetic retinopathy.[2] The prevalence of diabetic retinopathy is so high that it is estimated that at any time, 10.2% of diabetic patients have some form of vision threatening retinopathy.[3]

DIABETES MELLITUS: CLASSIFICATION, PATHOGENESIS, AND EPIDEMIOLOGY

DM is an imbalance of the body's ability to make insulin or to respond appropriately to insulin. This imbalance leads to an elevated level of glucose in the blood, leading to systemic complications. More than 29 million individuals in the United States and 422 million people worldwide have diabetes.[1,4] Classically three types of diabetes are described: type 1 (insulin dependent), type 2 (insulin resistance or non–insulin dependent), and gestational DM.

Type 1 diabetes typically presents in childhood or early adulthood and is caused by the destruction of the β cells in the pancreas. This destruction leads to low insulin levels, resulting in elevated blood glucose. These individuals require exogenous supplementation of insulin to lower blood glucose. Type 1 diabetes accounts for approximately 5% of diabetes in the United States.[1] It is the most common form of diabetes in childhood, with approximately 167,000 children under 20 years of age with this disorder in 2009. More than 18,000 new cases are expected to develop each year in this age group. This is compared with 20,000 individuals younger than 20 years being diagnosed with type 2 diabetes with an estimated 5000 new type 2 cases developing yearly.[1] There is currently no way to prevent type I diabetes. A variety of racial, geographic, environmental, and genetic factors may contribute to its development, including Caucasian race, cold weather, viruses, and early diet.[5]

Type 2 diabetes accounts for 90%–95% of all patients with diabetes in the United States as well as worldwide. Type 2 diabetes is characterized by resistance to insulin. The amount of insulin the body produces is no longer sufficient to keep blood glucose in a physiologic range. The strongest risk factors for developing type 2 diabetes are physical inactivity and obesity, which also play a major role in the current worldwide diabetes epidemic.[4,6] Other risk factors include family history, genetics, and maternal diabetes.[4] In 2014, 9.3% of adults over 18 years of age were estimated to have diabetes in the United States, comprising 21 million with the clinical diagnosis and 8 million undiagnosed.[1] It is estimated that 90% of the 422 million people worldwide with diabetes, 380 million people, have type 2 diabetes.[4] There is geographic variation in diabetes prevalence both in the United States and worldwide.

During pregnancy, there are many hormonal changes in the mother that ensure that the fetus receives enough nutrients. Gestational diabetes occurs when the mother's insulin is insufficient and excessive blood glucose develops. Approximately 5%–6% of pregnancies in the

United States are complicated by gestational diabetes.[1] Gestational diabetes varies between regions and ethnic groups, and its prevalence tends to parallel that of type 2 diabetes.[1,4]

SYSTEMIC MANIFESTATIONS OF DIABETES

Elevated blood glucose has a chronic effect on the systemic micro- and macrovasculature. Diabetes contributes to systemic morbidities, such as renal failure, heart attack, neuropathy, and stroke. These complications have resulted in diabetes being the number one cause of kidney failure, lower limb amputation, and blindness in adults in the United States.[1] The vascular and metabolic complications of diabetes can be fatal and were the direct cause of death of 1.5 million people worldwide in 2012.[4]

ECONOMIC BURDEN OF DIABETES

There has been a growing economic burden related to diabetes worldwide. In the United States, diabetes contributes to more than 20% of the total healthcare costs, and the direct annual cost worldwide is greater than US $827B.[1,4] Between 2007 and 2012, there was a 41% increase in the healthcare cost in the United States, resulting in a $245 billion dollar economic burden.[7] These costs are a combination of reduced productivity ($69B) and direct medical expenses ($176B) and are expected to increase with the rising prevalence. The categories that result in the largest costs are inpatient hospital care (42%), prescription medications (18%), and physician office visits (9%), among others. The majority of these costs are covered by the government (Medicare, Medicaid, and military coverage), but patients with diabetes can expect to pay over two times more than their counterparts without diabetes. Patients with diabetes can expect to pay roughly $13,700 per year in medical expenditures and $3640 on eye care alone if retinal disease is present.[7,8]

EPIDEMIOLOGY OF DIABETIC RETINOPATHY

Diabetes is the leading cause of blindness in working-age adults in the United States.[9] The main ocular complication is diabetic retinopathy, although it can affect elsewhere in the eye, including the anterior segment and optic nerve. The three forms of diabetic retinopathy are nonproliferative diabetic retinopathy (NPDR), proliferative diabetic retinopathy (PDR), and diabetic macular edema (DME). In 2000, 4.06 million Americans were diagnosed with diabetic retinopathy. This increased to 7.69 million in 2010 and is projected to increase to over 14 million people by 2050.[9] Worldwide, diabetic retinopathy is estimated to affect roughly 93 million people.[10] One-third of the global population with diabetic retinopathy, approximately 28 million people, are estimated to have vision-threatening diabetic retinopathy defined as severe NPDR, PDR, or the presence of DME.[10,11]

Natural History of Diabetic Retinopathy

Over the past 40 years there have been a multitude of studies evaluating the risk factors, progression, and intervention impact of diabetic retinopathy. Although the natural history of type I and type 2 diabetes was initially studied independently, similar risk factors were noted between the two diseases. In general, more advanced retinal disease was found in patients with diabetes with worse glycemic and blood pressure control and longer duration of diabetes. Improvement in the control of blood pressure and glycemic control can have a beneficial effect on the ocular complications at any stage of retinopathy.

Natural History of Retinopathy in Type I DM

The Wisconsin Epidemiologic Study of Diabetic Retinopathy (WESDR) evaluated individuals diagnosed with type I (and type 2) diabetes in a single geographic area beginning in 1979 and then followed up this cohort for up to 25 years. The prevalence and severity of retinopathy was strongly related to the duration of diabetes in different age groups. Diabetic retinopathy was present in 17%–29% of patients with type I diabetes with less than 5 years diabetes duration and in 78%–97.5% who had diabetes for greater than 15 years.[12] Proliferative diabetic retinopathy was present in 1.2%–2% with less than 10 years diabetes duration and in 67% who had type 1 diabetes for over 35 years.[12] The WESDR 25-year data showed a progression of NPDR in 83%, progression to PDR in 42%, and improvement of retinopathy in 18% of patients.[13] Factors associated with the progression of retinopathy included less severe diabetic retinopathy, male sex, higher or increasing hemoglobin A1c (HbA1c level), and increased diastolic blood pressure (BP) from baseline to 4-year follow-up.[13] The risk of progression to PDR was associated with worse control of systemic diabetic disease higher or increased HbA1c, higher systolic BP, increased HbA1C, and greater body mass index at baseline).[13] Fortunately, improvement of retinopathy was associated with better control of these systemic factors (lower HbA1c, male sex, decreased HbA1c and diastolic BP).[13]

The more recent Wisconsin Diabetes Registry Study (WDRS) followed up a cohort of patients with type I diabetes in the same geographic region as the WESDR for 20 years. Newly diagnosed patients with diabetes between 1987 and 1992 who were less than 30 years old living in specific counties in Wisconsin were eligible.[14] The WDRS found the prevalence of NPDR was 6% at 4 years, 73% at 14 years, and 92% after 20 years of diabetes duration.[14,15] Compared with WESDR results, the WDRS showed an overall decrease in PDR (10% vs. 36%) and vision-threatening retinopathy (18% vs. 43%) at 20 years. Similar risk factors for the increased severity of retinopathy included longer duration of diabetes, lower education, and poor glycemic control.[14] The improved control of diabetes and hypertension during the later era of the WDRS was thought to be responsible for the reduced degree of vision-threatening diabetic retinopathy.[14,15]

Both the WESDR and WDRS supported that improved blood sugar control decreased the development and progression of diabetic retinopathy. This was also confirmed by the multicenter Diabetes Control and Complications Trial (DCCT), which assessed the link between glycemic control and the level of retinopathy, among other complications in patients with type I diabetes.[16] The DCCT showed for each decrease of mean HbA1c by 10% there was a 39% decrease in the progression of retinopathy over the range of HbA1c values.

The Epidemiology of Diabetes Interventions and Complications (EDIC) studies enrolled patients from the DCCT following its completion.[16–18] The EDIC study confirmed a prolonged benefit of intensive blood sugar control, showing a 71% and 50% odds reduction in the progression of retinopathy over a 4- and 10-year period following the DCCT, respectively.[17,18]

Natural History of Retinopathy in Type II DM
The effect of glycemic control on the level of retinopathy and the natural history of patients with type 2 diabetes is similar to that of patients with type I diabetes, and poor control of diabetes, blood glucose, blood pressure, and obesity has been associated with more severe diabetic retinopathy and poorer visual outcomes. These studies were also consistent in showing that improved management of systemic risk factors reduced retinopathy progression as well as the need for treatment of retinopathy.

The United Kingdom Prospective Diabetes Study (UKPDS) enrolled patients with newly diagnosed type II DM and separated them into "intensive" and "conventional" glucose control groups.[19] At the time of diagnosis, ~40% of patients had retinopathy consisting of microaneurysms or worse in one eye.[20] Patients with intensive glucose control showed a 21% reduction in retinopathy

and a decreased need for panretinal photocoagulation by 29% compared with the conventional group.[17,19]

The UKPDS-Hypertension in Diabetes Study (UKPDS-HDS) analyzed the progression of retinopathy and vision loss related to blood pressure control in the setting of type II diabetes. Newly diagnosed patients with type II diabetes were divided into a tightly controlled hypertension group (blood pressure less than 150/85) and a less tightly controlled group (blood pressure less than 180/105). The HbA1c was similar in each group at intervals of less than 5 years and greater than 5 years. There were significant differences in the prevalence of microaneurysms in the tight versus conventional controlled hypertension groups at 4.5 years (23.3% vs. 33.5%, p=0.003) and hard exudates at 7.5 years (11.2% vs. 18.3%, p<0.001). Of note, fewer patients in the tight blood pressure control group showed two-step deterioration of retinopathy compared to the less tightly controlled group (RR 0.66; p<0.01). Twice as many subjects in the conventional BP controlled group changed by more than 10 steps on the ETDRS scale.[21] The UKPDS-HDS was critical in showing the natural history of blood pressure on progression of retinopathy and the need for hypertension treatment in patients with diabetes.

It is important to note that studies such as the ETDRS help establish the natural history of diabetes regardless of type 1 or type 2 and the risk of progression to proliferative disease. The ETDRS suggested a 15% risk of progressing to high-risk PDR within a 1-year period if severe NPDR is present, which increases to more than 50% if very severe NPDR is present.[17,22]

PREVALENCE OF DME
The WESDR showed an incidence over a 10-year period of 20.1% and a 25-year cumulative incidence of 29% for patients with type I diabetes.[23,24] This peaked at 14 years and had a minimal increase from years 14 to 25.[23] The incidence of DME in type 2 DM is inconsistent.[25] In various population-based studies, the prevalence of DME ranges between 4.2% and 7.9% for type 1 and 1.4%–12.8% in type 2 DM.[25] It is currently estimated that 750,000 people with diabetes are affected by DME.[11]

MANAGEMENT OF NPDR AND PDR
The management of diabetic retinopathy includes prevention via glycemic and hypertensive control at any stage of eye disease, which has a beneficial effect on patients with type 1 and type 2 diabetes. The modifiable and nonmodifiable risk factors that affect diabetic retinopathy progression are reviewed in Chapter 6.

The treatment of PDR and DME is focused on inducing regression of retinal neovascularization and macular thickening, respectively, inhibiting recurrences and preventing complications such as vitreous hemorrhage and tractional retinal detachments to prevent vision loss. Historically, laser had been the first-line treatment for both PDR and DME (see Chapter 9). An expansion of potential treatment options, including anti–vascular endothelial growth factor (VEGF) agents (Chapter 7) and corticosteroids (Chapter 8), has led to a more patient-based treatment plan. The Diabetic Retinopathy Study found that panretinal laser photocoagulation (PRP) reduced the risk of severe vision loss by 50%–60% in eyes with high-risk PDR.[26] The results were less definitive regarding the efficacy of PRP for severe NPDR or PDR without high-risk features. This study led to the recommendation for timely PRP in eyes with PDR with specific high-risk features. More recently, Protocol S from the DRCR.net studies (Appendix A) showed noninferiority of ranibizumab injections compared with PRP with regards to progression of PDR.[27] Results suggest that visual results may be superior with ranibizumab compared to PRP in eyes with both PDR and DME at 2 years. Those eyes with PDR without DME seem to have similar results with either PRP laser or repeated ranibizumab injections.[27] Repeated ranibizumab injections could be considered as the sole management of PDR with potential benefits over PRP, including a reduction in visual field loss, reduced risk of vitreous hemorrhage, and reduced need for vitrectomy surgery.[27] In the setting of vitreous hemorrhage or tractional retinal detachment, surgical intervention may be required (Chapter 10). In real-world clinical scenarios, the choice of anti-VEGF injections, PRP, or a combination of both modalities depends on multiple factors, including patient compliance, ability to return for follow-up, treatment availability, laterality, and cost. It is critical to be aware of the potential issues surrounding the various treatment options to offer patients the highest level of success.

MANAGEMENT OF DME

Anti-VEGF agents are currently the treatment of choice for center-involved DME (CI-DME), with intravitreal corticosteroid and focal macular laser photocoagulation as secondary options. There has been an explosion in clinical studies of new agents and combination therapies for DME in recent years. The ETDRS study defined clinically significant macular edema (CSME) and demonstrated that focal laser reduced moderate vision loss by approximately 50%, making this modality the mainstay of DME therapy for decades.[22] CSME was defined as one

of the following: (1) retinal thickening within 500 μm of the macular center, (2) hard exudates within 500 μm of the macular center with adjacent retinal thickening, or (3) one or more disc diameters of retinal thickening within one disc diameter from the fovea center (Chapter 3).[22] The ETDRS had established focal macular laser as the standard of care; however, anti-VEGF agents have surpassed focal macular laser because of the superior anatomic effects and visual improvements. The focus has also changed as currently OCT is utilized to assess whether DME involves the center of the fovea (CI-DME), compared to prior emphasis on clinical determination of CSME (Chapter 2). The three anti-VEGF agents that are most often used in the United States include bevacizumab (off label), ranibizumab, and aflibercept, with support from multiple studies such as the RIDE/RISE, VIVID/VISTA, BOLT, DRCR trials and others outlined in Chapter 7, which confirm the superiority of anti-VEGF injection over macular laser for visual improvement.

SUMMARY

Diabetes is a longitudinal systemic condition that has become a healthcare epidemic worldwide. Systemic management of diabetes and hypertension is critical. First-line therapy for CI-DME is currently intravitreal anti-VEGF injection. Laser and intravitreal corticosteroid injection remain as other treatment options for DME. Treatment options for PDR may include one or combination of the following: PRP, injection of intravitreal anti-VEGF agent, surgery, or a combination of therapies. Close management and longitudinal as-needed treatment can prevent vision loss and help regain a substantial amount of vision in the majority of patients. Patients should be prepared for long-term, frequent evaluation and potential for episodic or continual treatment to improve vision and reduce complications from diabetic retinopathy.

REFERENCES

1. Centers for Disease Control and Prevention. *2014 National Diabetes Report Card*. Atlanta, GA: US Department of Health and Human Services, Centers for Disease Control and Prevention; 2014.
2. Wong TY, Klein R, Islam FMA, et al. Diabetic retinopathy in a multi-ethnic cohort in the United States. *Am J Ophthalmol*. 2006;141(3):446–455.
3. Centers for Disease Control and Prevention. *National Diabetes Fact Sheet: National Estimates and General Information on Diabetes and Prediabetes in the United States*. Atlanta, GA: U.S. Department of Health and Human Services, Centers for Disease Control and Prevention; 2011.

4. World Health Organization. *Global Report on Diabetes*. Geneva; 2016.

5. *Genetics of Diabetes*. American Diabetes Association; March 8, 2017. www.diabetes.org/diabetes-basics/genetics-of-diabetes.html.

6. Forouzanfar MH, et al. Global, regional, and national comparative risk assessment of 79 behavioural, environmental and occupational, and metabolic risks or clusters of risks in 188 countries, 1990–2013: a systematic analysis for the Global Burden of Disease Study 2013. *Lancet*. 2015;386:2287–2323.

7. American Diabetes Association. Economic costs of diabetes in the US in 2012. *Diabetes Care*. 2013;36:1033–1046.

8. Wittenborn JS, et al. The economic burden of vision loss and eye disorders among the United States population younger than 40 years. *Ophthalmology*. 2013;120(9):1728–1735.

9. *Diabetic Retinopathy*. National Eye Institute. U.S. Department of Health and Human Services; (n.d.).

10. Yau JW, Rogers SL, Kawasaki R, et al. Global prevalence and major risk factors of diabetic retinopathy. *Diabetes Care*. 2012;35(3):556–564.

11. *Facts About Macular Edema*. National Eye Institute. U.S. Department of Health and Human Services; October 01, 2015.

12. Klein R, Klein BE, Moss SE, et al. The Wisconsin Epidemiologic Study of Diabetic Retinopathy. II. Prevalence and risk of diabetic retinopathy when age at diagnosis is less than 30 years. *Arch Ophthalmol*. 1984;102:520–526.

13. Klein R, et al. The Wisconsin epidemiologic study of diabetic retinopathy XXII: the twenty-five-year progression of retinopathy in persons with type 1 diabetes. *Ophthalmology*. 2008;115(11):1859–1868.

14. LeCaire T, Palta M, Klein R, et al. Assessing progress in retinopathy outcomes in type 1 diabetes. *Diabetes Care*. 2013;36(3):631–637.

15. Lecaire T, Palta M, Zhang H, et al. Lower-than-expected prevalence and severity of retinopathy in an incident cohort followed during the first 4–14 years of type 1 diabetes the Wisconsin diabetes Registry study. *Am J Epidemiol*. 2006;164(2):143–150.

16. Diabetes Control and Complications Trial/Epidemiology of Diabetes Interventions and Complications Research Group. Retinopathy and nephropathy in patients with type 1 diabetes four years after a trial of intensive therapy. *N Engl J Med*. 2000;342:381–389.

17. Preferred Practice Committee. *Diabetic Retinopathy PPP–Updated 2016*. American Academy Ophthalmology; 2014.

18. Diabetes Control and Complications Trial, and Epidemiology of Diabetes Interventions and Complications Research Group. Prolonged effect of intensive therapy on the risk of retinopathy complications in patients with type 1 diabetes mellitus: 10 years after the Diabetes Control and Complications Trial. *Arch Ophthalmol*. 2008;126(12):1707.

19. UK Prospective Diabetes Study (UKPDS) Group. Intensive blood-glucose control with sulphonylureas or insulin compared with conventional treatment and risk of complications in patients with type 2 diabetes (UKPDS 33). *Lancet*. 1998;352:837–853.

20. Kohner EM, Aldington SJ, Stratton IM, et al. United Kingdom Prospective Diabetes Study, 30: diabetic retinopathy at diagnosis of non–insulin-dependent diabetes mellitus and associated risk factors. *Arch Ophthalmol*. 1998;116(3):297–303.

21. UK Prospective Diabetes Study (UKPDS) Group. Risks of progression of retinopathy and vision loss related to tight blood pressure control in type 2 diabetes mellitus: UKPDS 69. *Arch Ophthalmol*. 2004;122(11):1631.

22. Early Treatment Diabetic Retinopathy Study Research Group. Early-treatment diabetic retinopathy study. *JAMA*. 1981;245(6):566.

23. Klein R, Knudston M, Lee K, Gangnon R, Klein B. The Wisconsin epidemiologic study of diabetic retinopathy XXIII: the twenty-five-year incidence of macular edema in persons with type 1 diabetes. *Ophthalmology*. 2009;116(3):497–503.

24. Klein R, Klein BE, Moss SE, Cruickshanks KJ. The Wisconsin Epidemiologic Study of Diabetic Retinopathy. XV. The long-term incidence of macular edema. *Ophthalmology*. 1995;102(1):7–16.

25. Lee R, Wong TY, Sabanayagam C. Epidemiology of diabetic retinopathy, diabetic macular edema and related vision loss. *Eye Vis (Lond)*. 2015;2:17. Published online September 30, 2015.

26. The Diabetic Retinopathy Study Research Group. Photocoagulation treatment of proliferative diabetic retinopathy. Clinical application of Diabetic Retinopathy Study (DRS) findings, DRS report number 8. *Ophthalmology*. 1981;88:583–600.

27. Diabetic Retinopathy Clinical Research Network. Panretinal photocoagulation vs intravitreous ranibizumab for proliferative diabetic retinopathy: a randomized trial. *JAMA*. 2015;314(20):2137–2146.

CHAPTER 2

Clinical Diagnosis of Diabetic Retinopathy

RANDEE M. WATSON, MD • LINDSAY MACHEN, MD • YANNEK I. LEIDERMAN, MD, PHD

INTRODUCTION

Diabetes is a leading cause of morbidity including vision loss in the United States in working age adults.[1,2] According to the Centers for Disease Control and Prevention (CDC), diabetes mellitus (DM) affected 29.1 million Americans in 2014—about 9.3% of the population.[3] This estimate includes 21.0 million persons diagnosed with diabetes and 8.1 million people with undiagnosed disease.[1] Diabetic retinopathy (DR) may affect up to half of the diabetic population and is the leading cause of vision loss in the United States.[4]

The American Diabetes Association (ADA) and the National Eye Institute (NEI) recommend that patients with diabetes undergo a dilated eye examination at least once per year, with more frequent examinations in individuals with DR[5,6]. Despite these guidelines, a significant proportion of patients with diabetes do not receive annual dilated fundus examination (DFE).[3] It is estimated that only 50%–70% of diabetics in the United States receive annual DFEs.[7] Persons under age 18 years have even lower rates of yearly comprehensive eye examinations compared with their adult counterparts.[8] Factors associated with a decreased likelihood of receiving annual diabetic eye examinations include younger age, lower income, lower education level, lack of health insurance, lack of access to diabetic education classes, and non-insulin-dependent disease.[9]

The estimated prevalence of DR among persons with known type 2 diabetes based on a pooled analysis of data from eight large population-based eye surveys was 40.3%.[2] The estimated prevalence of vision-threatening retinopathy (defined as proliferative diabetic retinopathy [PDR], severe nonproliferative diabetic retinopathy [NPDR], and/or macular edema) was 8.2%, with macular edema being the most frequent cause of vision loss in diabetes.[2,10] Given the morbidity of vision loss associated with undetected DR, and the availability of treatment modalities effective in preventing or retarding the progression of vision loss from diabetic eye disease, timely and effective ophthalmic screening examinations in diabetic patients are imperative.

SCREENING RECOMMENDATIONS

The timing of the recommended initial screening examination for DR (Table 2.1) is based on the age at onset and type of DM, whereas the frequency of follow-up examinations is based on the level of DR (Table 2.2). Systemic risk factors that may exacerbate DR (such as hypertension, poor or fluctuating glycemic control, renal failure), as well as patient adherence to the treatment regimen, should be taken into account and may lead to more frequent eye examinations. [11,12]

Children with type 1 DM should commence annual dilated eye examinations at the start of puberty or at 10 years of age, whichever is earlier, once the child has had diabetes for 3–5 years. Children and adolescents with type 2 DM should have yearly dilated eye examinations commencing at the time of diagnosis.[13]

Adults with type 2 diabetes should have a prompt examination at the time of diagnosis. As the onset of type 2 diabetes is often not well defined, many patients have had elevated blood glucose for years preceding the formal diagnosis. Up to 30% of newly diagnosed patients with diabetes have some clinical sign of DR at the initial eye examination.[14,15] If there is no retinopathy by clinical examination, yearly examination is recommended. More frequent examinations are based on the level of retinopathy and potential need for treatment.

Women with preexisting diabetes (type 1 or type 2) who become pregnant should have a baseline dilated eye examination early in the first trimester with further monitoring as indicated based on the extent of retinopathy because of the increased risk of progression of preexisting DR.[16–19] If no DR is found, then an examination each trimester is indicated unless the patient develops symptoms, which should prompt earlier follow-up care. Pregnant patients with preexisting NPDR or PDR should be reexamined every 1–2 months. Women who develop gestational diabetes do not require an eye examination during pregnancy and do not appear to be at increased risk of developing DR during pregnancy. However, it is important to be aware that these women are at increased risk for developing nongestational DM later in life and

TABLE 2.1
Timing of Initial Ophthalmic Examination in Diabetes

Patient Population	Recommended Initial Evaluation
Adults > 18 years of age	At time of diagnosis of diabetes
Pregnant women with preexisting diabetes mellitus	
Type 1 or type 2	Early in first trimester
Children < 18 years of age	
Type 1	At puberty, or age 10 years, whichever is earlier (after duration of diabetes 3–5 years)
Type 2	At time of diagnosis of diabetes

TABLE 2.2
Examination Intervals and Treatment Options in Diabetic Eye Disease

Degree of Retinopathy	Follow-Up (months)	Treatment Options
No diabetic retinopathy	12	Observation
Mild NPDR	9–12	Observation
Moderate NPDR	6–9	Observation
Severe NPDR	3–4	Observation May consider early PRP or anti-VEGF in some situations
Very severe NPDR	3–4	Observation May consider early PRP or anti-VEGF in some situations
Early PDR, no high-risk features	2–4	Observation Consider early PRP and/or anti-VEGF injection
PDR, with high-risk features[a]	1–3	PRP and/or anti-VEGF injection
WITH DME PRESENT		
Center-involving DME and NPDR[a]	1–3	Anti-VEGF injection, Focal macular laser, Intravitreal steroid
Non-center-involving DME and NPDR	2–4	Observation May consider focal macular laser or anti-VEGF in some cases
DME and PDR[a]	1–2	Anti-VEGF injection, PRP laser Focal macular laser Combination focal macular laser and PRP Combination anti-VEGF and PRP Other treatment combinations possible

DME, diabetic macular edema; *NPDR*, nonproliferative diabetic retinopathy; *PDR*, proliferative diabetic retinopathy; *PRP*, panretinal laser photocoagulation; *VEGF*, vascular endothelial growth factor. The above-suggested examination intervals are broadly representative of each disease stage; some patients may require more intensive monitoring, and examination intervals should be determined individually for each patient. The recommended interval for follow-up may vary based on the proposed therapy. The therapeutic options are outlined in the upcoming chapters.
[a]In the setting of ongoing treatment for PDR and/or DME.

that they should have ophthalmic examinations as described earlier if this occurs.

HISTORY AND EXAMINATION

Components of a complete diabetic eye examination include a detailed medical and ocular history and ophthalmic examination with dilated funduscopy. High-quality fundus photographs have been utilized for telemedicine screening for retinopathy in patients with diabetes who have not had previous treatment or other eye disease.[20–24] However, screening via fundus photography does not obviate the need for ophthalmic examinations, particularly in the setting of retinopathy or other eye disease.

A thorough diabetic history should be obtained as part of the detailed medical history. Salient items include the duration and type of diabetes, the presence and historic degree of blood glucose control as assessed by the percentage of glycosylated hemoglobin (HbA1C%), whether the patient is receiving insulin, and the presence of other diabetes-associated conditions, such as hypertension, dyslipidemia, kidney disease, and peripheral neuropathy, as these factors may be correlated with the progression of retinopathy. The patient should be specifically questioned about any previous diagnosis of or treatment for diabetic eye disease, including prior intravitreal injection and laser photocoagulation, in addition to standard queries regarding previous ocular surgery, trauma, amblyopia, or presence of concomitant eye disease.

The complete diabetic ocular examination includes, at a minimum, the assessment of the best-corrected visual acuity in each eye, measurement of intraocular pressure, pupillary evaluation, evaluation of the anterior chamber via slit-lamp biomicroscopy, and stereoscopic DFE. The iris should be examined before pupillary dilation to assess for anterior segment neovascularization. If *rubeosis iridis* is detected or suspected, gonioscopy should also be performed to assess for neovascularization of the angle. Additional ocular findings related to in diabetes include cataract, reduced corneal sensation, corneal epithelial defect, glaucoma, and optic nerve abnormalities.

DFE should include stereoscopic evaluation of the posterior pole, peripheral retina, and vitreous. Attention is given to identifying signs of nonproliferative retinopathy, PDR, and macular edema. Evaluation of the macula and postequatorial retina is best performed with noncontact or contact lens stereoscopic biomicroscopy. Binocular indirect ophthalmoscopy or wide-field contact lens slit-lamp biomicroscopy is utilized to examine the peripheral retina. Table 2.3 summarizes the key components of the complete ocular examination in diabetes.

The earliest clinically evident ocular manifestation is NPDR. Clinical signs of NPDR include microaneurysms, dot and blot intraretinal hemorrhages, cotton wool spots, intraretinal microvascular abnormalities (IRMAs), retinal edema, retinal exudate, and dilation and beading of retinal veins. Microaneurysms, small saccular outpouchings of retinal capillaries, usually represent the first clinical sign of NPDR. They appear as small, 25- to 100-μm deep red round dots in the posterior pole. Breakdown of the blood-retinal barrier occurs early in the disease process and may result in focal areas of retinal thickening with or without the deposition of hard exudates, visible as intraretinal, extravascular, yellow deposits of lipid-laden material (Fig. 2.1). The clinical appearance of intraretinal hemorrhage depends on the layer of the retina in which the focal bleeding occurs (Fig. 2.2). Hemorrhages in the nerve fiber layer assume a flame shape as blood dissects among the axons in the superficial retina. Conversely, hemorrhages emanating from the deep capillary plexuses appear dot or blot shaped. Blot hemorrhages refer to foci of blood that appear larger than microaneurysms. Focal nerve fiber layer infarcts, or cotton wool spots, appear as white, fluffy, superficial inner retinal lesions. These represent acute obstruction of axoplasmic transport from compromised perfusion of the affected retina. Intraretinal microvascular abnormalities (IRMA) are abnormal branching, sinuous shunt

TABLE 2.3
Diabetic History and Examination Components

Complete Medical History	Components
Medical history	• Duration and type of diabetes • Glycemic control/HbA1C% • Blood pressure control • Cardiovascular disease assessment • Other diabetic complications, including neuropathy, nephropathy, peripheral vascular disease
Ocular history	• Previous diagnosis of diabetic eye disease • Prior treatment for diabetic retinopathy • Presence of other ocular disorders
Ophthalmoscopic Examination	• Visual acuity • Pupillary examination • Intraocular pressure
Anterior segment biomicroscopy	• Nondilated pupil examination for iris neovascularization • Cataract assessment • Cornea
Gonioscopy	• If iris neovascularization present/suspected • If other signs of proliferative diabetic retinopathy are present, such as retinal neovascularization, vitreous hemorrhage, or tractional retinal detachment
Dilated fundus examination	• Assess for nonproliferative diabetic retinopathy, proliferative diabetic retinopathy, diabetic macular edema
Slit-lamp biomicroscopy of posterior segment	• High-magnification examination of vitreous, optic nerve, macula, retina
Indirect ophthalmoscopy	• Peripheral retinal examination

vessels that typically develop adjacent to areas of capillary nonperfusion or cotton wool spots. IRMAs are by definition within the plane of the retina (intraretinal) and are thought to represent either new vessel growth or remodeling of preexisting vessels. Retinal venous dilation and beading is associated with progressive capillary disruption and retinal ischemia, frequently

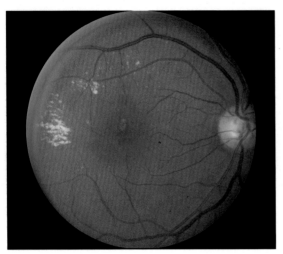

FIG. 2.1 Hard exudates. Intraretinal, extravascular, yellow deposits of lipid-laden material are present temporal and superior to the macula.

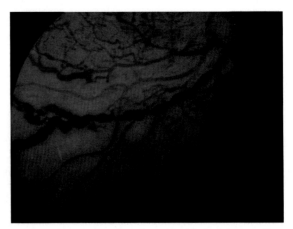

FIG. 2.3 Venous beading. Segmental foci of venous dilatation give the appearance of a "string-of-sausage" in this prominent example of venous beading. Diffuse retinal neovascularization is present in the superior half of the image.

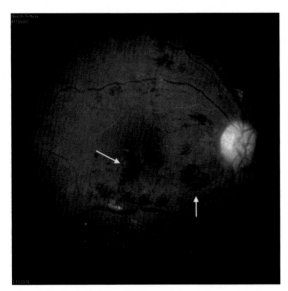

FIG. 2.2 Diabetic intraretinal hemorrhage. Nerve fiber layer hemorrhage exhibits a flame shape as blood dissects among the axons in the superficial retina (*white arrow*). Blot and dot hemorrhages (*yellow arrow*) are scattered about the macula. Sclerotic retinal arteries are apparent as white vessels.

occurring within the presence of significant intraretinal hemorrhages and IRMAs (Fig. 2.3).

Evidence of PDR includes neovascularization of the optic disc (NVD) or affecting the retina (termed neovascularization elsewhere, NVE), preretinal or vitreous hemorrhage arising from neovascularization of

the posterior segment, neovascularization of the iris or anterior chamber angle not associated with other disease entities, and tractional retinal detachment (TRD). Binocular indirect ophthalmoscopy may fail to reveal subtle retinal neovascularization; slit-lamp biomicroscopy is thus recommended in the evaluation for proliferative retinopathy. Fluorescein angiography may reveal leakage from retinal neovascular complexes, aiding in the detection of retinal neovascularization. With the advent of wide-field fluorescein angiography, investigations that strive to correlate quantitation of retinal nonperfusion with risk of progression to PDR are under way; the goal of this research is to provide an imaging-based biomarker of risk of progression to vision-threatening retinopathy.[25,26]

Posterior segment neovascularization often originates within 45 degrees of the optic disc or from the optic disc itself[20]; however, more anterior retinal neovascularization is not uncommon. NVE arises from existing retinal vessels, typically adjacent to areas of nonperfusion, and is commonly located in the superotemporal or inferonasal quadrants. NVD arises from vessels on the optic disc and generally occurs in the setting of significant peripheral nonperfusion. Early-stage NVD often appears as small loops or a fine vascular network on the surface of the optic nerve or juxtapapillary retina (Fig. 2.4). These small-caliber vessels may remain undetected if the optic disc is not carefully examined using slit-lamp biomicroscopy. Maturation of an optic disc neovascular complex may proceed by organization into a radial, spoke-like pattern, although asymmetric complexes

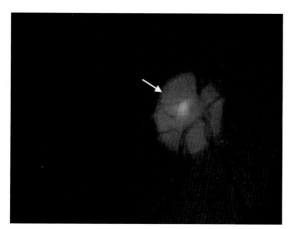

FIG. 2.4 Early neovascularization of the optic disc (NVD). Early NVD are fine vessels detected during slit-lamp biomicroscopy of the optic nerve head (ONH). These vessels are best appreciated overlying the rim of the ONH (*white arrow*) in normally avascular-appearing disc segments between the larger retinal vessels coursing over the ONH rim.

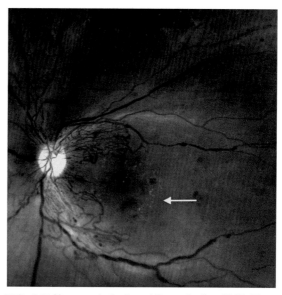

FIG. 2.5 Neovascularization of the optic disc (NVD). The mature NVD complex exhibits organization into a radial, spoke-like pattern with interconnections among the spokes and extension of the neovascular complex to the juxtapapillary retina. Intraretinal hemorrhage and hard exudates are present within the macula (*yellow arrow*).

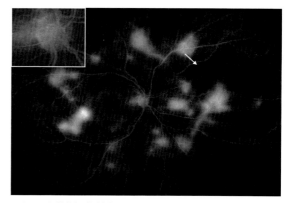

FIG. 2.6 Wide-field fluorescein angiogram in proliferative diabetic retinopathy (PDR) with neovascularization of the disc and retina. Multiple foci of leakage from retinal neovascular complexes are present. There is leakage from neovascular tissue involving the superotemporal aspect of the optic disc (inset) illustrated in the color photo in Fig. 2.4. Large patchy areas of nonperfusion are present (*white arrow*).

are frequent (Fig. 2.5). Neovascular complexes may be associated with both underlying retinal arteries and veins, a feature unique to diabetic eye disease. Distinguishing early retinal neovascularization (NVE) from IRMA can be challenging. Fluorescein angiography may be a helpful adjunct in corroborating the presence of NVD (Fig. 2.6) and distinguishing NVE from IRMAs, which generally do not leak dye to the same extent as neovascular tissue. In addition, IRMAs are in the plane of the retina, whereas neovascular vessels are generally of lesser caliber than IRMA and located at the interface between the posterior hyaloid and retina.

Vitreous hemorrhage may occur in association with several factors. Vitreous traction may cause bleeding from a direct mechanical effect on neovascular tissue. For example, evolving posterior vitreous detachment may induce an avulsion of neovascular or preexisting retinal vessels with associated hemorrhage. Hemorrhage can also be associated with Valsalva maneuvers, such as coughing or vomiting, in eyes with neovascularization. The onset of vitreous hemorrhage may occur during sleep without an obvious inciting factor. Preretinal hemorrhage results when bleeding occurs in the setting of an attached or partially detached posterior hyaloid. Loculated blood may assume a boat-shaped configuration, resulting from the effect of gravity in an upright patient (Fig. 2.7).

Maturation of a retinal neovascular complex refers to clinically visible proliferation of fibroglial elements manifested as a white fibrotic tissue component of the neovascular frond, concurrent with growth of the neovascular tissue with invasion of the overlying posterior hyaloid (Fig. 2.8). This process is referred to as

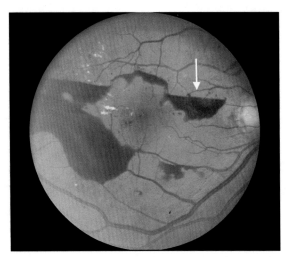

FIG. 2.7 Preretinal hemorrhage. Multiple foci of loculated hemorrhage are present between the posterior hyaloid and the retina. The discrete borders and relatively flat appearance of the subhyaloid hemorrhage contrasts with the more diffuse appearance of hemorrhage within the vitreous. The boat-shaped hemorrhage (*white arrow*) represents settling of pooled blood from the effects of gravity in an upright patient.

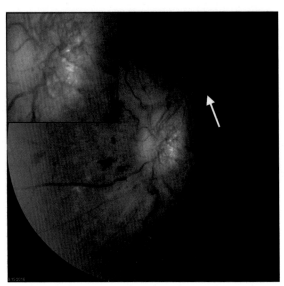

FIG. 2.8 Maturation of optic disc- and retinal neovascularization. As the neovascularization of the disc complex matures, there is an increase in the lesion area, increased fibroglial component, and progressive invasion of the vitreous (inset). The white arcuate lesion (*white arrow*) is the fibroglial component of a large retinal neovascular complex overlying the superotemporal vascular arcade.

fibrovascular proliferation (FVP). The fibroglial component may remain in the presence of decreased perfusion or "regression" of the neovascular element, e.g., following pharmacologic or laser photocoagulation treatment of PDR with a significant FVP component. Contraction of FVP or vitreous traction may induce distortion of the underlying retinal architecture and progress to TRD. Fibrous proliferation is most prominent overlying the temporal vascular arcades (Fig. 2.8), and the retina in this area is often preferentially affected by tractional pathology, which can progress to involve the fovea. Features of diabetic TRD include a concave or flat configuration, localization to the posterior fundus, and taut retinal surface in the area of detachment, lacking corrugations or shifting fluid. Further progression of tractional forces may induce a retinal break, leading to combined tractional-rhegmatogenous retinal detachment (CTRRD). Progression to rhegmatogenous detachment is often associated with a rapid reduction in vision if the fovea is involved. The retinal breaks are often located posterior to the equator. In most cases, only partial separation of the posterior hyaloid is present, and some cases exhibit complete attachment of the posterior hyaloid. It is important to recognize when a previously stable extrafoveal diabetic TRD develops new rhegmatogenous features, as these eyes often require prompt surgery and carry a worse prognosis.

TABLE 2.4
Examination Findings in the Assessment of NPDR Versus PDR

NPDR	PDR
Microaneurysms	Neovascularization
Hard/lipid exudate	of the optic nerve,
Retinal hemorrhage (dot/blot)	retina, iris
Cotton wool spot	Vitreous hemorrhage
Venous beading	Tractional retinal
Retinal nonperfusion	detachment
Intraretinal microvascular	
abnormalities	
Retinal Edema	
Diabetic macular edema	

NPDR, nonproliferative diabetic retinopathy; *PDR*, proliferative diabetic retinopathy.

Retinoschisis may also be a consequence of progressive traction. The examination features associated with NPDR and PDR are summarized in Table 2.4.

Diabetic macular edema (DME) is defined by the presence of retinal thickening or fluid-filled cysts within the macula and may also be associated with focal submacular fluid. It is a consequence of retinal vascular hyperpermeability with exudation of fluid from incompetent macular retinal capillaries and occurs in eyes along a wide spectrum of retinopathy, from mild NPDR to PDR. On clinical examination, edema is often observed as focal retinal thickening adjacent to prominent microaneurysms and may be encountered adjacent to hard exudates in a ring or circinate pattern. DME is frequently categorized as center-involving, when affecting the central macula, or non-center-involving, in cases of extrafoveal thickening. These descriptors are generally applied to differentiate DME that requires treatment in the case of center-involving DME from non-center-involving DME, which may not require ophthalmic intervention; the latter is an area of active investigation.[27] DME has also been described as focal or diffuse; however, this terminology may not be useful in clinical practice or research, as no standardized definitions have been formulated, and evidence is lacking that this distinction aids in guiding treatment.[28]

The Early Treatment Diabetic Retinopathy Study (ETDRS) defined clinically significant diabetic macular edema (CSME) as edema fulfilling any one of the following three criteria: (1) retinal thickening within 500 μm of the center of the macula, (2) hard exudates within 500 μm of the center of the macula with adjacent retinal thickening, or (3) retinal thickening at least one disc area in size, any part of which is within one disc diameter of the center of the macula (ETDRS Report 2).[29] CSME was defined as meeting the threshold of disease at which treatment with macular laser photocoagulation was implemented. Identification of CSME was initially based on clinical examination using slit-lamp biomicroscopy with a contact or noncontact fundus lens. Biomicroscopy has been largely supplanted by optical coherence tomography (OCT) in the assessment of DME, as OCT is more sensitive than clinical examination and allows for quantitative measures that greatly facilitate interval comparisons for clinical and research purposes.[30,31,32]

CONCLUSION

Given the prevalence of undetected DR and the existence of effective modalities for the prevention and treatment of vision loss, timely and effective screening examinations of patients with diabetes are imperative. Accepted methods include either a complete diabetic eye examination that includes dilated funduscopy or assessment of high-quality fundus images in patients without previous treatment for DR or other eye disease. The components of a complete diabetic eye examination include detailed medical and ocular histories and ophthalmic examination with dilated funduscopy. Ophthalmic imaging with OCT or FA may be indicated based upon the clinical findings. Patients should be informed that progressive diabetic eye disease is often asymptomatic until is it advanced and that prevention of visual loss is the primary goal, facilitated by timely screening examinations.

ACKNOWLEDGMENTS

The authors wish to thank Mark Janowicz and Andrea Degillio, CRA, CDOS in the Ophthalmic Imaging Division of the UIC Department of Ophthalmology and Visual Sciences for their expert abilities in performing the imaging studies and any processing of ophthalmic images included in this chapter.

REFERENCES

1. Sherrod CE, Vitale S, Frick KD, Ramulu PY. Association of vision loss and work status in the United States. *JAMA Ophthalmol.* 2014;132:1239–1242.
2. Kempen JH, O'Colmain BJ, Leske MC, et al. The prevalence of diabetic retinopathy among adults in the United States. *Arch Ophthalmol.* 2004;122:552–563.
3. Centers for Disease Control and Prevention. *National Diabetes Statistics Report: Estimates of Diabetes and Its Burden in the United States, 2014.* Atlanta, GA: US Department of Health and Human Services; 2014.
4. Zhang X, Saaddine JB, Chou CF, et al. Prevalence of diabetic retinopathy in the United States, 2005-2008. *JAMA.* 2010;304:649–656.
5. American Diabetes Association. Eye Care. Available from: http://www.diabetes.org/living-with-diabetes/complications/eye-complications/eye-care.html.
6. National Eye Institute. Diabetic Eye Disease. Available from: https://nei.nih.gov/diabetes.
7. Brechner RJ, Cowie CC, Howie LJ, et al. Ophthalmic examination among adults with diagnosed diabetes mellitus. *JAMA.* 1993;270:1714–1718.
8. Tapley JL, McGwin Jr G, Ashraf AP, et al. Feasibility and efficacy of diabetic retinopathy screening among youth with diabetes in a pediatric endocrinology clinic: a cross-sectional study. *Diabetol Metab Syndr.* 2015;7:56.
9. Paskin-Hall A, Dent ML, Dong F, Ablah E. Factors contributing to diabetes patients not receiving annual dilated eye examinations. *Ophthalmic Epidemiol.* 2013;20:281–287.
10. Arevalo JF. Diabetic macular edema: current management 2013. *World J Diabetes.* 2013;4(6):231–233.
11. Klein R, Knudtson MD, Lee KE, Gangnon R, Klein BE. The Wisconsin epidemiologic study of diabetic retinopathy: XXII the twenty-five-year progression of retinopathy in persons with type 1 diabetes. *Ophthalmology.* 2008;115:1859–1868.

12. Aiello LP, Cahill MT, Wong JS. Systemic considerations in the management of diabetic retinopathy. *Am J Ophthalmol*. 2001;132(5):760–776.

13. American Diabetes Association. Children and adolescents. *Diabetes Care*. 2015;38(suppl 1):S70–S76. Available from: http://care.diabetesjournals.org/content/38/Supplement_1/S70.

14. Owsley C, McGwin Jr G, Lee DJ, et al. Diabetes eye screening in urban settings serving minority populations: detection of diabetic retinopathy and other ocular findings using telemedicine. *JAMA Ophthalmol*. 2015;133:174–181.

15. Sprafka JM, Fritsche TL, Baker R, Kurth D, Whipple D. Prevalence of undiagnosed eye disease in high-risk diabetic individuals. *Arch Intern Med*. 1990;150:857–861.

16. Klein BE, Moss SE, Klein R. Effect of pregnancy on progression of diabetic retinopathy. *Diabetes Care*. 1990;13:34–40.

17. Morrison JL, Hodgson LA, Lim LL, Al-Qureshi S. Diabetic retinopathy in pregnancy: a review. *Clin Exp Ophthalmol*. 2016;44:321–334.

18. Chew EY, Mills JL, Metzger BE, et al. Metabolic control and progression of retinopathy. The diabetes in early pregnancy study. National Institute of child health and human development diabetes in early pregnancy study. *Diabetes Care*. 1995;18:631–637.

19. Toda J, Kato S, Sanaka M, Kitano S. The effect of pregnancy on the progression of diabetic retinopathy. *Jpn J Ophthalmol*. 2016;60:454–458.

20. Silva PS, Cavallerano JD, Sun JK, et al. Non-mydriatic ultrawide field retinal imaging compared with dilated standard 7-field 35-mm photography and retinal specialist examination for evaluation of diabetic retinopathy. *Am J Ophthalmol*. 2012;154:549–559.

21. Silva PS, Aiello LP. Telemedicine and eye examinations for diabetic retinopathy: a time to maximize real-world outcomes. *JAMA Ophthalmol*. 2015;133:525–526.

22. Silva PS, Cavallerano JD, Sun JK, et al. Peripheral lesions identified by mydriatic ultrawide field imaging: distribution and potential impact on diabetic retinopathy severity. *Ophthalmology*. 2013;120:2587–2595.

23. Tozer K, Woodward MA, Newman-Casey PA. Telemedicine, diabetic retinopathy: review of published screening programs. *J Endocrinol Diabetes*. 2015;2(4).

24. Mansberger SL, Sheppler C, Barker G, et al. Long-term comparative effectiveness of telemedicine in providing diabetic retinopathy screening examinations: a randomized clinical trial. *JAMA Ophthalmol*. 2015;133: 518–525.

25. Falavarjani KG, Wang K, Khadamy J, Sadda SR. Ultra-wide-field imaging in diabetic retinopathy; an overview. *J Curr Ophthalmol*. 2016;28:57–60.

26. Wessel MM, Aaker GD, Parlitsis G, et al. Ultra-wide-field angiography improves the detection and classification of diabetic retinopathy. *Retina*. 2012;32:785–791.

27. Treatment for center-involving-diabetic macular edema in eyes with very good VA study. Sponsor: Jaeb Center for Health Research. ClinicalTrials.gov Identifier: NCT01190979.

28. Browning DJ, Altaweel MM, Bressler NM, Bressler SB, Scott IU, Diabetic Retinopathy Clinical Research Network. Diabetic macular edema: what is focal and what is diffuse? *Am J Ophthalmol*. 2008;146(5):649–655.

29. Early Treatment Diabetic Retinopathy Study Research Group. Treatment techniques and clinical guidelines for photocoagulation of diabetic macular edema. Early Treatment Diabetic Retinopathy Study Report Number 2. *Ophthalmology*. 1987;94:761–774.

30. Browning DJ, Glassman AR, Aiello LP, et al. Optical coherence tomography measurements and analysis methods in optical coherence tomography studies of diabetic macular edema. *Ophthalmology*. 2008;115:1366–1371.

31. Browning DJ, McOwen MD, Bowen Jr RM, O'Marah TL. Comparison of the clinical diagnosis of diabetic macular edema with diagnosis by optical coherence tomography. *Ophthalmology*. 2004;111:712–715.

32. Virgili G, Menchini F, Casazza G, et al. Optical coherence tomography (OCT) for detection of macular oedema in patients with diabetic retinopathy (review). *Cochrane Database Syst Rev*. 2011;7:1–47.

CHAPTER 3

Classification of Diabetic Retinopathy

GERALDINE R. SLEAN, MS, MD • RAHUL N. KHURANA, MD

INTRODUCTION

An early classification of diabetic retinopathy (DR) was developed after a group of experts met at Airlie House, Virginia in 1968.[1] This "Airlie House" classification was later modified in the Diabetic Retinopathy Study (DRS), which used standard retinal photographic fields as benchmarks.[2] An extension of the "modified Airlie House classification" was used in the Early Treatment of Diabetic Retinopathy Study (ETDRS), which defined 13 complex levels of DR ranging from no retinopathy (level 10) to severe vitreous hemorrhage (level 85). As in the DRS, examiners graded stereophotographs of seven standard 30-degree fields with field one focused on the optic disc and field two centered on the macula (Fig. 3.1).[3] These studies helped reveal the natural history of DR as well as the impact of treatment on the progression of DR. The ETDRS also introduced the definition for clinically significant macular edema (CSME) and was instrumental in highlighting the effectiveness of photocoagulation to treat CSME.[4] Although definitions of DR stages based on the ETDRS severity scale are heavily relied upon in research, this classification system is not commonly used in clinical settings because of its grading complexity. There has been a recent interest in this classification, however, in clinical trials focused on evaluating the improvement of DR after anti-VEGF (vascular endothelial growth factor) or intravitreal steroid therapy.[5-7] The more recent International Clinical Diabetic Retinopathy Disease Severity Scale consists of only five levels, ranging from no apparent DR to proliferative DR. It is more commonly used in practice scenarios as well as recent studies. It is a simpler, easy-to-use scale that was developed to improve communication between ophthalmologists and other physicians internationally. It relies on information obtained from clinical examination; thus, no special instrumentation or imaging is required. This severity scale is also based on scientific information from the ETDRS and Wisconsin Epidemiologic Study of Diabetic Retinopathy (WESDR).[8]

This chapter focuses on presenting the ETDRS classification and the International Clinical Diabetic Retinopathy Disease Severity Scale and their stepwise correlation to the progression of DR. Classification of DR serves to categorize the progression of DR by stages as a means to better report incidence and prevalence, meaningfully communicate with other ophthalmologists as well as primary care physicians, and measure treatment efficacy. Moreover, classification serves an important role in informing practice patterns and treatment decision making.

PATHOGENESIS

DR is multifactorial and involves multiple biochemical changes, inflammatory processes, and genetic factors. Hyperglycemia causes an increased activation and upregulation of VEGF, erythropoietin, growth factors, oxidative stress, protein kinase C, the polyol pathway, and advanced glycation end-products, among other factors and pathways.[9,10] Through these multiple mechanisms, hyperglycemia induces apoptosis, inflammation, vascular changes, and angiogenesis.[11,12]

ABSENCE OF DIABETIC RETINOPATHY

Individuals with diabetes without visible evidence of DR are labeled as having no apparent retinopathy by both the ETDRS and International Clinical Diabetic Retinopathy Disease Severity Scale. However, these patients likely have some degree of subtle vascular and neural retinal damage. Even patients without retinopathy have demonstrated retinal arteriolar vasoconstriction and reductions in total retinal blood flow.[13] Optical coherence tomography angiography (OCTA) has demonstrated changes in vascular perfusion before clinical detection of DR.[14] Neuroretinal function may become compromised perhaps even before vessel damage.[15] Studies have shown degeneration and death of retinal ganglion cells, Müller cells, retinal pigment epithelium, and photoreceptors.[16-25]

NONPROLIFERATIVE DIABETIC RETINOPATHY

Nonproliferative diabetic retinopathy (NPDR) involves basement membrane (BM) thickening, pericyte loss, microaneurysms, intraretinal hemorrhages, cotton wool

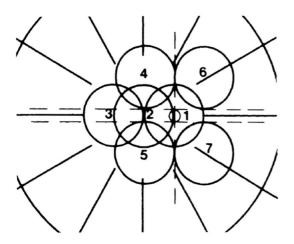

FIG. 3.1 Seven standard 30-degree fields used in grading from the Airlie House classification and Early Treatment of Diabetic Retinopathy Study. (From Grading diabetic retinopathy from stereoscopic color fundus photographs—an extension of the modified Airlie House classification, ETDRS report number 10 with permission.)

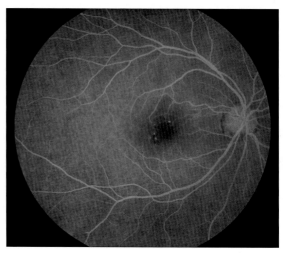

FIG. 3.2 Microaneurysms on fluorescein angiography appear as multiple hyperfluorescent dots around the fovea.

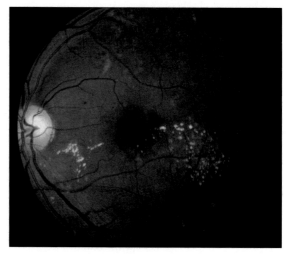

FIG. 3.3 Hard exudates appear as yellow lipid exudates in the posterior pole on fundus photography.

spots (CWS), hard exudates, venous beading, venous dilation, capillary acellularity, capillary nonperfusion, and intraretinal microvascular abnormalities (IRMAs). Early on, capillary BM thickening is seen with increased levels of collagen and laminin.[26] BM thickening may affect capillary autoregulation as well as interactions with proteins and neighboring pericytes.[27] Pericyte loss is hypothesized to be one of the initial pathologic alterations in DR, and their loss leads to altered microvascular autoregulation, a disrupted blood-retinal barrier, and proliferation of endothelial cells.[28]

Microaneurysms in the inner retina, representing the initial clinical evidence of NPDR, are thought to result from a combination of pericyte death, decreased vascular intercellular contact, BM thickening, endothelial cell proliferation, and thrombus formation.[27] Microaneurysms represent a distension of the capillary wall, which can remain patent, can become plugged by erythrocytes or thrombus, and also may become acellular. On clinical examination and fundus photos, microaneurysms appear as red dots measuring 25–125 μm. On fluorescein angiography (FA), patent microaneurysms appear as hyperfluorescent dots with potential for leakage in the late-phase FA (Fig. 3.2).[29] Intraretinal hemorrhages include dot-blot hemorrhages and flame hemorrhages. In contrast to microaneurysms, intraretinal hemorrhages are hypofluorescent on FA.[29]

Retinal capillary nonperfusion of the neural retina produces CWS, which are also hypofluorescent on FA. Hard exudates are sharply defined white-yellow

deposits (Fig. 3.3). Unlike drusen in age-related macular degeneration, which are subretinal on optical coherence tomography (OCT), hard exudates are usually intraretinal. They can often be found near areas of increased permeability and correspond to hypofluorescent foci on FA. Venous beading consists of vessels with alternating constriction and dilation.[29]

Capillary acellularity is present in more advanced DR and corresponds to retinal capillary nonperfusion on FA. IRMAs have an unusual curved and contorted

TABLE 3.1
ETDRS Classification of Diabetic Retinopathy

ETDRS Severity	ETDRS Level	ETDRS Definition
No diabetic retinopathy	10	• No evidence of diabetic retinopathy
Mild NPDR	20, 35	• At least one microaneurysm
Moderate NPDR	43, 47	• Microaneurysms and/or hemorrhages ≥ standard photograph 2A AND/OR • The presence of CWS, venous beading, or IRMA
Severe NPDR	53A-E	• CWS, venous beading, and IRMA in at least two of the 30-degree photographic fields 4–7 OR • Two of the aforementioned features (CWS, venous beading, IRMA) in at least two of photographic fields 4–7 plus microaneurysms and hemorrhages ≥ standard photograph 2A in at least one photographic field 4–7 OR • IRMAs in each of the photographic fields 4–7 with IRMAs ≥ standard photograph 8A in at least two of the photographic fields 4–7
Early PDR	61, 65	• New vessels
High-risk PDR	71, 75, 81, 85	• Neovascularization of the disc (NVD) ≥ standard photograph 10A (showing one-fourth to one-third disc area of NVD) on or within one disc diameter of the optic disc with or without vitreous hemorrhage or preretinal hemorrhage OR • vitreous and/or preretinal hemorrhage, plus NVD < standard photograph 10A or neovascularization elsewhere ≥ ¼ disc area
Apparently present DME		• Retinal thickening within one disc diameter of the fovea AND/OR • Hard exudates ≥ standard photograph 3 in the 30-degree photographic field 2 (centered on the macula) with some exudates within one disc diameter of the fovea
CSME		• Retinal thickening at or within 500 μm of the fovea OR • Hard exudates at or within 500 μm of the fovea that is associated with adjacent retinal thickening OR • Retinal thickening within one disc diameter of the fovea that is greater than or equal to one disc area

CSME, clinically significant macular edema; *CWS*, cotton wool spots; *DME*, diabetic macular edema; *ETDRS*, Early Treatment of Diabetic Retinopathy Study; *IRMA*, intraretinal microvascular abnormality; *NPDR*, nonproliferative diabetic retinopathy; *NVD*, neovascularization of the disc; *PDR*, proliferative diabetic retinopathy.

appearance, and they are intraretinal in location. This differentiates IRMA from neovascularization in proliferative diabetic retinopathy (PDR), which is on the surface of the retina. IRMAs are typically present at the edges of nonperfused areas and may demonstrate fluorescein leakage on late-phase FA. IRMA may represent a response to ischemic neural retina by connecting precapillary arterioles with postcapillary venules.[27] Foveal nonperfusion appears as an enlarged and often irregular foveal avascular zone (FAZ). Variations in the FAZ anatomy in normal and diabetic eyes may be better illustrated using OCTA.[14]

The ETDRS classification (Table 3.1) assumes that DR worsens in a discrete stepwise fashion and divides NPDR into mild, moderate, and severe. **Mild NPDR** consists of at least one microaneurysm. **Moderate NPDR** is defined as microaneurysms and/or hemorrhages ≥ standard photograph 2A (Fig. 3.4) and/or the presence of CWS, venous beading, or IRMA. **Severe NPDR** involves:

1. CWS, venous beading, and IRMA in at least two of the 30-degree photographic fields four to seven; or
2. two of the aforementioned features (CWS, venous beading, IRMA) in at least two of the photographic fields four to seven plus microaneurysms and hemorrhages ≥ standard photograph 2A in at least one photographic field four to seven; or
3. IRMAs in each of the photographic fields four to seven with IRMAs ≥ standard photograph 8A (Fig. 3.5) in at least two of the photographic fields four to seven.[3,30]

The International Clinical Diabetic Retinopathy Disease Severity Scale (Table 3.2) divides NPDR into three

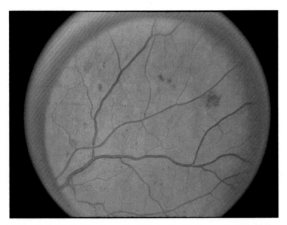

FIG. 3.4 Early Treatment of Diabetic Retinopathy Study standard photograph 2A showing microaneurysms and intraretinal hemorrhages. (From Grading diabetic retinopathy from stereoscopic color fundus photographs—an extension of the modified Airlie House classification, ETDRS report number 10 with permission.)

TABLE 3.2
International Clinical Diabetic Retinopathy Disease Severity Scale

Mild NPDR	• Microaneurysms only
Moderate NPDR	• More than just microaneurysms present, but less findings than severe NPDR
Severe NPDR	• Twenty intraretinal hemorrhages in each of the 4 quadrants OR • Venous beading in ≥ 2 quadrants OR • Prominent IRMAs in ≥ 1 quadrant
PDR	• Neovascularization, vitreous hemorrhage, or preretinal hemorrhage
Mild DME	• Retinal thickening or hard exudates removed from the fovea
Moderate DME	• Retinal thickening or hard exudates approaching the fovea
Severe DME	• Retinal thickening or hard exudates involving the fovea

DME, diabetic macular edema; NPDR, nonproliferative diabetic retinopathy; PDR, proliferative diabetic retinopathy.

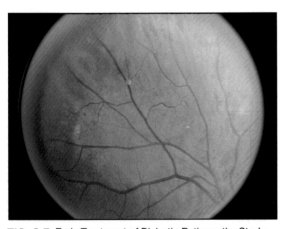

FIG. 3.5 Early Treatment of Diabetic Retinopathy Study standard photograph 8A showing intraretinal microvascular abnormalities. (From Grading diabetic retinopathy from stereoscopic color fundus photographs—an extension of the modified Airlie House classification, ETDRS report number 10 with permission.)

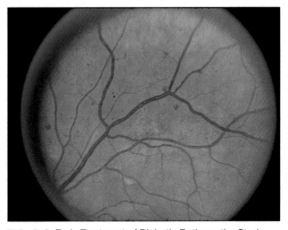

FIG. 3.6 Early Treatment of Diabetic Retinopathy Study standard photograph 6A showing venous beading. (From Grading diabetic retinopathy from stereoscopic color fundus photographs—an extension of the modified Airlie House classification, ETDRS report number 10 with permission.)

categories: (1) mild NPDR, (2) moderate NPDR, and (3) severe NPDR. Mild NPDR consists of microaneurysms only. Severe NPDR is defined as:
• twenty intraretinal hemorrhages in each of the four quadrants, or
• venous beading in ≥ 2 quadrants, or
• prominent IRMA in ≥ 1 quadrant.
Moderate NPDR lies between the aforementioned two categories with more than just microaneurysms present but less findings than severe NPDR.[8]

For purposes of simplification, severe NPDR has popularly been defined using the 4-2-1 rule:
• Microaneurysms and intraretinal hemorrhages in all *four* quadrants (≥ standard photograph 2A), or
• venous beading in at least *two* quadrants (≥ standard photograph 6A, Fig. 3.6), or
• IRMA in at least *one* quadrant (≥ standard photograph 8A).

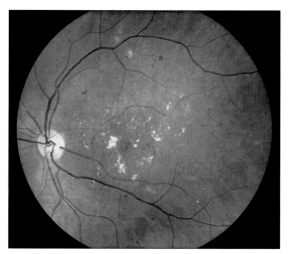

FIG. 3.7 Diabetic macular edema with lipid exudate, microaneurysms, and intraretinal hemorrhages on color fundus photography.

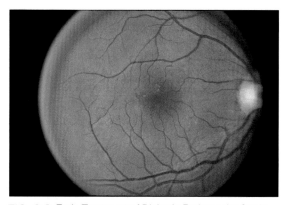

FIG. 3.8 Early Treatment of Diabetic Retinopathy Study standard photograph 3 showing hard exudates in the macula. (From Grading diabetic retinopathy from stereoscopic color fundus photographs—an extension of the modified Airlie House classification, ETDRS report number 10 with permission.)

Very severe NPDR is classified as the presence of two or more of the aforementioned severe NPDR features.[8,31] Half of patients with severe NPDR develop PDR within 1 year, and 15% are high-risk PDR. For patients with very severe NPDR, the risk of developing PDR within 1 year is 75%, and 45% are high-risk PDR.[32]

DIABETIC MACULAR EDEMA

Diabetic macular edema (DME) is due to vascular leakage and blood-retinal barrier breakdown. Note that macular edema can also occur in other settings such as vitreous traction or epiretinal membrane pulling on the retina.[29] DME involves thickening of the retina, and it has been subclassified by a variety of methodologies including clinical examination, stereophotographs, FA, and OCT. DME has been divided into focal or diffuse subtypes.[33] Focal DME is due to leakage from microaneurysms.[33] Lipid exudation is often associated with hard exudate that can be found beneath the sensory retina or in the plexiform layers (Fig. 3.7). Diffuse DME indicates more extensive inner blood-retinal barrier breakdown from disruption of vascular endothelial tight junctions.[34] In the ETDRS, FA was used to distinguish DME subtypes such that if two-thirds or more of leakage was attributed to microaneurysms, then this constituted focal DME. Leakage in which one-third to two-thirds of leakage was from microaneurysms was labeled as intermediate DME. Eyes with one-third or less of overall leakage because of microaneurysms were considered to have diffuse DME, attributed to dilated capillaries.[35] Over time, there have been differing definitions of what comprises focal and diffuse subtypes of DME, and this terminology is not ideal because of a lack of clear consensus.

According to the ETDRS (Table 3.1), apparently present DME consists of retinal thickening within one disc diameter of the fovea and/or hard exudates ≥ standard photograph 3 (Fig. 3.8) in the 30-degree photographic field two (centered on the macula) with some exudates within one disc diameter of the fovea. CSME describes thickening that is eminently threatening or currently affecting the fovea and defined on biomicroscopic examination as:

- retinal thickening at or within 500 μm of the fovea, or
- hard exudates at or within 500 μm of the fovea that is associated with adjacent retinal thickening, or
- retinal thickening within one disc diameter of the fovea that is greater than or equal to one disc area.[3,36]

According to the International Clinical Diabetic Retinopathy Disease Severity Scale (Table 3.2), apparently present DME is defined as some hard exudates or retinal thickening located in the posterior pole. Mild DME is defined as retinal thickening of hard exudates removed from the fovea, whereas moderate DME involves retinal thickening or hard exudates approaching the fovea, and severe DME consists of retinal thickening or hard exudates involving the fovea.[8]

There is a trend to use OCT to classify DME in research studies as well as clinically when deciding on whether anti-VEGF therapy is indicated. OCT is a fast, noninvasive way to evaluate DME and reproducibly measure its location in relation to the fovea. OCT has demonstrated subtle retinal thickening that may not be clinically apparent.

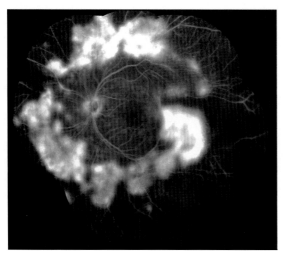

FIG. 3.9 Neovascularization demonstrated by extensive leakage on fluorescein angiography in proliferative diabetic retinopathy.

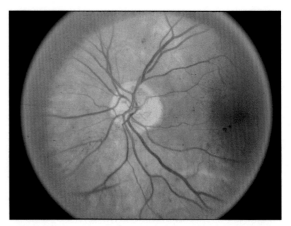

FIG. 3.10 Early Treatment of Diabetic Retinopathy Study standard photograph 10A showing neovascularization of the optic disc covering one-fourth to one-third of the disc area used to differentiate eyes with high-risk PDR. (From Grading diabetic retinopathy from stereoscopic color fundus photographs—an extension of the modified Airlie House classification, ETDRS report number 10 with permission.)

It has also proved useful to differentiate CSME as either center-involving or non-center-involving, with center-involving CSME defined as ETDRS visual acuity between 20/32 and 20/320 in the presence of central retinal thickening (specifically central subfield thickness ≥ 250 μm on a Zeiss Stratus).[37] Given its importance in central vision, center-involving CSME has been allocated an increasingly important role in studies and treatment decisions and will likely soon become an important classification. Several studies,[38–40] including the DRCR.net protocol T,[41] have examined the impact of anti-VEGF injections (bevacizumab, ranibizumab, and aflibercept) in center-involving CSME and found these treatments to be very effective. Future studies will likely continue to rely on OCT for further evaluations of center-involving CSME. Although OCT retinal thickness measurements show only a modest correlation with visual acuity,[42] these measurements are easily available as longitudinal markers. As such, they are widely used in studies as outcome measurements and in decisions about retreatment.

PROLIFERATIVE DIABETIC RETINOPATHY

Progression of DR and capillary nonperfusion leads to ischemia, which generally starts in the periphery and encroaches centrally to the macula and nerve.[43] VEGF and other vasoproliferative factors are released with retinal ischemia, causing the development of new vessels and fibrovascular proliferation.[44] Initially, new vessels grow beyond the inner limiting membrane in radial arrangements and leak profusely on FA (Fig. 3.9).[29]

These vessels then expand and extend and are accompanied by fibrovascular growth. Eventually these vessels regress, leaving behind the fibrovascular tissue. Traction from attachments of the fibrovascular tissue to the hyaloid can lead to vitreous hemorrhage, tractional retinal detachment, macular heterotopia, retinal schisis, retinal tear, and rhegmatogenous retinal detachment. Moreover, vitreous shrinkage is escalated in PDR because of the leakage of serum components from leaky, new vessels.[43] Contraction of fibrovascular proliferation can distort the retina, with the macula often being shifted nasally and vertically.[45] Increasing retinal ischemia also leads to neovascularization in the anterior segment referred to as neovascularization of the iris or neovascularization of the angle.

According to the ETDRS (Table 3.1), PDR is classified as early PDR (also known as PDR without high-risk characteristics) and high-risk PDR. Early PDR consists merely of new vessels that do not reach high-risk criteria. High-risk PDR is defined by:

- neovascularization of the disc (NVD) ≥ standard photograph 10A (showing one-fourth to one-third disc area with NVD, Fig. 3.10) on or within one disc diameter of the optic disc with or without vitreous hemorrhage or preretinal hemorrhage; or
- vitreous and/or preretinal hemorrhage, plus NVD < standard photograph 10A or neovascularization elsewhere (NVE) ≥ ¼ disc area.[3,30]

TABLE 3.3
ETDRS Severity Scale

ETDRS Severity	ETDRS Level	ETDRS Definition
No diabetic retinopathy	10	• No evidence of diabetic retinopathy
Very mild NPDR	20	• Only microaneurysms
Mild NPDR	35	• CWS, hard exudates, and/or mild intraretinal hemorrhages
Moderate NPDR	43	• 43A: Moderate intraretinal hemorrhages > standard photograph 1A in four quadrants or severe intraretinal hemorrhages ≥ standard photograph 2A in one quadrant • 43B: Mild IRMA < standard photograph 8A in 1–3 quadrants
Moderate NPDR	47	• 47A: Exhibiting both characteristics for level 43 • 47B: Mild IRMA in four quadrants • 47C: Severe intraretinal hemorrhages in two to three quadrants • 47D: Venous beading in one quadrant
Severe NPDR	53A–D	• 53A: Exhibiting ≥ 2 characteristics for level 47 • 53B: Severe intraretinal hemorrhages in four quadrants • 53C: Moderate to severe IRMA ≥ standard photographs 8A in ≥ 1 quadrant • 53D: Venous beading in ≥ 2 quadrants
Very severe NPDR	53E	• Exhibiting ≥ 2 characteristics for level 53A–D
Mild PDR	61	• NVE < ½ disk area in ≥ 1 quadrant
Moderate PDR	65	• 65A: NVE ≥ ½ disc area in ≥ 1 quadrant • 65B: NVD < standard photograph 10A
High-risk PDR	71, 75	• NVD ≥ standard photograph 10A, OR • NVD < standard photograph 10A or NVE ≥ ½ disc area plus VH OR preretinal hemorrhage, OR • VH or preretinal hemorrhage obscuring ≥ 1 disc area
Advanced PDR	81, 85	• Fundus partially obscured by vitreous hemorrhage, and • Ungradable NV or retinal detachment at the center of the macula

CWS, cotton wool spots; *ETDRS*, Early Treatment of Diabetic Retinopathy Study; *IRMA*, intraretinal microvascular abnormality; *NPDR*, nonproliferative diabetic retinopathy; *NV*, neovascularization; *NVD*, neovascularization of the disc; *NVE*, neovascularization elsewhere; *PDR*, proliferative diabetic retinopathy.

Per the International Clinical Diabetic Retinopathy Disease Severity Scale (Table 3.2), PDR is defined as neovascularization, vitreous hemorrhage, or preretinal hemorrhage.[8]

Renewed interest in the Early Treatment of Diabetic Retinopathy Study (ETDRS) severity score has generated a better understanding of the subtle progression in cases of DR. Evaluators carefully examine seven standard 30-degree stereoscopic color fundus photographs and then assign a grade. The standard scale (Table 3.3) includes no retinopathy (10), mild NPDR (20, 35), moderate NPDR (43, 47), severe NPDR (53A–D), very severe NPDR (53E), mild PDR (61), moderate PDR (65), high-risk PDR (71, 75), and advanced PDR (81, 85).[3] Additional levels can be included to tease out further differences in presentation and progression. Although this complex grading system is difficult to implement in clinical settings, it allows for more subtle distinctions in classification that are beneficial to answering research questions. One such study showed that eyes treated with ranibizumab are less likely to progress two or three levels along the ETDRS scale and more likely to regress two or three levels along the scale at 24 months as compared with the sham group.[5]

CONCLUSION

DR is a complex disease with diverse clinical findings. Looking forward, it is of the utmost importance to continue to standardize our usage of DR classification to be able to communicate effectively between practitioners who take care of diabetic individuals. It will also enable comparison of the incidence and prevalence of the various stages of DR worldwide and help to determine the therapeutic benefit of treatment modalities across nations.

REFERENCES

1. Goldberg M, Fine S. *Symposium on the Treatment of Diabetic Retinopathy*. Arlington, VA: US Department of Health, Education, and Welfare; 1968.
2. Diabetic retinopathy study. Report Number 6. Design, methods, and baseline results. Report Number 7. A modification of the Airlie House classification of diabetic retinopathy. Prepared by the Diabetic Retinopathy. *Invest Ophthalmol Vis Sci*. 1981;21(1 Pt 2):1–226.
3. Grading diabetic retinopathy from stereoscopic color fundus photographs–an extension of the modified Airlie House classification. ETDRS report number 10. Early Treatment Diabetic Retinopathy Study Research Group. *Ophthalmology*. 1991;98(suppl 5):786–806.
4. Aiello LM. Perspectives on diabetic retinopathy. *Am J Ophthalmol*. 2003;136:122–135. United States.
5. Ip MS, Domalpally A, Hopkins JJ, Wong P, Ehrlich JS. Long-term effects of ranibizumab on diabetic retinopathy severity and progression. *Arch Ophthalmol*. 2012;130(9):1145–1152.
6. Ip MS, Domalpally A, Sun JK, Ehrlich JS. Long-term effects of therapy with ranibizumab on diabetic retinopathy severity and baseline risk factors for worsening retinopathy. *Ophthalmology*. 2015;122(2):367–374.
7. Bressler SB, Qin H, Melia M, et al. Exploratory analysis of the effect of intravitreal ranibizumab or triamcinolone on worsening of diabetic retinopathy in a randomized clinical trial. *JAMA Ophthalmol*. 2013;131(8):1033–1040.
8. Wilkinson CP, Ferris 3rd FL, Klein RE, et al. Proposed international clinical diabetic retinopathy and diabetic macular edema disease severity scales. *Ophthalmology*. 2003;110(9):1677–1682.
9. Cheung N, Mitchell P, Wong TY. Diabetic retinopathy. *Lancet*. 2010;376(9735):124–136.
10. Brownlee M. Biochemistry and molecular cell biology of diabetic complications. *Nature*. 2001;414(6865):813–820.
11. Cohen SR, Gardner TW. Diabetic retinopathy and diabetic macular edema. *Dev Ophthalmol*. 2016;55:137–146.
12. Ahsan H. Diabetic retinopathy–biomolecules and multiple pathophysiology. *Diabetes Metab Syndr*. 2015;9(1):51–54.
13. Bursell SE, Clermont AC, Kinsley BT, Simonson DC, Aiello LM, Wolpert HA. Retinal blood flow changes in patients with insulin-dependent diabetes mellitus and no diabetic retinopathy. *Invest Ophthalmol Vis Sci*. 1996;37(5):886–897.
14. Takase N, Nozaki M, Kato A, Ozeki H, Yoshida M, Ogura Y. Enlargement of foveal avascular zone in diabetic eyes evaluated by en face optical coherence tomography angiography. *Retina*. 2015;35(11):2377–2383.
15. Antonetti DA, Barber AJ, Bronson SK, et al. Diabetic retinopathy: seeing beyond glucose-induced microvascular disease. *Diabetes*. 2006;55(9):2401–2411.
16. Barber AJ, Lieth E, Khin SA, Antonetti DA, Buchanan AG, Gardner TW. Neural apoptosis in the retina during experimental and human diabetes. Early onset and effect of insulin. *J Clin Invest*. 1998;102(4):783–791.
17. Barber AJ. A new view of diabetic retinopathy: a neurodegenerative disease of the eye. *Prog Neuro-psychopharmacol Biol Psychiatry*. 2003;27(2):283–290.
18. Kern TS, Barber AJ. Retinal ganglion cells in diabetes. *J Physiol*. 2008;586(18):4401–4408.
19. Lieth E, Gardner TW, Barber AJ, Antonetti DA. Retinal neurodegeneration: early pathology in diabetes. *Clin Exp Ophthalmol*. 2000;28(1):3–8.
20. Martin PM, Roon P, Van Ells TK, Ganapathy V, Smith SB. Death of retinal neurons in streptozotocin-induced diabetic mice. *Invest Ophthalmol Vis Sci*. 2004;45(9):3330–3336.
21. Mizutani M, Gerhardinger C, Lorenzi M. Muller cell changes in human diabetic retinopathy. *Diabetes*. 1998;47(3):445–449.
22. Decanini A, Karunadharma PR, Nordgaard CL, Feng X, Olsen TW, Ferrington DA. Human retinal pigment epithelium proteome changes in early diabetes. *Diabetologia*. 2008;51(6):1051–1061.
23. Puro DG. Diabetes-induced dysfunction of retinal Muller cells. *Trans Am Ophthalmol Soc*. 2002;100:339–352.
24. Park SH, Park JW, Park SJ, et al. Apoptotic death of photoreceptors in the streptozotocin-induced diabetic rat retina. *Diabetologia*. 2003;46(9):1260–1268.
25. Phipps JA, Fletcher EL, Vingrys AJ. Paired-flash identification of rod and cone dysfunction in the diabetic rat. *Invest Ophthalmol Vis Sci*. 2004;45(12):4592–4600.
26. Cagliero E, Roth T, Roy S, Lorenzi M. Characteristics and mechanisms of high-glucose-induced overexpression of basement membrane components in cultured human endothelial cells. *Diabetes*. 1991;40(1):102–110.
27. Stitt AW, Lois N, Medina RJ, Adamson P, Curtis TM. Advances in our understanding of diabetic retinopathy. *Clin Sci*. 2013;125(1):1–17.
28. Shepro D, Morel NM. Pericyte physiology. *FASEB J*. 1993;7(11):1031–1038.
29. Ryan SJ. *Retina*. 5th ed. London: Saunders/Elsevier; 2013.
30. Fundus photographic risk factors for progression of diabetic retinopathy. ETDRS report number 12. Early Treatment Diabetic Retinopathy Study Research Group. *Ophthalmology*. 1991;98(suppl 5):823–833.
31. Murphy RP. Management of diabetic retinopathy. *Am Fam Physician*. 1995;51(4):785–796.
32. Early photocoagulation for diabetic retinopathy. ETDRS report number 9. Early Treatment Diabetic Retinopathy Study Research Group. *Ophthalmology*. 1991;98(suppl 5):766–785.
33. Bresnick GH. Diabetic macular edema. A review. *Ophthalmology*. 1986;93(7):989–997.
34. Wallow IH, Engerman RL. Permeability and patency of retinal blood vessels in experimental diabetes. *Invest Ophthalmol Vis Sci*. 1977;16(5):447–461.

35. Focal photocoagulation treatment of diabetic macular edema. Relationship of treatment effect to fluorescein angiographic and other retinal characteristics at baseline: ETDRS report no. 19. Early Treatment Diabetic Retinopathy Study Research Group. *Arch Ophthalmol*. 1995;113(9): 1144–1155.

36. Photocoagulation for diabetic macular edema. Early treatment diabetic retinopathy study report number 1. Early Treatment Diabetic Retinopathy Study Research Group. *Arch Ophthalmol*. 1985;103(12):1796–1806.

37. Maturi RK, Walker JD, Chambers RB. *Diabetic Retinopathy for the Comprehensive Ophthalmologist*. 2nd ed. Fort Wayne, IN: Deluma Medical Publishing; 2016.

38. Elman MJ, Qin H, Aiello LP, et al. Intravitreal ranibizumab for diabetic macular edema with prompt versus deferred laser treatment: three-year randomized trial results. *Ophthalmology*. 2012;119(11):2312–2318.

39. Rajendram R, Fraser-Bell S, Kaines A, et al. A 2-year prospective randomized controlled trial of intravitreal bevacizumab or laser therapy (BOLT) in the management of diabetic macular edema: 24-month data: report 3. *Arch Ophthalmol*. 2012;130(8):972–979.

40. Do DV, Schmidt-Erfurth U, Gonzalez VH, et al. The DA VINCI Study: phase 2 primary results of VEGF Trap-Eye in patients with diabetic macular edema. *Ophthalmology*. 2011;118(9):1819–1826.

41. Wells JA, Glassman AR, Ayala AR, et al. Aflibercept, bevacizumab, or ranibizumab for diabetic macular edema. *N Engl J Med*. 2015;372(13):1193–1203.

42. Browning DJ, Glassman AR, Aiello LP, et al. Relationship between optical coherence tomography-measured central retinal thickness and visual acuity in diabetic macular edema. *Ophthalmology*. 2006;114(3):525–536.

43. Maturi RK, Walker JD, Chambers RB. *Diabetic Retinopathy for the Comprehensive Ophthalmologist*. 2nd ed. Fort Wayne, IN: Deluma Medical Publishers; 2015.

44. Aiello LP, Avery RL, Arrigg PG, et al. Vascular endothelial growth factor in ocular fluid of patients with diabetic retinopathy and other retinal disorders. *N Engl J Med*. 1994;331(22):1480–1487.

45. Bresnick GH, Haight B, de Venecia G. Retinal wrinkling and macular heterotopia in diabetic retinopathy. *Arch Ophthalmol*. 1979;97(10):1890–1895.

CHAPTER 4

Imaging in Diabetic Retinopathy

CAROLINE R. BAUMAL, MD

INTRODUCTION

Imaging of the posterior pole plays a key role in the management of diabetic retinopathy (DR). Retinal imaging in diabetes has been utilized for population screening, telemedicine, natural history studies, and assessment of response to therapy. Technologic advances in the last decade have improved image acquisition, processing, reproducibility, and comparability between sequential retinal examinations. Fundus photography and fluorescein angiography (FA) had previously been the main modalities used to study DR. Optical coherence tomography (OCT) imaging for commercial use was introduced in 2001 and provides a superior, noninvasive modality to evaluate diabetic macular edema (DME). New imaging techniques are continually being introduced, whereas established ones are updated. OCT angiography (OCTA) is a relatively new, novel modality to image flow in the retinal and choroidal vasculature. OCT angiography (OCTA) provides more detailed information about the vascular changes in DR, as it can segment the retinal circulation into individual vascular plexuses.

The information provided by retinal imaging techniques can be classified as structural, functional, or a combination of these. Multimodal imaging, which describes the use of more than one technologic system to acquire complementary images for the purpose of diagnosis, prognostication, disease monitoring, and therapy, may provide greater insight into DR.[1] To interpret images, knowledge of the clinical features and the sequence of progression as outlined by the diabetic retinopathy severity score (DRSS) (Chapter 3) is required.[2,3] The DRSS presumes that microaneurysm formation secondary to pericyte dysfunction is the earliest visible clinical change in DR and that progression of retinopathy occurs in discrete levels. However, OCT of the retinal nerve fiber layer (RNFL) and OCTA have demonstrated subtle abnormalities in diabetics before the development of any visible DR, such as microaneurysms.[4,5] This chapter outlines the current imaging techniques used to evaluate DR.

FUNDUS PHOTOGRAPHY

Fundus photography provides a color or red-free image of the retina. It is primarily digital, which has many advantages compared with its predecessor, color photographic film. Digital retinal imaging provides rapidly acquired, high-resolution, reproducible images that are available immediately and easily amenable to image enhancement. Fundus photography is most often used for disease documentation and clinical studies, with potential use for telemedicine and patient education. Types of fundus photography include standard view and wide field.

Standard fundus photography provides a 30- to 50-degree image that includes the macula and optic nerve. This modality is widely available, so it is often used in clinical trials and provides relatively good documentation of DR when the findings are not subtle. For example, lipid exudate and microaneurysms are well visualized on color and red-free images, respectively (Fig. 4.1A). Multiple images may be manually overlapped to create a montage, such as when the 7 standard 30-degree fundus images are combined to create a 75-degree field of view (Fig. 4.1B). However, standard fundus photography is not able to accurately establish the presence of macular edema without stereoscopic imaging and viewing, which is labor intensive, time consuming, and limited in accuracy. The field of view in single standard fundus photograph may be restricted by coexisting media opacities, such as cataract or vitreous hemorrhage.

Ultrawide field (UWF) imaging can produce up to a 200-degree retinal view extending beyond the macula to the peripheral retina. Over 80% of the total surface retinal area can be imaged. The amount of peripheral retina imaged and need for pupil dilation depends on which camera is used. UWF imaging is available for fundus photography, as well as FA, indocyanine green (ICG) angiography, and fundus autofluorescence (FAF) (Fig. 4.1C–E). The theoretical advantage of the larger field of view is to allow for more thorough documentation and detection of peripheral retinal pathology in a minimally invasive fashion. Some of the disadvantages include distortion of images caused by the spherical

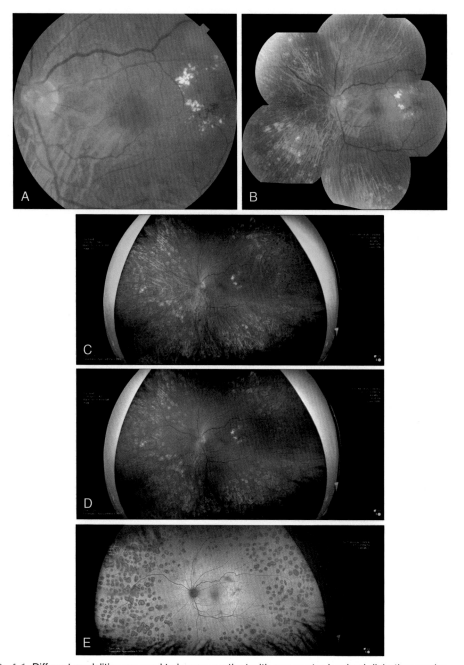

FIG. 4.1 Different modalities are used to image a patient with non-center-involved diabetic macular edema and proliferative diabetic retinopathy who is status post panretinal laser photocoagulation (PRP) in his left eye. Single fundus photograph **(A)** (Topcon, NJ, USA). Note the regressing fibrovascular tissue on the optic nerve head. There is lipid exudate temporal to the fovea surrounding dot and blot hemorrhages. Montage of 7 standard fields **(B)** including figure 4.1A. PRP peripheral to the arcades is now apparent. Ultrawide-field color photograph **(C)** (Optos California, MA, USA) and red-free photograph **(D)** reveal a wider view of peripheral laser. Note the eye lashes obscuring the inferior retina. Ultrawide-field fundus autofluorescence **(E)** (FAF, Optos) demonstrates the peripheral hypoautofluorescent laser spots.

shape of the globe, eyelash artifacts, false color representation of fundus findings, continued inability to view the far peripheral retina, and much higher equipment costs. Owing to these limitations, traditional 30-degree fundus photography continues to be the standard method to photograph the fundus.

TELEMEDICINE

There are realistic concerns that there may not be enough eye care specialists to meet the demand for diabetic eye examination and treatment as the number of diabetic patients increases.[6] It is projected that the prevalence of diabetes mellitus will increase from 14% in 2010 to 33% by 2050 in the United States.[7] Less than 50% of diabetics currently receive the recommended annual diabetic eye examinations. Telemedicine involves utilization of remote retinal imaging, typically fundus photography, to screen for DR. The imaging could be performed in a location other than the ophthalmologist's office in an effort to screen a large number of patients with diabetes and capture those patients with diabetes who do not present for eye examination. The result would be to focus diabetic eye care and resources to those in need of closer monitoring and therapy. Automated computerized grading of telemedicine images may be possible, as deep learning algorithms have shown high sensitivity and specificity to manual grading by ophthalmologists.[8]

Advantages of telemedicine include its ability to capture more patients with diabetes in locations such as the primary physician's office, improved patient compliance, efficiency, cost-effectiveness, potential access in remote areas with limited eye specialists, and the ability to establish reading centers with trained graders or automated software to detect retinopathy with high sensitivity.[9] Telemedicine models have been shown to increase the percentage of annual DR screening examinations, reduce wait times for screening, and have potential to monitor for disease worsening over a long time.[10] The American Academy of Ophthalmology concluded there is level I evidence that single-field digital fundus photography can serve as a screening tool to identify patients with diabetes with retinopathy for ophthalmic referral, although it currently maintains this is not a substitute for a comprehensive eye examination, as issues such as cataract, intraocular pressure, complete peripheral retinal examination, and refraction are not evaluated.[11] Issues with nonmydriatic fundus imaging include image quality and artifacts that are compounded with small pupils and media opacity. In addition, monocular fundus photographs are not accurate when compared with OCT to screen for retinal thickening in DME.[12]

DYE-BASED ANGIOGRAPHY
Fluorescein Angiography

FA is a two-dimensional, dye-based technique in which fluorescein dye is injected intravenously with simultaneous retinal imaging using filters to transmit specific wavelengths (490 nm excitation and 530 nm emission) to show dynamic changes in the retinal and choroidal circulation. After its initial description in humans in 1961, FA has been the gold standard to evaluate retinal microvasculature changes in DR, including microaneurysms, retinal capillary nonperfusion (ischemia), neovascularization, and breakdown of the blood-retinal barrier evident as leakage or edema.[13] FA is still used, although less frequently for DME subsequent to the widespread availability of OCT. Although FA is very sensitive to identify signs of early nonproliferative diabetic retinopathy, its use as a screening tool for minimal retinopathy is not indicated. Most of the common classifications for DR severity do not consider FA in their criteria, and FA was not part of the Early Treatment Diabetic Retinopathy Study (ETDRS) definition of clinically significant macular edema (CSME). FA is not very useful in evaluating success of macular edema therapy, limiting its use in DME clinical trials. In clinical practice, FA is useful in specific circumstances, including for the detection of subtle suspected neovascularization and differentiation of early neovascularization from IRMA. FA can evaluate for macular ischemia and capillary nonperfusion as a cause of visual impairment, although OCTA may be more sensitive because of its higher resolution and ability to image both the superficial and deep retinal vascular plexus.[5] FA may distinguish DME associated with retinal microvascular irregularities from pseudophakic cystoid macular edema, which features a petalloid pattern and optic nerve dye leakage.

Standard FA covers a 30- to 55-degree field of retina, although peripheral images in different stages of the FA can be taken by directing the camera peripherally. UWF FA is a more recent development that has improved visualization of the peripheral retinal vasculature with utility to reveal peripheral capillary nonperfusion that is otherwise clinically undetectable in patients with diabetes. Both Optos and Heidelberg Spectralis feature UWF FA imaging of 200 and 102 degrees of field, respectively. UWF FA can better demonstrate peripheral diabeic pathology, such as capillary nonperfusion,

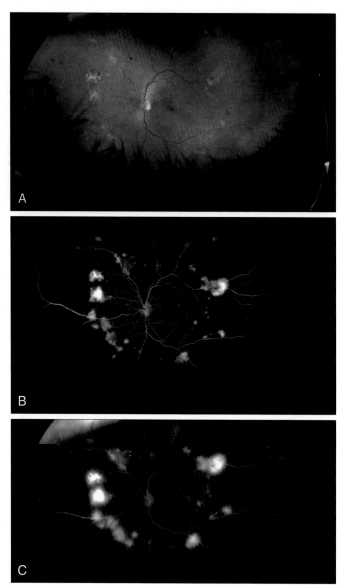

FIG. 4.2 Ultrawide-field (UWF) color photo **(A)** of the patient from Fig. 4.1 before PRP laser showed fibrovascular tufts nasally and along the arcades. UWF fluorescein angiography **(B,** 1.07 min) and laer **(C,** 3 min) highlighting foci of retinal neovascularization with active late leakage and peripheral capillary nonperfusion.

neovascularization, and vessel leakage, compared with standard imaging, and software is available to quantify zones of nonperfusion (Fig. 4.2).[14] Several studies have shown an association between peripheral retinal nonperfusion and the occurrence of neovascularization and DME. The presence of peripheral diabetic lesions identified with UWF imaging was associated with an increased risk of DR progression over a 4-year study period.[15] Further studies with UWF FA imaging are necessary to determine if recognition or treatment of peripheral capillary nonperfusion can alter the development of proliferative diabetic retinopathy (PDR) or reduce the treatment burden of intravitreal injections for DME.

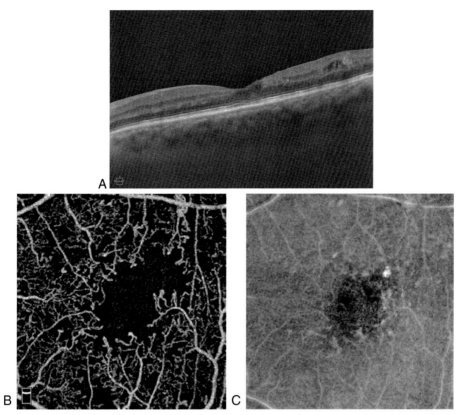

FIG. 4.3 Optical coherence tomography (OCT) B scan **(A)** from the patient in Figs. 4.1 and 4.2. There are small cysts temporal to the fovea with hyperreflective dots, likely corresponding to hard exudate. There is loss of distinction of the inner retinal layers temporal to the fovea. OCT angiography **(B)** shows enlarged foveal avascular zone, microaneurysms, and prominent capillary drop out superotemporal to the fovea. The corresponding en face image **(C)** shows subtle cystic change and microaneurysms.

Another type of dye-based angiography uses ICG dye, which fluoresces in the near-infrared range (790–805 nm). The longer wavelength of ICG angiography optimizes visualization of the choroidal circulation, and thus it has utility to image vascular and inflammatory disorders that affect the choroid. ICG angiography has demonstrated irregular choroidal filling defects as well as microaneurysms in DR, although current studies of the diabetic choroidal circulation primarily concentrate on OCT and OCTA.[16]

OPTICAL COHERENCE TOMOGRAPHY

OCT has become the gold standard imaging modality to diagnose and monitor DME. Current commercial spectral-domain OCT technology allows for the rapid, noninvasive acquisition of real-time, high-resolution, cross-sectional, and en face images of the

retina with axial resolution up to 1 μm.[17] Automated software provides quantitative and reproducible measurement of retinal thickness, whereas the interpretation of anatomy depends on a trained reader. OCT findings in DME may include intraretinal cystic spaces, diffuse retinal thickening, and loss of the foveal depression (Fig. 4.3A). Severe DME may be associated with subretinal fluid and focal neurosensory retinal detachment seen as dark spaces or voids between the retina and retinal pigment epithelium (RPE) (Fig. 4.4A). When present, hard exudates are evident as punctate foci of high reflectivity, often in the outer plexiform layer. Hemorrhage in the retinal layers and cotton wool spots in the superficial retina may be imaged. Retinal neovascularization may be imaged with OCT as a highly reflective lesion in association with the inner retinal surface, although clinical correlation with biomicroscopy or other

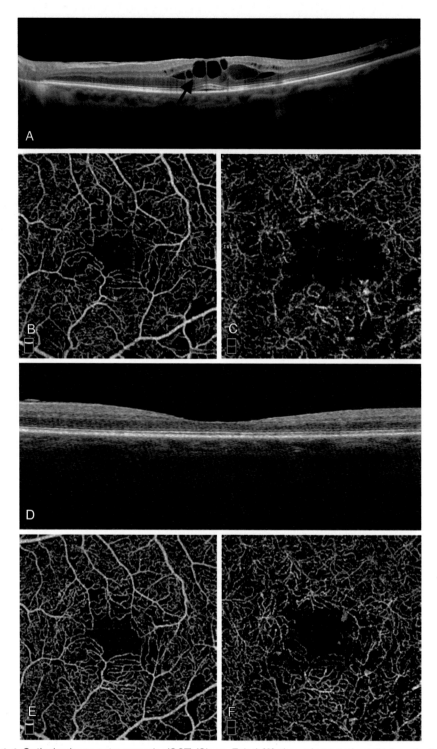

FIG. 4.4 Optical coherence tomography (OCT) (Cirrus, Zeiss) **(A)** shows large and small intraretinal cysts (red arrows) and a small amount of subretinal fluid (blue arrow) in a man with center-involving diabetic macular edema (DME). Vision measured 20/60. OCT angiography (OCTA) (3×3 mm, Optovue AngioVue) of the superficial **(B)** retinal plexus shows an irregular foveal avascular zone (FAZ) and very faint central cysts. OCTA of the deep retinal plexus **(C)** more prominently reveals dark oval voids from cystoid DME. Resolution of DME **(A)** 4 weeks after anti-VEGF injection for DME. Note the small extrafoveal preretinal membrane on OCT. The FAZ is larger in the deep compared with the superficial retinal plexus **(E)**. The cysts have resolved from the deep retinal plexus **(F)**.

imaging modalities is usually necessary. OCT may demonstrate distortion of the retinal architecture from hyaloid traction or preretinal membranes. Eyes with this traction may not respond to medical therapy and may ultimately require surgery for the resolution of macular edema. In addition to an OCT line scan, retinal thickness maps are generated. Increased central foveal thickness on OCT has been correlated with fluorescein leakage and thickening on clinical examination and has moderate correlation with visual acuity.[18]

One shortcoming is that OCT cannot diagnose macular ischemia, which has traditionally been diagnosed with FA. This limits the ability of OCT to correlate structure to function (visual acuity). Certain parameters such as disorganization of the retinal inner layers (DRIL) identified within 1 mm with OCT have been evaluated as a potential marker for visual acuity in eyes with current or resolved DME.[19,20] OCTA is a more recent imaging modality that may serve to link structural anatomy with circulation in the posterior pole.

Some of the most important uses of OCT are to detect and localize subtle DME, for DME classification schemata, and to evaluate pharmacotherapy. OCT permits earlier and more sensitive diagnosis and localization of retinal thickening compared with other imaging modalities and is more accurate than clinical examination. This has led to the use of OCT as a parameter in all clinical studies to determine if DME involves the fovea center (center-involved DME, CI-DME) or not (non-center-involved DME, non-CI-DME). This is in contrast to the term CSME, which is based on clinical examination. One important reason for the use of an OCT-based definition is to evaluate the best treatment for DME based on its location and the level of visual acuity. Preliminary studies support that focal laser may be the preferred initial treatment for non-CI-DME.[21] Protocol V from the DRCR.net (see Appendix A) is currently comparing treatment options for eyes with CI-DME and good visual acuity.

The central subfield thickness (CST) is a reproducible measure of central macular thickness, whereas macular volume may better assess extrafoveal DME. The parameters to define CI-DME and OCT reproducibility and a conversion factor to compare results with different OCT machines have been assessed because the numeric values for CST and volumes differ between time domain and spectral domain OCT devices.[22] For example, in Protocol S from the DRCR.net study, development of CI-DME with visual impairment (visual acuity letter score 78 or less)

was defined as the following: CST ≥305 for women and ≥320 for men with Heidelberg Spectralis spectral domain OCT, CST ≥290 for women and ≥305 for men with Zeiss Cirrus and Optovue RTVue spectral domain OCT, or CST ≥250 with Zeiss Stratus time domain OCT (www.drcr.net).

There have been various classifications proposed for DME based on OCT morphology. The patterns of DME have been described as diffuse (or sponge-like) retinal thickening, diabetic cystoid macular edema, serous subretinal fluid without posterior hyaloid traction, DME with posterior hyaloid traction, and mixed patterns.[23,24] These patterns have been used to prognosticate and in some cases to direct treatment. For example, eyes with posterior hyaloid traction may not respond to anti-VEGF injections and ultimately require vitrectomy for the resolution of retinal thickening. The cystoid variety of DME has been associated with worse visual acuity than with diffuse retinal thickening. OCT can also help differentiate DME from imitators such as macular telangiectasia.

OCT is used for sequential imaging and to gauge success of the therapeutic modality whether medical, surgical, or laser. Because OCT is more reliable for the detection of retinal thickening than clinical examination, it enables more precise treatment decisions and is a standard for all DME therapeutic research (Fig. 4.4A and B). OCT in DR has also been used to study choroid thickness with enhanced-depth imaging, as well as the vitreoretinal interface and peripapillary retina in patients with diabetes.[25] Focal and widespread peripapillary RNFL thinning has been noted in patients with prediabetes and type 2 diabetes, respectively, before clinical detection of clinical retinopathy.[26]

Enhancements of OCT technology are being investigated to further define imaging. Functional OCT uses OCT to give a physiologic assessment of the retina, such as metabolism.[27] Doppler OCT uses Doppler phase shift to measure and quantify the total blood flow.[28] Intraoperative OCT pairs OCT with the operating microscope for real-time micrometer-resolution imaging.[29]

OPTICAL COHERENCE TOMOGRAPHY ANGIOGRAPHY

OCTA is a novel, noninvasive technique to image flow in the retinal and choroidal vasculature without dye injection. OCTA denotes progression of OCT technology, whereby motion contrast is utilized to create high-resolution, depth-resolved, volumetric, angiographic flow images in minutes. The OCTA software compares the decorrelation signal or phase variance between consecutive OCT B scans taken at the same retinal location to detect scatter or motion and differentiates this from the static background. Differences between repeat B scans are caused by erythrocyte movement in vessels, thus identifying flow. OCTA can be performed with either a spectral domain or a swept source platform, and a variety of OCTA devices are available for commercial and research use. A segmented, en face depiction of blood flow and the OCT B scan corresponding to the segmented flow image are produced. Most devices have automated segmentation of the retina, with optional manual adjustment of automated lines. The Angiovue (Avanti OCT, Optovue, Fremont, CA, USA) displays segmented images in four layers: superficial capillary plexus, deep capillary plexus, outer retinal layer, and choroidal circulation.[30] The ability of OCTA to depict blood vessel flow details will continue to improve with software enhancements. Compared with FA, OCTA is much faster, requiring only minutes to perform, and it produces images with higher resolution and greater detail that are quantifiable and reproducible. OCTA lacks the risks of fluorescein dye injection, such as intravenous access and allergic reaction. FA evaluates only the superficial retinal plexus, whereas OCTA identifies the superficial and deep retinal vascular plexuses and the choroidal circulation. On the other hand, current OCTA imaging is limited to small scan areas and is prone to various motion and projection artifacts that need to be considered when interpreting OCTA images. OCTA can characterize the abnormal presence or absence of flow and irregular vessel geometry, which manifests in DR as retinal neovascularization, capillary nonperfusion, and microaneurysms, respectively. OCTA is currently finding its clinical role, and an enormous amount of research and data is rapidly being generated. OCTA is a formidable challenger with potential to replace FA for imaging macular vasculature in DR.

OCTA has been used to qualitatively demonstrate features of DR. In patients with diabetes without clinical signs of retinopathy, OCTA imaging reveals subtle changes in the perifoveal vasculature, including foci of capillary nonperfusion, microaneurysms, remodeling of the foveal avascular zone (FAZ), and a larger mean FAZ size in patients with diabetes compared with nondiabetic control eyes (Fig. 4.3B).[5] Similar findings from other studies confirm that OCTA imaging of retinovascular changes may precede clinical detection, with potential for OCTA to be a screening tool for individuals at risk for DR. OCTA has been directly compared with FA imaging in patients with diabetes with and without retinopathy (Fig. 4.5)[31] OCTA delineates the foveal nonflow zone (FAZ) as well as areas of capillary nonperfusion and can detect preretinal neovascularization in the posterior pole by adjusting segmentation to include the retina-vitreous interface above the internal limiting membrane.[32] OCTA can precisely localize the intraretinal depth of microaneurysms, although it appears to be less sensitive than FA in identifying the presence of microaneurysms[33] This may be related to flow characteristics in the microaneurysm being below the threshold of OCTA detection and/or pooling of blood within a microaneurysm without flow. Microaneurysms, which are hyperfluorescent spots with FA, may be apparent as capillary loops, dilated capillary segments, small foci of neovascularization, or focal dilations in areas bordering capillary nonperfusion on OCTA.[33] Arteriole wall staining with fluorescein appears as vascular attenuation on OCTA. Intraretinal cystoid spaces appear as dark oblong spaces with smooth borders and should be differentiated from foci of capillary nonperfusion, which have a grayer hue and irregular border (Fig. 4.4B and C).[34]

OCTA can also generate quantitative measures of the fovea avascular (nonflow) zone, capillary nonperfusion, flow maps, and vessel density analysis. OCTA data are more detailed and precise than data from FA, in which dynamic fluorescein dye leakage obscures images thus precluding accurate measurement. Automated algorithms have been developed demonstrating the reduction of both the superficial and deep parafoveal retinal vessel density in patients with diabetes without retinopathy compared with age-matched healthy controls.[35] A progressive reduction in capillary density and branching complexity and an increased average vascular caliber have been found in eyes with different stages of DR.[36–38] Quantitative changes in vascular density correlate with the severity of DR: specifically, the capillary density index decreased with worsening DR severity and systemic vascular and metabolic risk factors were associated with quantifiable structural changes on OCTA.[39]

Novel methods are being developed to assess relative blood flow speeds using OCTA, reduce artifacts, and increase the scanning area. Overall, OCTA combined with the OCT B scan provides both structural and functional imaging with potential to stage retinopathy, evaluate macular flow, and produce quantitative parameters that may eventually be used for clinical trials.

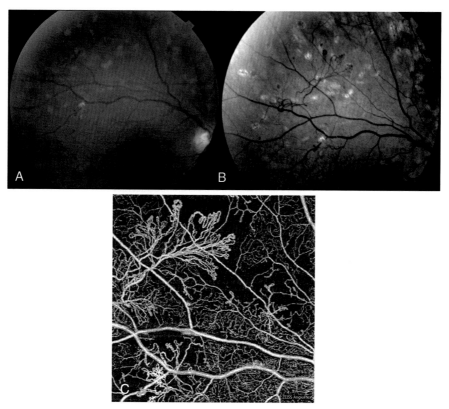

FIG. 4.5 Color standard **(A)** and red-free **(B)** photographs directed along the superotemporal arcade where there is neovascularization of the retina surrounded by panretinal laser. Note that the new blood vessels are more apparent on red-free images. Optical coherence tomography angiography **(C)** directed to this area segmented to include the superficial and deep retinal plexus reveals that the neovascularization is surrounded by capillary nonperfusion.

ADAPTIVE OPTICS

Adaptive optics (AO) is a technology that has been adapted to scanning laser ophthalmoscopy (SLO) and OCT to resolve optical aberrations from retinal imaging. AO can produce high-resolution images of foveal cones, as well as dynamic images of the retinal vasculature, and measure arterial wall dimensions and the speed of blood flow. However, AO is limited by its very small field of view, typically in the range of 1–2 degrees, which impedes its clinical utility.

In diabetic eyes, AO-SLO has demonstrated irregular branching of blood vessels, shunt vessels, capillary sprouts, and narrowed perifoveal capillaries.[40,41] One study demonstrated that OCTA is comparable with AO-SLO FA to image the fine foveal vessels, with very small differences in FAZ area and lumen diameter between these techniques. The authors concluded that OCTA is technically easier to

perform and more widely available, whereas AO remains primarily a research tool.[42] Decreased regularity of the cone photoreceptor arrangement demonstrated with AO-SLO has been associated with increasing DR severity and DME.[43] A study using both AO-SLO and OCTA found an association between capillary nonperfusion in the deep capillary plexus and abnormalities in the photoreceptor layer in DR. These authors hypothesized this was secondary to reduced oxygen delivery from the deep capillary plexus to the photoreceptors.[44]

FUNDUS AUTOFLUORESCENCE

FAF is a noninvasive imaging modality that has been used to characterize the status of the RPE in various retinal disorders. Short-wave FAF derives its signal from lipofuscin in the RPE, and patterns of increased FAF have been described in eyes with DME, which correlate to structural (OCT, FA) and functional (visual acuity) impairment.[45,46] As FAF depends on the status of the RPE, it can delineate the location of prior laser photocoagulation (Fig. 4.1E). However, the current role of FAF in the management of DR is minimal because OCT provides more robust qualitative and quantitative data and is also more widely available.

ULTRASOUND IMAGING

Ophthalmic ultrasound imaging uses the acoustic wave technology to generate reflections or "echos" at tissue interfaces of differential acoustic impedance. In DR, B scan ultrasound imaging is used to determine the status of the retina when visualization is obscured by vitreous hemorrhage or dense cataract. It can also help characterize diabetic retinal detachment as tractional, rhegmatogenous, or combined. It may play a role in determining whether vitreous traction is present or in surgical planning. B scan ultrasound imaging is not sensitive enough to evaluate for DME, and it has limited utility when the ocular media are clear.

SUMMARY

Retinal imaging characterizes the features of DR, with potential to demonstrate more precise details than clinical examination. Modifications of established imaging techniques and development of new ones will improve our knowledge of the pathogenesis of DR. The future holds innovations in technology, such as automated image interpretation, mobile applications, quantification of large data sets, ischemia analysis, and further exploration into the relationship between retinal function and structure.

REFERENCES

1. Novais EA, Baumal CR, Sarraf D, Freund KB, Duker JS. Multimodal imaging in retinal disease. A consensus definition. *Ophthal Surg Lasers Imaging Retina.* 2016;47(3):201–205.
2. Early Treatment Diabetic Retinopathy Study Research Group. Grading diabetic retinopathy from stereoscopic color fundus photographs–an extension of the modified Airlie House classification. ETDRS report number 10 *Ophthalmology.* 1991;98(suppl 5):786–806.
3. Wilkinson CP, Ferris 3rd FL, Klein RE, et al. Proposed international clinical diabetic retinopathy and diabetic macular edema disease severity scales. *Ophthalmology.* 2003;110(9):1677–1682.
4. Sohn EH, van Dijk HW, Jiao C, et al. Retinal neurodegeneration may precede microvascular changes characteristic of diabetic retinopathy in diabetes mellitus. *Proc Natl Acad Sci USA.* 2016;113:E2655–E2664.
5. de Carlo TE, Chin AT, Bonini Filho MA, et al. Detection of microvascular changes in eyes of patients with diabetes but not clinical diabetic retinopathy using optical coherence tomography angiography. *Retina.* 2015;35:2364–2370.
6. Silva PS, Aiello LP. Telemedicine and eye examinations for diabetic retinopathy. A time to maximize real-world outcomes. *JAMA Ophthalmol.* 2015;113:525–526.
7. Boyle JP, Thompson TJ, Gregg EW, Barker LE, Williamson DF. Projection of the year 2050 burden of diabetes in the US adult population: dynamic modeling of incidence, mortality, and prediabetes prevalence. *Popul Health Metr.* 2010;8:29.
8. Gulshan V, Peng L, Coram M, et al. Development and validation of a deep learning algorithm for detection of diabetic retinopathy in retinal fundus photographs. *JAMA.* 2016;316:2402–2410.
9. Tozer K, Woodward MA, Newman-Casey PA. Telemedicine and diabetic retinopathy: review of published screening programs. *J Endocrinol Diabetes.* 2015;2(4).
10. Mansberger SL, Sheppler C, Barker G, et al. Long-term comparative effectiveness of telemedicine in providing diabetic retinopathy screening examinations A Randomized clinical trial. *JAMA Ophthalmol.* 2015;133:518–525.
11. Williams GA, Scott IU, Haller JA, Maguire AM, Marcus D, McDonald HR. Single-field fundus photography for diabetic retinopathy screening: a report by the American Academy of Ophthalmology. *Ophthalmology.* 2004;111(5):1055–1062.
12. Wang YT, Tadarati M, Wolfson Y, Bressler SB, Bressler NM. Comparison of prevalence of diabetic macular edema based on monocular fundus photography vs. optical coherence tomography. *JAMA Ophthalmol.* 2016;134:222–228.

Fluorescein Angiography
13. Novotny HR, Alvis DL. A method of photographing fluorescence in circulating blood in the human retina. *Circulation.* 1961;24:82–86.
14. Wessel MM, Aaker GD, Parlitsis G, et al. Ultra-wide-field angiography improved detection and classification of diabetic retinopathy. *Retina.* 2012;32:785–791.
15. Silva PS, Cavallerano JD, Haddad NM, et al. Peripheral lesions identified on ultrawide field imaging predict increased risk of diabetic retinopathy progression over 4 years. *Ophthalmology.* 2015;122:949–956.
16. Weinberger D, Kramer M, Priel E, et al. Indocyanine green angiographic findings in nonproliferative diabetic retinopathy. *Am J Ophthalmol.* 1998;126:238–247.

OCT
17. Huang D, Swanson EA, Lin CP, et al. Optical coherence tomography. *Science.* 1991;254:1178–1181.

18. Ou WC, Brown DM, Payne JF, Wykoff CC. Relationship between visual acuity and retinal thickness during anti-vascular endothelial growth factor therapy for retinal diseases. *Am J Ophthalmol.* 2017;180.

19. Sun JK, Lin MM, Lammer J, et al. Disorganization of the retinal inner layers as a predictor of visual acuity in eyes with center-involved diabetic macular edema. *JAMA Ophthalmol.* 2014;132:1309–1316.

20. Nicholson L, Ramu J, Triantafyllopoulou I et al. Diagnostic accuracy of disorganization of the retinal inner layers in detecting macular capillary non-perfusion in diabetic retinopathy. Clin Exp Ophthalmol, 43.

21. Scott IU, Danis RP, Bressler SB, et al. Effect of focal/grid photocoagulation on visual acuity and retinal thickening in eyes with non-center–involved diabetic macular edema. *Retina.* 2009;29:613–617.

22. Diabetic Retinopathy Clinical Research Network Writing Group. Reproducibility of spectral-domain optical coherence tomography retinal thickness measurements and conversion to equivalent time-domain metrics in diabetic macular edema. *JAMA Ophthalmol.* 2014;132:1113–1122.

23. Otani T, Kishi S, Maruyama Y. Patterns of diabetic macular edema with optical coherence tomography. *Am J Ophthalmol.* 1999;127:688–693.

24. Kim NR, Kim YJ, Chin HS, Moon YS. Optical coherence tomographic patterns in diabetic macular oedema: prediction of visual outcome after focal alser photocoagulation. *Br J Ophthalmol.* 2009;93:901–905.

25. Adhi M, Badaro E, Liu JJ, et al. Three-dimensional enhanced imaging of vitreoretinal interface in diabetic retinopathy using swept-source optical coherence tomography. *Am J Ophthalmol.* 2016;162. 140–149.e1.

26. De Clerck EEB, Schouten JSAG, Berendschot TTJM, et al. Loss of temporal peripapillary retinal nerve fibers in prediabetes or type 2 diabetes without diabetic retinopathy: the Maastricht Study. *Invest Ophthalmol Vis Sci.* 2017;58:1017–1027.

27. Zhang Q, Lu R, Wang B, et al. Functional optical coherence tomography enables in vivo physiological assessment of retinal rod and cone photoreceptors. *Sci Rep.* 2015;5:9595.

28. Lee B, Novais EA, Waheed NK, et al. En face Doppler optical coherence tomography measurement of total retinal blood flow in diabetic retinopathy and diabetic macular edema. *JAMA Ophthalmol.* 2017;135:244–251.

29. Ehlers JP, Goshe J, Dupps WJ, et al. Determination of feasibility and utility of microscope – integrated optical coherence tomography during ophthalmic surgery: the DISCOVER Study RESCAN results. *JAMA Ophthalmol.* 2015;133:1124–1132.

OCT Angiography
30. Spaide RF, Klancnik Jr JM, Cooney MJ. Retinal vascular layers imaged by fluorescein angiography and optical coherence tomography angiography. *JAMA Ophthalmol.* 2015;133(1):45–50.

31. Hwang TS, Jia Y, Gao SS, et al. Optical coherence tomography angiography features of diabetic retinopathy. *Retina.* 2015;35(11):2371–2376.

32. de Carlo TE, Bonini Filho MA, Baumal CR, et al. Evaluation of preretinal neovascularization in proliferative diabetic retinopathy using optical coherence tomography angiography. *Ophthal Surg Lasers Imaging Retina.* 2016;47(2):115–119.

33. Salz DA, de Carlo TE, Adhi M, et al. Select features of diabetic retinopathy on swept-source optical coherence tomographic angiography compared with fluorescein angiography and normal eyes. *JAMA Ophthalmol.* 2016;134(6):644–650.

34. de Carlo TE, Chin AT, Joseph T, et al. Distinguishing diabetic macular edema from capillary nonperfusion using optical coherence tomography angiography. *Ophthal Surg Lasers Imaging Retina.* 2016;47(2):108–114.

35. Dimitrova G, Chihara E, Takahashi H, Amano H, Okazaki K. Quantitative retinal optical coherence tomography angiography in patients with diabetes without diabetic retinopathy. *Invest Ophthalmol Vis Sci.* 2017;58:190–196.

36. Kim AY, Chu Z, Shahidzadeh A, et al. Quantifying microvascular density and morphology in diabetic retinopathy using spectral-domain optical coherence tomography angiography. *Invest Ophthalmol Vis Sci.* 2016;57:OCT362–OCT370.

37. Hwang TS, Gao SS, Liu L, et al. Automated quantification of capillary nonperfusion using optical coherence tomography angiography in diabetic retinopathy. *JAMA Ophthalmol.* 2016;134(4):367–373.

38. Agemy SA, Scripsema NK, Shah CM et al. Retinal vascular perfusion density mapping using optical coherence tomography angiography in normal and diabetic retinopathy patients Retina, 35.

39. Ting DSW, Tan GSW, Agawal R, et al. Optical coherence tomography angiography in type 2 diabetes and diabetic retinopathy. *JAMA Ophthalmol.* 2017;135:306–312.

Adaptive Optics
40. Burns SA, Elsner AE, Chui TY, et al. In vivo adaptive optics microvascular imaging in diabetic patients without clinically severe diabetic retinopathy. *Biomed Optics Express.* 2014;5(3):961–974.

41. Lombardo M, Parravano M, Serrao S, et al. Analysis of retinal capillaries in patients with type 1 diabetes and non-proliferative diabetic retinopathy using adaptive optics imaging. *Reina.* 2013;33:1630–1639.

42. Mo S, Krawitz B, Efstathiadis E, et al. Imaging foveal microvasculature: optical coherence tomography angiography versus adaptive optics scanning light ophthalmoscope fluorescein angiography. *IOVS.* 2016;57:OCT130–OCT140.

43. Lammer J, Prager SG, Cheney MC, et al. Cone photoreceptor irregularity on adaptive optics scanning laser ophthalmoscopy correlates with severity of diabetic retinopathy and macular edema. *Invest Ophthalmol Vis Sci.* 2016;1(57):6624–6632.

44. Nesper PL, Scarinci F, Fawzi AA. Adaptive optics reveals photoreceptor abnormalities in diabetic macular ischemia. *PLoS One.* 2017;12(1):e0169926.

Fundus autofluorescence

45. Vujosevic S, Casciano M, Pilotto E, et al. Diabetic macular edema: fundus autofluorescence and functional correlations. *Invest Ophthalmol Vis Sci.* 2011;52:442–448.

46. Chung H, Park B, Shin HJ, Kim HC. Correlation of fundus autofluorescence with spectral-domain optical coherence tomography and vision in diabetic macular edema. *Ophthalmology.* 2012;119:1056–1065.

CHAPTER 5

Genetics of Diabetic Retinopathy

KAREN W. JENG-MILLER, MD, MPH • CAROLINE R. BAUMAL, MD

While certain risk factors such as duration of diabetes mellitus and glycemic control have been shown to correlate with an increased risk of developing diabetic retinopathy (DR), there are circumstances when individuals with similar metabolic factors demonstrate disparate degrees of diabetic retinopathy.[1,2] Diabetic retinopathy disproportionately affects Hispanics and African-Americans in the United States.[3,4] Worldwide, Latin Americans and South Asians are among groups that have relatively higher rates of diabetic retinopathy.[5] This clustering of DR among different ethnic groups, as well as findings from twin and familial studies suggest a possible genetic component in determining the phenotype of diabetic retinopathy. Methodologies thus far to identify the genetic factors that may play a role in DR include familial studies, candidate gene studies, linkage studies, and systematic genome-wide scans. The study of epigenetic factors that may alter an individual's genetic expression is a new compelling topic that may also affect the phenotype of diabetic retinopathy.

FAMILIAL STUDIES

Familial studies aim to evaluate risk factors causing familial aggregation of disease traits and attempt to identify genetic mechanisms in these diseases. This principle has been employed to understand the genetic factors that may exist in DR. In 1982, Leslie and Pyke found that 95% of concordant type 2 diabetic identical twins versus 68% of concordant type 1 diabetic identical twins had the same degree of diabetic retinopathy.[6] Subsequently, other familial studies with siblings and relatives of diabetics demonstrated varying degrees of familial clustering of DR.[7–9] Notably the Family Investigation of Nephropathy and Diabetes (FIND) Eye study demonstrated heritability of DR to be as high as 24% in a population of Mexican-Americans with type 2 diabetes.[4]

CANDIDATE GENES

Candidate genes refer to genes that may play a key role in the biochemical pathogenesis of diabetic retinopathy. The most prominent genes studied include genes encoding aldose reductase (ALR2), angiotensin-1 converting enzyme (ACE), endothelial nitric oxide synthase (eNOS), receptor for advanced glycation end products (RAGE) and vascular endothelial growth factor (VEGF).

Aldose Reductase

Aldose reductase is part of the rate-limiting step in the polyol pathway, which converts glucose to sorbitol. Due to glucose excess, sorbitol accumulates and results in intracellular osmotic stress. In mice models, this osmotic stress was associated with retinal microaneurysm formations and pericyte loss.[10] As a result, the aldose reductase gene has been associated with diabetic retinopathy in various population studies.[11,12] A recent meta-analysis of over 3000 patients from China, Brazil, Australia, and Japan with diabetic retinopathy concluded that there was a genetic association between the ALR2 C106T polymorphism among type 1 diabetics (OR 1.78, 95% CI = 1.39–2.28) but not in type 2 diabetes.[13]

Angiotensin-1 Converting Enzyme

ACE is an integral component of the renin-angiotensin system (RAS) that converts angiotensin I to angiotensin II (ATII). ATII functions to promote vascular remodeling and proliferation, mainly through the angiotensin type I (AT1) receptor, and can result in increased capillary growth, enhanced vascular permeability, and oxidative stress.[14,15] Therefore, blockade of the renin-angiotensin system theoretically decreases vascular proliferation. Many human and animal studies have corroborated that ACE inhibitors or angiotensin receptor-1 blockers may result in delayed progression of diabetic retinopathy.[16,17]

Endothelial Nitric Oxide Synthase

Endothelial nitric oxide synthase is a key enzyme in production of the vasodilator, nitric oxide (NO) which is an important factor resulting in increased blood flow to the retina. In many studies, eNOS has been shown to play an essential role in retinal vascular function.[15,18] While a recent 2014 meta-analysis of 15 studies did not demonstrate a significant association between eNOS and diabetic retinopathy,[19] this was in contrast to a previous 2012 meta-analysis that demonstrated eNOS may be a protective factor against diabetic retinopathy as well as a 2014 meta-analysis suggesting a decreased risk of diabetic retinopathy with eNOS, specifically in African patients.[20,21]

Receptor for Advanced Glycation End Products

Advanced glycation end products (AGEs) are derived from nonenzymatic glycation of proteins and lipids secondary to prolonged exposure to hyperglycemia.[2] AGEs have the potential to contribute to diabetic retinopathy through (1) accumulation in tissues resulting in direct tissue damage[22] and (2) activation of specific receptors for advanced glycation end products (RAGE), resulting in cytokine secretion that can increase endothelial permeability and accelerate progression of diabetic retinopathy.[23,24] Various meta analyses demonstrate the association of DR with the 1704T allele but not polymorphisms −429T/C, −374T/A, and Gly82Ser.[25,26] In contrast, a 2012 meta-analysis concluded that the −374T/A polymorphism was a protective factor for DR in type 2 diabetics (OR = 0.64, 95% CI = 0.42–0.99, $P = .05$).[27]

Vascular Endothelial Growth Factor

The VEGF gene is the best-studied candidate gene in the context of DR. It is an important cytokine in angiogenesis and microvascular permeability.[28,29] Increased VEGF levels are stimulated through hypoxia from diabetic microvascular changes, and thus significantly contribute to the pathology of DR by stimulating neovascularization and breakdown of the blood-retinal barrier.[30,31] As a result, anti-VEGF drugs have been widely employed in the treatment of diabetic retinopathy. Polymorphisms of interest include rs833061 (−460T/C), rs699947 (−2578C/A), rs2010963 ([405G/C] and [634G/C]), rs3025039 (+936C/T), and rs2146323.[32] These polymorphisms have been extensively examined in various meta-analyses but there is no clear consensus on their role in susceptibility to diabetic retinopathy.[15,33,34]

Other less well-studied candidate genes include adiponectin, complement factors H and B, intercellular adhesion molecule-1, erythropoietin, P selectin, transforming growth factor β, toll-like receptor 4, and tumor necrosis factor α.[32] However, candidate gene approaches to determine genetic markers for diabetic retinopathy have been limited by small sample sizes and incorrect hypotheses regarding genes involved in the disease pathways. The Candidate Gene Association Resource (CARe) performed a large, comprehensive candidate gene study for diabetic retinopathy with comprehensive inclusion of genes associated with cardiovascular and inflammatory pathways in attempt to address these limitations.[35] By examining pathways rather than specific genes, this study was less dependent on the accuracy of a priori hypotheses regarding the causality of certain genes in diabetic retinopathy. The study findings only supported three single nucleotide polymorphisms (SNPs) in P selectin to be associated with diabetic retinopathy.

LINKAGE STUDIES

Linkage studies are driven by chromosomal location identification in diseases through familial inheritance patterns and do not rely on biochemical or pathophysiological pathway hypotheses. These studies identify specific genetic markers, usually single nucleotide polymorphisms (SNPs), inherited by large families with a disease affecting several generations and are able to narrow down the chromosomal region until a gene or gene variant of interest is detected. Studies in Pima Indians[36] and Mexican-Americans[37] identified regions on chromosomes 3, 9 and 12 leading to potential candidate genes in these locations.

GENOME-WIDE ASSOCIATION STUDIES

Genome-wide association studies (GWAS) allow for numerous SNPs to be tested against specific traits and diseases, like diabetic retinopathy. This methodology also bypasses a priori hypotheses limiting candidate gene studies. A 2010 GWAS of Mexican-Americans found two potential SNPs associated with severe diabetic retinopathy in the calcium/calmodulin-dependent protein kinase IV and formin 1 genes.[38] In 2011, a meta-analysis of genome-wide association data did not find any significant associations at a genome-wide level; however, the most significant variant identified was rs476141 on chromosome 1.[39]

EPIGENETICS AND DIABETIC RETINOPATHY

Epigenetics are heritable changes in gene activity and expression secondary to environment, lifestyle, and even disease states, which occur without any changes in DNA sequence. DNA methylation and histone modifications are major mechanisms of epigenetic modification.[40] A 2015 case-control study of type 2 diabetes patients found that global DNA methylation levels were significantly higher in those with diabetic retinopathy than those without, leading investigators to conclude higher DNA methylation was predictive for retinopathy.[41] Furthermore, a 2015 genome wide analysis of DNA methylation in type 1 diabetics concluded that differential DNA methylation in over 200 genes was associated with development of proliferative diabetic retinopathy and that epigenetic markers have the potential to predict proliferative DR.[42]

CONCLUSIONS

Genetics factors potentially play a role in development and progression of diabetic retinopathy. To date, the results of studies evaluating associations between genes and diabetic retinopathy are inconsistent, with many studies failing to substantiate these associations. Further research is needed to understand the genotype to phenotype relationships as well as the role of epigenetic modifications in diabetic retinopathy.

REFERENCES

1. Keenan HA, Costacou T, Sun JK, et al. Clinical factors associated with resistance to microvascular complications in diabetic patients of extreme disease duration: the 50-year medalist study. *Diabetes Care*. 2007;30(8):1995–1997.
2. Liew G, Klein R, Wong TY. The role of genetics in susceptibility to diabetic retinopathy. *Int Ophthalmol Clin*. 2009;49(2):35–52.
3. Wong TY, Klein R, Islam FMA, et al. Diabetic retinopathy in a multi-ethnic cohort in the United States. *Am J Ophthalmol*. 2006;141(3):446–455.
4. Arar NH, Freedman BI, Adler SG, et al. Heritability of the severity of diabetic retinopathy: the FIND-eye study. *Invest Ophthalmol Vis Sci*. 2008;49(9):3839–3845.
5. Sivaprasad S, Gupta B, Crosby-Nwaobi R, Evans J. Prevalence of diabetic retinopathy in various ethnic groups: a worldwide perspective. *Surv Ophthalmol*. 2012;57(4):347–370.
6. Leslie RD, Pyke DA. Diabetic retinopathy in identical twins. *Diabetes*. 1982;31(1):19–21.
7. Hietala K, Forsblom C, Summanen P, Groop P-H. Heritability of proliferative diabetic retinopathy. *Diabetes*. 2008;57(8):2176–2180.
8. Looker HC, Nelson RG, Chew E, et al. Genome-wide linkage analyses to identify loci for diabetic retinopathy. *Diabetes*. 2007;56(4):1160–1166.
9. The Diabetes Control and Complications Trial Research Group. Clustering of long-term complications in families with diabetes in the diabetes control and complications trial. *Diabetes*. 1997;46(11):1829–1839.
10. Robison WG, Nagata M, Laver N, Hohman TC, Kinoshita JH. Diabetic-like retinopathy in rats prevented with an aldose reductase inhibitor. *Invest Ophthalmol Vis Sci*. 1989;30(11):2285–2292.
11. Wang Y, Ng MCY, Lee S-C, et al. Phenotypic heterogeneity and associations of two aldose reductase gene polymorphisms with nephropathy and retinopathy in type 2 diabetes. *Diabetes Care*. 2003;26(8):2410–2415.
12. Richeti F, Noronha RM, Waetge RTL, et al. Evaluation of AC(n) and C(-106)T polymorphisms of the aldose reductase gene in Brazilian patients with DM1 and susceptibility to diabetic retinopathy. *Mol Vis*. 2007;13:740–745.
13. Zhou M, Zhang P, Xu X, Sun X. The relationship between aldose reductase C106T polymorphism and diabetic retinopathy: an updated meta-analysis. *Invest Ophthalmol Vis Sci*. 2015;56(4):2279–2289.
14. Funatsu H, Yamashita H. Pathogenesis of diabetic retinopathy and the renin-angiotensin system. *Ophthal Physiol Opt*. 2003;23(6):495–501.
15. Abhary S, Hewitt AW, Burdon KP, Craig JE. A systematic meta-analysis of genetic association studies for diabetic retinopathy. *Diabetes*. 2009;58(9):2137–2147.
16. Chaturvedi N, Sjolie A-K, Stephenson JM, et al. Effect of lisinopril on progression of retinopathy in normotensive people with type 1 diabetes. *Lancet*. 1998;351(9095):28–31.
17. Sjølie AK, Klein R, Porta M, et al. Effect of candesartan on progression and regression of retinopathy in type 2 diabetes (DIRECT-Protect 2): a randomised placebo-controlled trial. *Lancet*. 2008;372(9647):1385–1393.
18. Li Q, Verma A, Han P-Y, et al. Diabetic eNOS-knockout mice develop accelerated retinopathy. *Invest Ophthalmol Vis Sci*. 2010;51(10):5240–5246.
19. Ma Z, Chen R, Ren H-Z, Guo X, Guo J, Chen L. Association between eNOS 4b/a polymorphism and the risk of diabetic retinopathy in type 2 diabetes mellitus: a meta-analysis. *J Diabetes Res*. 2014;2014:549747.
20. Zhao S, Li T, Zheng B, Zheng Z. Nitric oxide synthase 3 (NOS3) 4b/a, T-786C and G894T polymorphisms in association with diabetic retinopathy susceptibility: a meta-analysis. *Ophthal Genet*. 2012;33(4):200–207.
21. Qian-Qian Y, Yong Y, Jing Z, et al. Association between a 27-bp variable number of tandem repeat polymorphism in intron 4 of the eNOS gene and risk for diabetic retinopathy Type 2 diabetes mellitus: a meta-analysis. *Curr Eye Res*. 2014;39(10):1052–1058.
22. Stitt AW. AGEs and diabetic retinopathy. *Invest Ophthalmol Vis Sci*. 2010;51(10):4867–4874.
23. Fukami K, Yamagishi S-I, Ueda S, Okuda S. Role of AGEs in diabetic nephropathy. *Curr Pharm Des*. 2008;14(10):946–952.
24. Goldin A, Beckman JA, Schmidt AM, Creager MA. Advanced glycation end products: sparking the development of diabetic vascular injury. *Circulation*. 2006;114(6):597–605.
25. Niu W, Qi Y, Wu Z, Liu Y, Zhu D, Jin W. A meta-analysis of receptor for advanced glycation end products gene: four well-evaluated polymorphisms with diabetes mellitus. *Mol Cell Endocrinol*. 2012;358(1):9–17.
26. Ng ZX, Kuppusamy UR, Tajunisah I, Fong KCS, Chua KH. Association analysis of -429T/C and -374T/A polymorphisms of receptor of advanced glycation end products (RAGE) gene in Malaysian with type 2 diabetic retinopathy. *Diabetes Res Clin Pract*. 2012;95(3):372–377.

27. Yuan D, Yuan D, Liu Q. Association of the receptor for advanced glycation end products gene polymorphisms with diabetic retinopathy in type 2 diabetes: a meta-analysis. *Ophthalmologica.* 2012;227(4):223–232.

28. Aiello LP, Pierce EA, Foley ED, et al. Suppression of retinal neovascularization in vivo by inhibition of vascular endothelial growth factor (VEGF) using soluble VEGF-receptor chimeric proteins. *Proc Natl Acad Sci USA.* 1995;92(23):10457–10461.

29. Qaum T, Xu Q, Joussen AM, et al. VEGF-initiated blood-retinal barrier breakdown in early diabetes. *Invest Ophthalmol Vis Sci.* 2001;42(10):2408–2413.

30. Ribatti D. The crucial role of vascular permeability factor/vascular endothelial growth factor in angiogenesis: a historical review. *Br J Haematol.* 2005;128(3):303–309.

31. Schlingemann RO, van Hinsbergh VW. Role of vascular permeability factor/vascular endothelial growth factor in eye disease. *Br J Ophthalmol.* 1997;81(6):501–512.

32. Hampton BM, Schwartz SG, Brantley MA, Flynn HW. Update on genetics and diabetic retinopathy. *Clin Ophthalmol.* 2015;9:2175–2193.

33. Gong J-Y, Sun Y-H. Association of VEGF gene polymorphisms with diabetic retinopathy: a meta-analysis. *PLoS One.* 2013;8(12):e84069.

34. Han L, Zhang L, Xing W, et al. The associations between VEGF gene polymorphisms and diabetic retinopathy susceptibility: a meta-analysis of 11 case-control studies. *J Diabetes Res.* 2014;2014:805801.

35. Sobrin L, Green T, Sim X, et al. Candidate gene association study for diabetic retinopathy in persons with type 2 diabetes: the Candidate gene Association Resource (CARe). *Invest Ophthalmol Vis Sci.* 2011;52(10):7593–7602.

36. Imperatore G, Hanson RL, Pettitt DJ, Kobes S, Bennett PH, Knowler WC. Sib-pair linkage analysis for susceptibility genes for microvascular complications among Pima Indians with type 2 diabetes. Pima Diabetes Genes Group. *Diabetes.* 1998;47(5):821–830.

37. Hallman DM, Boerwinkle E, Gonzalez VH, Klein BEK, Klein R, Hanis CL. A genome-wide linkage scan for diabetic retinopathy susceptibility genes in Mexican Americans with type 2 diabetes from Starr County, Texas. *Diabetes.* 2007;56(4):1167–1173.

38. Fu Y-P, Hallman DM, Gonzalez VH, et al. Identification of diabetic retinopathy genes through a genome-wide association study among Mexican-Americans from Starr County. *Tex J Ophthalmol.* 2010;2010.

39. Grassi MA, Tikhomirov A, Ramalingam S, Below JE, Cox NJ, Nicolae DL. Genome-wide meta-analysis for severe diabetic retinopathy. *Hum Mol Genet.* 2011;20(12): 2472–2481.

40. Uribe-Lewis S, Woodfine K, Stojic L, Murrell A. Molecular mechanisms of genomic imprinting and clinical implications for cancer. *Expert Rev Mol Med.* 2011;13:e2. http://dx.doi.org/10.1017/S1462399410001717.

41. Maghbooli Z, Hossein-nezhad A, Larijani B, Amini M, Keshtkar A. Global DNA methylation as a possible biomarker for diabetic retinopathy. *Diabetes Metab Res Rev.* 2015;31(2):183–189. http://dx.doi.org/10.1002/dmrr.2584.

42. Agardh E, Lundstig A, Perfilyev A, et al. Genome-wide analysis of DNA methylation in subjects with type 1 diabetes identifies epigenetic modifications associated with proliferative diabetic retinopathy. *BMC Med.* 2015;13: 182.

CHAPTER 6

Effect of Modifiable Risk Factors on the Incidence and Progression of Diabetic Retinopathy

MICHAEL D. TIBBETTS, MD

INTRODUCTION

The identification of potential risk factors that affect the development and progression of diabetic retinopathy or response to therapy is an active area of investigation. Some of these risk factors are modifiable, such as lifestyle choices, whereas others, such as disease duration, are not. The duration of diabetes mellitus has been identified as a major risk factor associated with the development as well as the severity of diabetic retinopathy. This has been confirmed by multiple studies for individuals with both type 1 and type 2 diabetes. For patients with type 1 diabetes, after 5 years of diabetes duration, 25% will have some evidence of retinopathy, after 10 years, 60% have retinopathy, and after 15 years 80% have retinopathy.[1–3] Proliferative diabetic retinopathy (PDR) may be present in 50% of patients with type 1 diabetes (often 30 years and younger) who have the disease for 20 or more years.[2] PDR develops in 25% of individuals who have type 2 diabetes for 25 years or more and in only 2% of those with diabetes less than 5 years.[1] In patients with type 2 diabetes over the age of 30 years who have the diagnosis for less than 5 years, the risk of diabetic retinopathy increases for those patients who require insulin. Forty percent of such patients have retinopathy, whereas 24% of patients not taking insulin have retinopathy.

In the current era in which ophthalmologists have a variety of tools to treat diabetic macular edema (DME) and PDR, the assessment of the modifiable risk factors that can reduce the onset and severity of diabetic retinopathy may be overlooked. The anti–vascular endothelial growth factor (anti-VEGF) medications, in particular, can improve vision in patients with DME, induce regression of neovascularization, and also reduce the diabetic retinopathy severity score (DRSS).[4,5] Although anti-VEGFs may improve the retinopathy, these medications given by intravitreal injection do not affect the course

of nephropathy, neuropathy, and other systemic sites of microvascular injury nor do they mitigate the risks of myocardial infarction and stroke, which are the leading cause of death in diabetic patients. Eye care providers must communicate effectively with the patient's care team, including the primary care physician and endocrinologist, to encourage the management of systemic risk factors that can alter the course of the disease.

This chapter systematically reviews the evidence for modifiable risk factors that influence the onset and severity of retinopathy (Tables 6.1 and 6.2). The weight of the evidence varies for each factor and may not apply to every diabetic patient.

The modifiable risk factors for diabetic retinopathy include:

- Glycemic control
- Hypertension
- Inhibition of the renin-angiotensin system (RAS)
- Serum lipid levels
- Dietary intake of omega-3 fatty acids
- Physical activity and sedentary behavior
- Obesity
- Aspirin therapy
- Smoking

GLYCEMIC CONTROL

Glycemic control is the most important modifiable risk factor for diabetic retinopathy.[6] Numerous reports based on both clinical trials and epidemiologic studies have demonstrated that glycemic control forecasts the incidence and progression from earlier to later stages of diabetic retinopathy. In fact, glycemic control is a more important factor than the duration of diabetes to predict progression to more advanced stages of diabetic retinopathy.[7] The mechanism by which

TABLE 6.1
Risk Factors for Diabetic Retinopathy

Risk Factors	Modifiable Risk Factors
• Duration of diabetes mellitus	• Glycemic control
• Age	• Blood glucose
• Genetic predisposition	• Blood pressure
• Ethnicity	• Serum lipids
• Gender	• Diet
• Pregnancy	• Body mass index
• Diabetic end-organ disease (nephropathy, neuropathy)	• Physical inactivity
• Microalbuminuria	• Smoking

TABLE 6.2
Evidence Based Assessment of Modifiable Risk Factors for Diabetic Retinopathy

Modifiable Risk Factor	Association	Strength of Evidence	Key Studies
Glycemic control	Tighter glycemic control (HgbA1c <7%) associated with lower incidence and progression of retinopathy	Strong	Diabetes Control and Complications Trial (DCCT) for type 1 diabetic patients United Kingdom Prospective Diabetes Study (UKPDS) for type 2 diabetic patients
Hypertension	Blood pressure (BP) control under 150/85 mm Hg reduces risk of retinopathy but there may be floor effect for BP less than systolic 120 mm Hg	Strong	United Kingdom Prospective Diabetes Study (UKPDS) for type 2 diabetic patients The Action to Control Cardiovascular Risk in Diabetes (ACCORD)
Inhibition of the renin-angiotensin system	Angiotensin-converting enzyme (ACE) inhibitors and angiotensin receptor blockers can reduce the incidence and progression of retinopathy	Strong	Controlled Trial of Lisinopril in Insulin-Dependent Diabetes Mellitus Diabetic Retinopathy Candesartan Trials (DIRECT-Protect 1 and DIRECT-Protect 2)
Serum lipid levels	Elevated total serum cholesterol levels or serum low-density lipoprotein (LDL) levels increase the risk of retinal hard exudates Intense lipid lowering with fenofibrate was compared with control group	Moderate	Early Treatment Diabetic Retinopathy Study (ETDRS); Fenofibrate Intervention and Event Lowering in Diabetes (FIELD) study; The Action to Control Cardiovascular Risk in Diabetes (ACCORD)
Dietary intake of omega-3 fatty acids	Greater than 500 mg per day dietary intake of long-chain polyunsaturated fatty acids reduces the incidence of sight-threatening diabetic retinopathy	Limited	PREDIMED: Dietary Marine omega-3 Fatty Acids and Incident Sight-Threatening Retinopathy in Middle-Aged and Older Individuals With Type 2 Diabetes
Physical activity and sedentary behavior	Small studies showed a reduction in the risk of advanced retinopathy with increased physical activity and an increased risk of retinopathy with increases in sedentary behavior	Limited	NA
Obesity	Higher body mass index (BMI) (>30 kg/m) and higher waist-hip-ratio (WHR) increase the risk of retinopathy	Moderate	Diabetes Incidence Study in Sweden (DISS); Prospective Complications Study; Wisconsin Epidemiologic Study of Diabetic Retinopathy; The Hoorn Study

TABLE 6.2
Evidence Based Assessment of Modifiable Risk Factors for Diabetic Retinopathy—cont'd

Modifiable Risk Factor	Association	Strength of Evidence	Key Studies
Aspirin therapy	Neither helpful nor harmful to the incidence or progression of diabetic retinopathy	Limited	Early Treatment of Diabetic Retinopathy Study (ETDRS)
Smoking	Not a risk factor for increased risk of retinopathy	Limited	United Kingdom Prospective Diabetes Study (UKPDS) for type 2 diabetic patients

Strength of evidence:
Strong: Multiple large randomized controlled trials demonstrate benefit
Moderate: Randomized controlled trials demonstrate variable benefits
Limited: Randomized controlled studies with equivocal outcomes or no randomized studies available

hyperglycemia induces diabetic retinopathy is multifactorial, with glycosylated end products, oxidative stress, overactivation of protein kinase C, and upregulation of VEGF and other biochemical pathways disrupting vascular homeostasis and inducing retinal vascular injury. Chronic hyperglycemia causes retinal endothelial dysfunction and subsequent ischemia that can lead to proliferative vascular changes with neovascularization.

The pivotal clinical trials that supported better glycemic control to reduce the risk of retinopathy were the Diabetes Control and Complications Trial (DCCT) for type 1 diabetic patients and the United Kingdom Prospective Diabetes Study (UKPDS) for type 2 diabetic patients.[8,9] Both trials established the importance of optimizing metabolic control as early as possible and for as long as safely possible.[10] In the DCCT, 1441 patients with insulin-dependent type 1 diabetes (IDDM) between the ages of 13 and 39 years were randomized to conventional insulin dosing (median hemoglobin A1c [HgbA1c] 9.1%) or an intensive regimen (median HgbA1c 7.2%) that required more insulin injections as well as more intensive glucose monitoring.[11] The study evaluated two groups: a primary prevention cohort with IDDM for 1–5 years duration and no retinopathy and an intervention cohort with IDDM for 1–15 years who had minimal to moderate nonproliferative retinopathy at baseline. Intensive therapy included three or more daily insulin injections or a continuous subcutaneous insulin infusion versus standard therapy with one or two daily insulin injections. The DCCT demonstrated a 27% risk reduction in the development of any retinopathy in the intensive primary prevention cohort (70% risk of any retinopathy with intensive treatment vs. 90% with standard therapy). Patients who already had mild to moderate nonproliferative retinopathy also benefited from intensive glucose control and had

a 54% risk reduction of retinopathy progression. The DCCT also revealed a strong exponential relationship between HgbA1c and diabetic retinopathy progression. For every 10% decrease in HgbA1c there was a 43%–45% decrease in the risk of progression of diabetic retinopathy.[12]

After the DCCT ended with 6.5 years of follow-up, 95% of the subjects were followed up for a longer period in the Epidemiology of Diabetes Interventions and Complications (EDIC) study.[13] Patients who were previously in the intensive treatment group in the DCCT had a 66%–77% lower risk of retinopathy progression over 4 years.[13] This benefit included a reduced incidence of severe diabetic retinopathy as well as less frequent focal/grid or panretinal laser photocoagulation. The EDIC study also demonstrated that the effects of prior prolonged hyperglycemia are long-lasting, as better control in the conventional group (improved HgbA1c from 9% to 8%) after the DCCT study ended did not significantly reduce the progression of retinopathy in the following 4-year interval. This finding highlights that diabetic retinopathy caused by prolonged hyperglycemia (over 6 plus years in the DCCT) is not easily reversed. The EDIC study also suggests that the total glycemic exposure (comprising the degree and duration) may determine the degree of retinopathy at any one time.

The most significant drawback of intensive insulin therapy is the risk of hypoglycemic episodes. Patients in the DCCT intensive treatment group were three times more likely to have severe hypoglycemia than those in the conventional study arm and also have greater weight gain.[6,8] Risk factors for hypoglycemia include irregular food intake, failure to check blood glucose before planned or unplanned exercise, and excess alcohol intake. These risks can be mitigated by education and reinforcement provided by trained nurses and educators.

The other notable finding from the DCCT was that intensive treatment initially caused worsening of retinopathy, but these effects reversed by 18 months and did not result in serious long-term vision loss.[11] Based on these findings, tight glycemic control should be instituted by a primary care physician or endocrinologist under close supervision and ophthalmic examination should be performed at 3- to 6-month intervals until glycemic control stabilizes.[14]

In the UKPDS, 3867 patients with newly diagnosed type 2 diabetes who after 3 months of diet control had a mean of two fasting plasma glucose (FPG) concentrations of 6.1–15.0 mmol/L (110–270 mg/dL) were randomized to either "intensive blood glucose control" or conventional diet control.[9] "Intensive blood glucose control" was defined as a target FPG level of <6 mmol/L (108 mg/dL), and conventional diet control targeted an FPG level of <15 mmol/L (270 mg/dL) (note that the definition of "intensive control" differed between the UKPDS and the DCCT). This wide variance in the treatment targets was meant to ensure sufficient differences in the treatment groups to test the hypothesis that lowering blood glucose was beneficial in type 2 diabetic patients.

At the outset of the UKPDS, the "intensive blood glucose control" treatment groups included monotherapy with chlorpropamide, glyburide, or insulin. However, the investigators soon realized that none of the oral monotherapies provided sufficient glycemic control to meet the definition of intensive glucose control and therefore combination therapy with sulfonylureas, metformin, and insulin was then allowed. Medications were given to patients in the conventional diet control group only if they had symptoms of hyperglycemia or an FPG of greater than 15 mmol/L (270 mg/dL). However, 80% of the patients in the diet control group ultimately required one or more the same pharmacologic agents for which the group was to serve as the control. As a result, both the "intensive control" and "diet controlled" groups were confounded by crossovers. The final "intention to treat" comparison was between all patients originally assigned to intensive therapy (regardless of the original medication group assigned) and all patients originally assigned to diet treatment. In the intensive groups, the HgbA1c averaged 7.0%, and in the conventional diet group HgbA1c averaged 7.9%.[9] There was a 25% risk reduction in the intensive group for microvascular end points, including the need for panretinal photocoagulation. Intensive treatment reduced progression by 21% after 12 years of follow-up. However, patients in the intensive group had more hypoglycemic episodes.

More recently, the Action to Control Cardiovascular Risk in Diabetes (ACCORD) study evaluated intensive therapy (using both insulin and oral agents) in more than 10,000 patients with type 2 diabetes who were deemed to be at high risk for cardiovascular disease (CVD) events.[15] The goal of the study was to determine the best methodologies (intensive glucose control, intensive blood pressure control, and lipid lowering with both a statin and fibrate) to lower the risk of major CVD events, including nonfatal myocardial infarction, nonfatal stroke, or CVD death. The primary outcome for all three trials within ACCORD was the first occurrence after randomization of a major CVD event.

In the ACCORD glucose control trial, a target HgbA1c of less than 6.0% (median 6.4%) was set for the intensive group as compared with the conventional therapy group with a target HgbA1c of 7.0%–7.9% (median 7.5%).[16] Retinopathy progression was lower with intensive treatment (7.3% vs. 10.4%), but the rates of moderate vision loss were similar in both groups. The study was terminated early at 3.5 years because of increased all-cause mortality for patients treated in the extremely tightly controlled group.[17] There was a 22% higher rate of death in the intensive group compared with the conventional group, which equates to an excess death rate of three deaths per 1000 participants. The mortality end point was inconsistent with other outcomes, leading some to question the need for early termination; however, the study does provide caution about the potential risks of very tight glycemic control.

Based on these and other studies, the American Diabetes Association (ADA) recommends a target HgbA1c of less than 7% to lower the risk of diabetic retinopathy and also suggests that some patients may benefit from even tighter glycemic control with a HgbA1c less than 6.5%.[18] The ADA recommends that treatment be initiated with lifestyle modifications and oral metformin for type 2 diabetic patients.[19] Additional oral medications can be added to achieve the glycemic target and then insulin as needed.

Despite the well-established causation of glycemic control with diabetic retinopathy, more recent studies do not show a differential response to treatment with anti-VEGF intravitreal injection therapy based on HgbA1c control. In a post hoc analysis of the Ranibizumab Injection in Subjects with Clinically Significant Macular Edema with Center-Involvement Secondary to Diabetes Mellitus (RIDE/RISE) trials of ranibizumab, there was no difference between patients with a baseline HgbA1c of >7% or ≤7%.[4] In fact, there was no correlation of baseline HgbA1c with any visual or anatomic parameter. Given the similar response among treatment groups, it is perhaps not surprising that treating ophthalmologists may neglect to emphasize the importance of glycemic control with their patients. Notwithstanding the efficacy of intravitreal anti-VEGF agents, glycemic control is still critical to reduce microvascular damage that may not only worsen retinopathy, but also increase the risk of major CVD events and death.

Given the importance of glycemic control to reduce diabetic retinopathy incidence and progression, the Diabetic Retinopathy Clinical Research Network (DRCR.net) investigated whether augmented diabetes assessment and education would improve glycemic control in diabetic patients.[20] In this multicenter, randomized trial, 1746 adults with type 1 or 2 diabetes were enrolled into two cohorts: those with more frequent than annual follow-up and those with annual follow-up. These subjects were then randomized to standard care or an intervention group. The intervention included point-of-care measurements of HgbA1c and blood pressure and assessment of diabetic retinopathy severity at a routine follow-up visit with a retina specialist. The intervention group also received an individualized assessment of diabetic retinopathy progression, structured review of their ophthalmic clinical findings, and structured education with immediate feedback to assess the patient's understanding. The interventions were performed at enrollment and at routine ophthalmic follow-up visits at least 12 weeks apart. The investigators hypothesized that increased patient education and understanding of the need for glycemic control to reduce the risk of diabetic retinopathy would increase compliance with diet and medication regimens and therefore improve glycemic control. To the disappointment of the investigators, the intervention did not result in a reduction in HgbA1c over 1 year as compared with the standard care control. The study suggests that other measures are needed to improve glycemic control. These measures may include improved coordination and intervention by the treating primary care physician or endocrinologist to optimize the diabetic patient's medication regimen.

It should also be noted that some diabetic patients with excellent HgbA1c parameters (HgbA1c < 6%) nonetheless have progressive diabetic retinopathy with macular edema requiring ongoing therapy that does not appear to be explained by poor glucose control. This retinopathy progression may be related to other risk factors discussed later or perhaps as of yet unidentified risk factors.

HYPERTENSION

Hypertension is a primary risk factor for diabetic retinopathy.[21] An elevated blood pressure results in microvascular damage that may exacerbate the small vessel injury induced by elevated glucose levels. In some patients, the concomitant presence of hypertensive retinopathy and diabetic retinopathy increases macular edema and vision loss.

Epidemiological studies including the Wisconsin Epidemiological Study of Diabetic Retinopathy (WESDR) showed that the progression of retinopathy was associated with higher diastolic blood pressure at baseline and an increase in diastolic blood pressure over the first 4 years of the 14-year study.[22] In addition, the presence of hypertension at baseline was associated with an increased risk of PDR.[22]

Given the pathophysiology and clinical observations, the role of tight blood pressure control has been studied in multiple trials. Further evaluation of the UKPDS showed that type 2 diabetic patients who had tighter blood pressure control (less than 150/85 mm Hg as compared with less than 180/105 mm Hg in the control group) were less likely to develop diabetic retinopathy.[21] After 9 years of follow-up, the tight blood pressure control group had a 34% risk reduction for a two-step deterioration of the DRSS and 47% reduced risk of three or more lines of visual acuity loss.[21]

In contrast to the UKPDS trial, the Action to Control Cardiovascular Risk in Diabetes (ACCORD) study did not demonstrate reduced progression of diabetic retinopathy if the blood pressure target was less than systolic 120 mm Hg as compared with less than 140 mm Hg in the control group.[16] It is likely that there is a floor effect to lowering blood pressure below the normal range.[23] Clinicians should aim to reduce diabetic patients' systolic blood pressure to less than 130/85 mm Hg as recommended by the ADA, but further studies are needed to determine the optimal level of blood pressure control to reduce the risk of retinopathy.

INHIBITION OF THE RENIN-ANGIOTENSIN SYSTEM

There are multiple therapeutic options for blood pressure control, including β-blockers, calcium channel blockers, diuretics, and inhibitors of the RAS. No studies have shown a definitive advantage of one class of medications over another.[24] In the Appropriate Blood Pressure Control in Diabetes (ABCD) trial, a calcium-channel blocker (nisoldipine) was compared with an angiotensin-converting enzyme (ACE) inhibitor (enalapril).[25] There was no difference in the progression of retinopathy between the two medications over 5 years of follow-up. However, a multiple regression analysis pointed to a higher incidence of myocardial infarctions with the calcium-channel antagonist, and therefore this class of medications should be used cautiously in diabetic patients.[25]

Multiple studies have evaluated inhibitors of the RAS, including ACE inhibitors and angiotensin receptor blockers (ARBs), for their role in reducing the incidence or progression of diabetic retinopathy.[21,26–28] Given that ACE inhibitors and ARBs slow the progression of nephropathy even in normotensive diabetic patients, investigators reasoned that this class of therapeutic agents may have a similar effect on retinopathy. In a randomized, placebo-controlled study of the ACE inhibitor lisinopril conducted by the European EUCLID (EURODIAB Controlled Trial of Lisinopril in Insulin-Dependent Diabetes Mellitus) study group in normotensive patients with type 1 diabetes, the lisinopril-treated group had a significantly reduced progression of diabetic retinopathy by approximately 50% and this remained unchanged when adjusted for glycemic control.[29] A similar trial of the ARB candesartan (the Diabetic Retinopathy Candesartan Trials [DIRECT] Protect 1 study) also reduced the incidence of diabetic retinopathy in normotensive patients with type 1 diabetes with normal kidney function.[26] For patients treated with candesartan, there was an 18% reduction in a two-step ETDRS progression of retinopathy and a 34% reduction in the incidence of a three-step progression. However, there was no effect on the progression in patients with established retinopathy before candesartan treatment. In a parallel study (DIRECT-Protect 2) for patients with type 2 diabetes, there was a 34% increase in the regression of retinopathy but there was no significant difference in the percentage of patients with retinopathy progression.[28] Although the results were not statistically significant, there was also an overall trend toward less severe diabetic retinopathy in the candesartan group.[28] These studies suggest that RAS blockade may have a role in reducing retinopathy incidence in patients with type 1 and type 2 diabetes.[30]

The results of the DIRECT-Protect trials were affirmed by a multicenter study of 285 type 1 diabetic patients who were randomized to the ACE inhibitor enalapril, the ARB losartan, or placebo and followed up for 5 years.[27] The retinopathy end point was progression of two steps or more of the DRSS. The odds of retinopathy progression were significantly reduced by 65% with the ACE inhibitor and 70% with the ARB. These findings were apparently independent of changes in blood pressure. Some have argued that there is not definitive proof that these effects are due to RAS blockade as opposed to lower blood pressure, but the concordance of the evidence suggests that RAS blockade has a role in the medical management of diabetic retinopathy.[27] Eye care providers typically do not have a role in the selection of an antihypertensive regimen but may want to communicate to primary care providers that ACE inhibitors and ARBs are the preferred first-line antihypertensive therapies in diabetic patients.

SERUM LIPID LEVELS

Serum lipid levels are known risk factors for atherosclerosis and CVD. Medical management to lower serum lipids may reduce the risk of systemic morbidity and mortality even in some patients with lipids in the normal range. In addition, lipid-lowering therapy may reduce retinopathy progression and the risk of vision loss in diabetic patients. Multiple studies have suggested that lipid-lowering therapy can reduce hard exudates and microaneurysms in diabetic retinopathy.[31–33] Patients with elevated total serum cholesterol levels or serum low-density lipoprotein (LDL) levels at baseline are twice as likely to have or develop de novo retinal hard exudates as patients with normal levels of serum lipids.[31] A large cross-sectional study evaluated the association between atherosclerosis, vascular risk factors, and diabetic retinopathy in adults with type 2 diabetes.[34] The study did not find an association with the severity of diabetic retinopathy and coronary artery disease or stroke history but did find a positive association with plasma LDL if other risk factors affecting severity were controlled. Another population-based study found an odds ratio of 1.3 for increased risk of diabetic retinopathy per standard deviation increase in total cholesterol and an odds ratio of 1.2 for every 50% increase in triglyceride level.[33]

The class of medications that inhibit 3-hydroxy-3-methylglutaryl coenzyme A commonly called statins are the first-line agents for lipid lowering. Statins have been well studied for their role in reducing the risk of CVD. Small randomized controlled trials have shown a benefit of statins to reduce diabetic retinopathy severity.[35,36] Treatment with a statin may decrease hard exudates and reduce subfoveal lipid migration after laser photocoagulation for DME.[35] As a result, lipid-lowering medications have been hypothesized to decrease the risk of diabetic vision loss. However, these previous studies have their limitations and a large trial of 5144 patients is under way to evaluate standard therapy (target LDL-C ≥100 and <120 mg/dL) versus intensive therapy (target LDL-C < 70 mg/dL) with statins alone in patients with elevated cholesterol and diabetic retinopathy.[37] This study should help guide clinicians determine the optimal end point for lipid-lowering therapy. There are multiple approved statins currently in clinical use in the United States. To date, there is no evidence to suggest that one statin should be preferred over another for the management of diabetic patients with retinopathy.

If statin therapy alone is not adequate to control serum lipids, an alternate agent such as a fibrate may be recommended. The effect of long-term fenofibrate therapy for type 2 diabetic patients was evaluated in the Fenofibrate Intervention and Event Lowering in Diabetes (FIELD) study.[38] In this multinational randomized trial of almost 10,000 patients, there was a lower risk of requiring laser treatment in the fenofibrate group as compared with controls. However, the relative risk reduction was only 1.5%. There was a significant difference in patients with preexisting diabetic retinopathy, but the numbers were relatively small (3 patients vs. 14 patients). However, the findings were not correlated with the plasma concentration of lipids and there was uneven statin use among treated patients.[23] The results of the FIELD study may have been affected by the higher rate of starting statin therapy in the placebo group, which may have masked a larger treatment benefit.

A subgroup analysis of the ACCORD study evaluated the progression of retinopathy in patients treated with fenofibrate plus simvastatin versus placebo plus simvastatin.[39] In this better controlled study, subjects treated with fenofibrate had a 40% lower progression of retinopathy (6.5% in the treatment group vs. 10.2% with placebo, $P = .006$).[39] In multiple studies the effect of fenofibrate has been shown to be independent of lipid concentration, and therefore its mechanism of action is unclear.[10]

Overall, the management of serum lipids is an important step in reducing cardiovascular morbidity and mortality in diabetic patients. There is insufficient evidence to determine if lipid lowering should be advocated solely for the management of diabetic retinopathy, particularly in the new era of anti-VEGF therapy.

DIETARY INTAKE OF POLYUNSATURATED FATTY ACIDS

The retina contains long-chain polyunsaturated omega-3 fatty acids (LCω3PUFAs).[40] These fatty acids are the substrate for oxylipins and have antiangiogenic and antiinflammatory properties. Omega 3-fatty acids in the retina may modulate metabolic processes and have protective effects against environmental exposures that activate the pathogenesis of vasoproliferative and neurodegenerative disease.

Experimental models suggest that the dietary intake of LCω3PUFAs is protective against diabetic retinopathy. This hypothesis has been validated in studies of older adults (>55 years old) by examining dietary intake of greater than 500 mg per day of long-chain polyunsaturated fatty acids, which equates to approximately two meals of oily fish per week.[41] In a prospective study of 3482 individuals, those patients who met the criteria of 500 mg per day of LCω3PUFAs had a 48% decreased incidence of sight-threatening diabetic retinopathy (including a reduced need for laser photocoagulation, vitrectomy, and intravitreal antiangiogenic injections). Another dietary association study demonstrated that an increased PUFA intake in patients with well-controlled diabetes reduced the likelihood of the presence and severity of diabetic retinopathy.[42] Randomized prospective studies are needed to further evaluate the role of LCω3PUFAs in the management of diabetic patients and determine whether supplemental doses of LCω3PUFAs can alter the course of retinopathy.

PHYSICAL ACTIVITY AND SEDENTARY BEHAVIOR

Physical activity has well-documented benefits in the management of CVD. Given that physical activity benefits vascular endothelial function, it is possible that the effects are independent of other modifiable risk factors, such as glycemic control and hypertension. Questionnaire-based studies have demonstrated an inverse association between physical activity and diabetic retinopathy independent of the effects of HgbA1c and body mass index (BMI).[43] In one relatively small study of 292 participants who wore accelerometers to measure physical activity, only women demonstrated a significant reduction in advanced retinopathy but men had a nonsignificant reduction with increased activity.[44] A similar study also evaluated the effect of sedentary behavior on retinopathy as measured by a wearable accelerometer and demonstrated that for each 60-min per day increase in sedentary behavior, patients had 16% increased odds of mild or worse diabetic retinopathy.[45]

Prospective interventional studies are needed to assess whether physical activity can indeed protect against retinopathy and improve outcomes in patients with preexisting retinopathy independent of other modifiable factors. Notwithstanding additional evidence, eye care providers should encourage exercise and a reduction in sedentary behavior in all diabetic patients given the numerous systemic benefits.

OBESITY

Obese individuals have higher rates of dyslipidemia and hypertension, which increase the risk of retinopathy. However, obesity may also have a more direct role in the development of retinopathy as an independent, modifiable risk factor.[46] There are several pathogenic theories regarding the role of obesity, including the role of vasoproliferative factors such as VEGF and oxidative stress, which may be elevated in obese humans.[47,48]

Many studies have demonstrated a relationship between higher BMI (obesity is defined as BMI > 30 kg/m) and higher waist-hip-ratio (WHR) and increased risk of retinopathy.[49,50] In a study of patients with type 1 diabetes with 10-year follow-up, individuals with a higher BMI developed retinopathy at an earlier onset.[50] In another prospective study, WHR was an independent risk factor for retinopathy incidence.[49] Other studies suggest that individuals who are underweight (BMI <20 kg/m) have a threefold increased risk of retinopathy, as being underweight may indicative more severe diabetes with poor glycemic control.[51] Nondiabetic persons may develop signs of retinopathy, such as retinal hemorrhages, microaneurysms, and hard exudates, associated solely with obesity. In a large study from the Netherlands, WHR was associated with diabetic retinopathy but BMI was not statistically significant.[52]

Weight loss may be a particularly important step in managing glycemic control in type 2 diabetic patients.[53] It is reasoned that weight loss would reduce diabetic retinopathy, although it is difficult to parse this association from the effect on glycemic control.[46] As evidenced by the DCCT and follow-up EDIC studies, the effects of prolonged hyperglycemia are long lasting and diabetic retinopathy may progress even in patients who have undergone gastric bypass surgery and no longer need medical management of diabetes.

ASPIRIN THERAPY

Studies indicate that aspirin therapy is neither helpful nor harmful to the incidence or progression of diabetic retinopathy.[54] Early studies suggested that high doses of aspirin alone (330 mg three times daily) or in conjunction with dipyridamole (75 mg three times daily) reduced the progression of microaneurysms in subjects with diabetic retinopathy.[55] This high dose of 990 mg daily aspirin far exceeds the current recommended doses, and there are no subsequent studies that identified a similar association at standard doses of aspirin at 650 mg or less.

The Early Treatment of Diabetic Retinopathy Study (ETDRS) was a multicenter, randomized clinical trial of 3711 patients followed up for 4 years designed to evaluate argon laser photocoagulation and aspirin treatment in the management of patients with nonproliferative or early PDR.[56] Previous observations of diabetic patients who were taking large doses of aspirin for rheumatoid arthritis showed that the prevalence of diabetic retinopathy in this group was lower than the prevalence that would be expected in the diabetic population at large. Evidence suggested that diabetic patients have altered platelet aggregation and disaggregation, which may contribute to the capillary closure seen in retinopathy. Because aspirin can reverse these alterations in vitro, it was hypothesized that aspirin therapy could reduce the progression of retinopathy. However, the ETDRS did not demonstrate beneficial effects of aspirin (325 mg twice daily) on the progression of retinopathy. In addition, aspirin therapy did not increase the risk of vitreous or preretinal hemorrhages compared with placebo.[57] Therefore, diabetic patients may take aspirin as prescribed for other indications without an adverse effect on their risk of retinopathy. Other inhibitors of platelet aggregation, such as clopidogrel, have been shown to decrease the risk of ischemic events in patients with transient ischemic attacks, but there is no definitive evidence on their impact on diabetic retinopathy.

SMOKING

Smoking is a well-known risk factor for multiple ocular diseases, including cataract development and age-related macular degeneration.[58] Tobacco smoke contains as many as 4000 active compounds, some of which are toxic upon acute or chronic exposure. Despite these known toxicities, smoking has not been shown to be a risk factor for the increased incidence or progression of diabetic retinopathy.[54,59] The UKPDS actually showed a lower incidence and progression of retinopathy in smokers.[60] The inverse relationship is counterintuitive and has been debated. The effect of smoking may be due to the association of smoking with lower blood pressure. However, these equivocal findings on the risk of diabetic retinopathy do not justify advising patients to smoke given the numerous known deleterious effects, including CVD, cancer risk, and nephropathy progression in diabetic patients.

Ongoing and future studies may further elucidate risk factors that affect the development and progression of diabetic retinopathy. These investigations will guide the optimal therapeutic targets for the modifiable risk factors and may provide new therapeutic modalities.

SUMMARY OF KEY RECOMMENDATIONS FOR EYE CARE PROVIDERS

- Communicate frequently with primary care providers and endocrinologists with letters or reports on diabetic patients at least annually and more frequently in patients undergoing active treatment for vision-threatening retinopathy.
- Educate patients on their diabetic eye disease by showing fundus photographs, optical coherence tomography scans, or fluorescein angiograms, as these images may be the only evidence to an asymptomatic patient of the microvascular damage caused by their diabetes.
- Encourage glycemic control with a target HgbA1c <7.0%.
- Recommend a blood pressure control target of at least <140/80 mm Hg.
- Consider ACE inhibitors or ARBs as first-line antihypertensive therapy in diabetic patients.
- Consider advising patients to increase dietary intake of omega-3 fatty acids to at least 500 mg per day (equivalent to two meals of oily fish per week).
- Advise patients on the benefits of physical activity and weight loss that may be independent of glycemic control.
- Encourage smoking cessation in all patients given the many systemic benefits.
- Advise patients to take aspirin as prescribed, as there is no additional risk to retinopathy progression.

REFERENCES

1. Klein R, Klein BE, Moss SE, Davis MD, DeMets DL. The Wisconsin epidemiologic study of diabetic retinopathy. III. Prevalence and risk of diabetic retinopathy when age at diagnosis is 30 or more years. *Arch Ophthalmol.* 1984;102(4):527–532.
2. Klein R, Klein BE, Moss SE, Davis MD, DeMets DL. The Wisconsin epidemiologic study of diabetic retinopathy. II. Prevalence and risk of diabetic retinopathy when age at diagnosis is less than 30 years. *Arch Ophthalmol.* 1984;102(4):520–526.
3. Varma R, Torres M, Pena F, Klein R, Azen SP, Los Angeles Latino Eye Study G. Prevalence of diabetic retinopathy in adult Latinos: the Los Angeles Latino eye study. *Ophthalmology.* 2004;111(7):1298–1306.
4. Bansal AS, Khurana RN, Wieland MR, Wang PW, Van Everen SA, Tuomi L. Influence of glycosylated hemoglobin on the efficacy of ranibizumab for diabetic macular edema: a post hoc analysis of the RIDE/RISE trials. *Ophthalmology.* 2015;122(8):1573–1579.
5. Heier JS, Korobelnik JF, Brown DM, et al. Intravitreal aflibercept for diabetic macular edema: 148-week results from the VISTA and VIVID studies. *Ophthalmology.* 2016;123.
6. Fong DS, Aiello LP, Ferris 3rd FL, Klein R. Diabetic retinopathy. *Diabetes Care.* 2004;27(10):2540–2553.
7. Davis MD, Fisher MR, Gangnon RE, et al. Risk factors for high-risk proliferative diabetic retinopathy and severe visual loss: Early Treatment Diabetic Retinopathy Study Report #18. *Invest Ophthalmol Vis Sci.* 1998;39(2):233–252.
8. The Diabetes Control and Complications Trial Research Group. The effect of intensive treatment of diabetes on the development and progression of long-term complications in insulin-dependent diabetes mellitus. *N Engl J Med.* 1993;329(14):977–986.
9. Intensive blood-glucose control with sulphonylureas or insulin compared with conventional treatment and risk of complications in patients with type 2 diabetes (UKPDS 33). UK Prospective Diabetes Study (UKPDS) Group. *Lancet.* 1998;352(9131):837–853.
10. Kiire CA, Porta M, Chong V. Medical management for the prevention and treatment of diabetic macular edema. *Surv Ophthalmol.* 2013;58(5):459–465.
11. Diabetes Control and Complications Trial Research Group. Progression of retinopathy with intensive versus conventional treatment in the diabetes control and complications trial. *Ophthalmology.* 1995;102(4):647–661.
12. The relationship of glycemic exposure (HbA1c) to the risk of development and progression of retinopathy in the diabetes control and complications trial. *Diabetes.* 1995;44(8):968–983.
13. The Diabetes Control and Complications Trial/Epidemiology of Diabetes Interventions and Complications Research Group. Retinopathy and nephropathy in patients with type 1 diabetes four years after a trial of intensive therapy. *N Engl J Med.* 2000;342(6):381–389.
14. Shah CP, Chen C. Review of therapeutic advances in diabetic retinopathy. *Ther Adv Endocrinol Metab.* 2011;2(1):39–53.
15. Group AS, Buse JB, Bigger JT, et al. Action to control cardiovascular risk in diabetes (ACCORD) trial: design and methods. *Am J Cardiol.* 2007;99(12A):21i–33i.
16. Ismail-Beigi F, Craven T, Banerji MA, et al. Effect of intensive treatment of hyperglycaemia on microvascular outcomes in type 2 diabetes: an analysis of the ACCORD randomised trial. *Lancet.* 2010;376(9739):419–430.
17. Action to Control Cardiovascular Risk in Diabetes Study G, Gerstein HC, Miller ME, et al. Effects of intensive glucose lowering in type 2 diabetes. *N Engl J Med.* 2008;358(24):2545–2559.
18. American Diabetes A. Standards of medical care in diabetes–2013. *Diabetes Care.* 2013;36(suppl 1):S11–S66.
19. Nathan DM, Buse JB, Davidson MB, et al. Medical management of hyperglycemia in type 2 diabetes: a consensus algorithm for the initiation and adjustment of therapy: a consensus statement of the American Diabetes Association and the European Association for the Study of Diabetes. *Diabetes Care.* 2009;32(1):193–203.
20. Aiello LP, Ayala AR, Antoszyk AN, et al. Assessing the effect of personalized diabetes risk assessments during ophthalmologic visits on glycemic control: a randomized clinical trial. *JAMA Ophthalmol.* 2015;133(8):888–896.

21. Tight blood pressure control and risk of macrovascular and microvascular complications in type 2 diabetes: UKPDS 38. UK Prospective Diabetes Study Group. *BMJ.* 1998;317(7160):703–713.

22. Klein R, Klein BE, Moss SE, Cruickshanks KJ. The Wisconsin Epidemiologic Study of Diabetic Retinopathy: XVII. The 14-year incidence and progression of diabetic retinopathy and associated risk factors in type 1 diabetes. *Ophthalmology.* 1998;105(10):1801–1815.

23. Lim LS, Liew G, Cheung N, Mitchell P, Wong TY. Mixed messages on systemic therapies for diabetic retinopathy. *Lancet.* 2010;376(9751):1461. Author reply 1462.

24. Ockrim Z, Yorston D. Managing diabetic retinopathy. *BMJ.* 2010;341:c5400.

25. Estacio RO, Jeffers BW, Gifford N, Schrier RW. Effect of blood pressure control on diabetic microvascular complications in patients with hypertension and type 2 diabetes. *Diabetes Care.* 2000;23(suppl 2):B54–B64.

26. Chaturvedi N, Porta M, Klein R, et al. Effect of candesartan on prevention (DIRECT-Prevent 1) and progression (DIRECT-Protect 1) of retinopathy in type 1 diabetes: randomised, placebo-controlled trials. *Lancet.* 2008;372(9647):1394–1402.

27. Mauer M, Zinman B, Gardiner R, et al. Renal and retinal effects of enalapril and losartan in type 1 diabetes. *N Engl J Med.* 2009;361(1):40–51.

28. Sjolie AK, Klein R, Porta M, et al. Effect of candesartan on progression and regression of retinopathy in type 2 diabetes (DIRECT-Protect 2): a randomised placebo-controlled trial. *Lancet.* 2008;372(9647):1385–1393.

29. Chaturvedi N, Sjolie AK, Stephenson JM, et al. Effect of lisinopril on progression of retinopathy in normotensive people with type 1 diabetes. The EUCLID study group. EURODIAB controlled trial of lisinopril in insulin-dependent diabetes mellitus. *Lancet.* 1998;351(9095):28–31.

30. Wright AD, Dodson PM. Diabetic retinopathy and blockade of the renin-angiotensin system: new data from the DIRECT study programme. *Eye (Lond).* 2010;24(1):1–6.

31. Chew EY, Klein ML, Ferris 3rd FL, et al. Association of elevated serum lipid levels with retinal hard exudate in diabetic retinopathy. Early Treatment Diabetic Retinopathy Study (ETDRS) Report 22. *Arch Ophthalmol.* 1996;114(9):1079–1084.

32. Gordon B, Chang S, Kavanagh M, et al. The effects of lipid lowering on diabetic retinopathy. *Am J Ophthalmol.* 1991;112(4):385–391.

33. van Leiden HA, Dekker JM, Moll AC, et al. Blood pressure, lipids, and obesity are associated with retinopathy: the hoorn study. *Diabetes Care.* 2002;25(8):1320–1325.

34. Klein R, Sharrett AR, Klein BE, et al. The association of atherosclerosis, vascular risk factors, and retinopathy in adults with diabetes: the atherosclerosis risk in communities study. *Ophthalmology.* 2002;109(7):1225–1234.

35. Gupta A, Gupta V, Thapar S, Bhansali A. Lipid-lowering drug atorvastatin as an adjunct in the management of diabetic macular edema. *Am J Ophthalmol.* 2004;137(4):675–682.

36. Sen K, Misra A, Kumar A, Pandey RM. Simvastatin retards progression of retinopathy in diabetic patients with hypercholesterolemia. *Diabetes Res Clin Pract.* 2002;56(1):1–11.

37. Ueshima K, Itoh H, Kanazawa N, et al. Rationale and design of the standard versus intensive statin therapy for hypercholesterolemic patients with diabetic retinopathy (EMPATHY) study: a randomized controlled trial. *J Atheroscler Thromb.* 2016;23(8):976–990.

38. Keech AC, Mitchell P, Summanen PA, et al. Effect of fenofibrate on the need for laser treatment for diabetic retinopathy (FIELD study): a randomised controlled trial. *Lancet.* 2007;370(9600):1687–1697.

39. Group AS, Group AES, Chew EY, et al. Effects of medical therapies on retinopathy progression in type 2 diabetes. *N Engl J Med.* 2010;363(3):233–244.

40. SanGiovanni JP, Chew EY. The role of omega-3 long-chain polyunsaturated fatty acids in health and disease of the retina. *Prog Retin Eye Res.* 2005;24(1):87–138.

41. Sala-Vila A, Diaz-Lopez A, Valls-Pedret C, et al. Dietary marine omega-3 fatty acids and incident sight-threatening retinopathy in middle-aged and older individuals with type 2 diabetes: prospective investigation from the PREDIMED trial. *JAMA Ophthalmol.* 2016;134.

42. Sasaki M, Kawasaki R, Rogers S, et al. The associations of dietary intake of polyunsaturated fatty acids with diabetic retinopathy in well-controlled diabetes. *Invest Ophthalmol Vis Sci.* 2015;56(12):7473–7479.

43. Praidou A, Harris M, Niakas D, Labiris G. Physical activity and its correlation to diabetic retinopathy. *J Diabetes Complicat.* 2016.

44. Loprinzi PD, Brodowicz GR, Sengupta S, Solomon SD, Ramulu PY. Accelerometer-assessed physical activity and diabetic retinopathy in the United States. *JAMA Ophthalmol.* 2014;132(8):1017–1019.

45. Loprinzi PD. Association of accelerometer-assessed sedentary behavior with diabetic retinopathy in the United States. *JAMA Ophthalmol.* 2016.

46. Cheung N, Wong TY. Obesity and eye diseases. *Surv Ophthalmol.* 2007;52(2):180–195.

47. Miyazawa-Hoshimoto S, Takahashi K, Bujo H, Hashimoto N, Saito Y. Elevated serum vascular endothelial growth factor is associated with visceral fat accumulation in human obese subjects. *Diabetologia.* 2003;46(11):1483–1488.

48. Caldwell RB, Bartoli M, Behzadian MA, et al. Vascular endothelial growth factor and diabetic retinopathy: role of oxidative stress. *Curr Drug Targets.* 2005;6(4):511–524.

49. Chaturvedi N, Sjoelie AK, Porta M, et al. Markers of insulin resistance are strong risk factors for retinopathy incidence in type 1 diabetes. *Diabetes Care.* 2001;24(2):284–289.

50. Henricsson M, Nystrom L, Blohme G, et al. The incidence of retinopathy 10 years after diagnosis in young adult people with diabetes: results from the nationwide population-based Diabetes Incidence Study in Sweden (DISS). *Diabetes Care.* 2003;26(2):349–354.

51. Klein R, Klein BE, Moss SE. Is obesity related to microvascular and macrovascular complications in diabetes? The Wisconsin Epidemiologic Study of Diabetic Retinopathy. *Arch Intern Med.* 1997;157(6):650–656.

52. van Leiden HA, Dekker JM, Moll AC, et al. Risk factors for incident retinopathy in a diabetic and non-diabetic population: the Hoorn study. *Arch Ophthalmol.* 2003;121(2):245–251.

53. Sheard NF. Moderate changes in weight and physical activity can prevent or delay the development of type 2 diabetes mellitus in susceptible individuals. *Nutr Rev.* 2003;61(2):76–79.

54. Jain A, Sarraf D, Fong D. Preventing diabetic retinopathy through control of systemic factors. *Curr Opin Ophthalmol.* 2003;14(6):389–394.

55. The DAMAD Study Group. Effect of aspirin alone and aspirin plus dipyridamole in early diabetic retinopathy. A multicenter randomized controlled clinical trial. *Diabetes.* 1989;38(4):491–498.

56. ETDRS Investigators. Aspirin effects on mortality and morbidity in patients with diabetes mellitus. Early Treatment Diabetic Retinopathy Study report 14. *JAMA.* 1992;268(10):1292–1300.

57. Chew EY, Klein ML, Murphy RP, Remaley NA, Ferris 3rd FL. Effects of aspirin on vitreous/preretinal hemorrhage in patients with diabetes mellitus. Early Treatment Diabetic Retinopathy Study report no. 20. *Arch Ophthalmol.* 1995;113(1):52–55.

58. Solberg Y, Rosner M, Belkin M. The association between cigarette smoking and ocular diseases. *Surv Ophthalmol.* 1998;42(6):535–547.

59. Moss SE, Klein R, Klein BE. Cigarette smoking and ten-year progression of diabetic retinopathy. *Ophthalmology.* 1996;103(9):1438–1442.

60. Stratton IM, Kohner EM, Aldington SJ, et al. UKPDS 50: risk factors for incidence and progression of retinopathy in Type II diabetes over 6 years from diagnosis. *Diabetologia.* 2001;44(2):156–163.

Anti–Vascular Endothelial Growth Factor Therapy for Diabetic Eye Disease

KENDRA KLEIN, MD • MICHELLE C. LIANG, MD

HISTORY AND IMPACT OF ANTI–VASCULAR ENDOTHELIAL GROWTH FACTOR AGENTS

As far back as the late 1800s, scientists observed a relationship between tumor growth and increased vascularity. It was not until the 1970s, however, that more research was done to isolate this tumor-derived angiogenic factor. In 1989, two groups simultaneously reported on a possible agent that fit this description. One was an endothelial mitogen from pituitary follicular cells, which researchers termed "vascular endothelial growth factor" (VEGF). The other was named "vascular permeability factor," because of its ability to induce vascular permeability and leakage. Subsequent gene sequencing determined that these two factors were in fact identical, and it is now referred to as vascular endothelial growth factor in the current nomenclature.[1]

Similarly, eye researchers separately hypothesized that retinal ischemia produced a diffusible factor, so-called factor X, which was responsible for new vessel formation. This factor was later determined to be VEGF, and additional studies using ocular models supported the direct role of VEGF in ocular neovascularization (NV). In addition, injection of VEGF into eyes of nonhuman primates showed growth and increased permeability of new vessels in the retina as well as the development of neovascular glaucoma (NVG).[1] With the identification of this factor and the realization of its role in pathologic disease, thus began the era of using VEGF inhibitors to target both systemic malignancy and ophthalmic vascular diseases.

The development of antiangiogenesis therapies has been a monumental step in the treatment of neovascular ocular disease. Bevacizumab (Avastin; Genentech Inc., San Francisco, CA, USA) was the first clinically available antiangiogenesis agent in the United States. It is a full-length recombinant humanized anti-VEGF antibody active against all VEGF isoforms and was approved by the US Food and Drug Administration (FDA) in 2004 as a systemic infusion for the treatment of metastatic colorectal cancer.[1] It was later introduced into the field of ophthalmology and is now widely used for numerous ocular disorders, albeit in an off-label fashion.

ANTI-VEGF AGENTS: ROLE IN OPHTHALMOLOGY

Following the approval of bevacizumab for the treatment of systemic malignancy and the discovery of the role that VEGF has in ocular NV, it was realized that use of intravenous bevacizumab led to improved visual function in patients with neovascular age-related macular degeneration (AMD).[2] Clinical studies evaluating the intravitreal administration of bevacizumab began after this breakthrough finding, and it quickly became a common off-label treatment for neovascular AMD. Table 7.1 summarizes the features of the common anti-VEGF agents used in ophthalmology.

One of the first anti-VEGF agents developed for intraocular use was pegaptanib (Macugen; Eyetech Inc, Cedar Knolls, NJ, USA), a 28-nucleotide RNA aptamer that binds and specifically neutralizes the $VEGF_{165}$ isoform, the major pathologic VEGF protein in the eye. Two large Phase II and III clinical trials showed that intravitreal pegaptanib (IVP) was able to reduce progressive vision loss related to neovascular AMD. Following these studies, IVP gained FDA approval in December 2004, making it the first approved antiangiogenic therapy for ocular NV from AMD.[1]

Ranibizumab (Lucentis; Genentech USA, Inc., San Francisco, CA, USA/Novartis ophthalmics, Basel, Switzerland) is a recombinant humanized antibody fragment (Fab) also designed specifically for ocular use but, unlike pegaptanib, is active against all VEGF-A isoforms. As a small antibody fragment that lacks an Fc domain, it has a shorter half-life than the other anti-VEGF agents. Intravitreal ranibizumab (IVR) was the second anti-VEGF agent licensed as an intravitreal agent to treat neovascular AMD.[3]

TABLE 7.1
Comparison of Anti-VEGF Agents in Ophthalmology

Drug	Ranibizumab (Lucentis)	Aflibercept (Eylea)	Bevacizumab (Avastin)	Pegaptanib (Macugen)
Molecular weight (kDa)	48	115	149	50
Half-life in vitreous after intravitreal injection (days)	2.9 for 0.5 mg (rabbits) 2.6 for 0.5 mg, 3.9 for 2 mg (monkeys)	4.8 (rabbits)	4.3–6.6 for 1.25 mg (rabbits) 6.7 for 1.25 mg (humans)	3.9 (monkeys)
Binding specificity	All isoforms of human VEGF-A	VEGF-A, VEGF-B, PlGF	All isoforms of human VEGF-A	VEGF 165 isoform
Structure	Recombinant human-ized monoclonal IgG antibody fragment (Fab), specifically designed for ophthalmic use	Human recombinant fusion protein: domain 2 of VEGFR-1 & domain 3 of VEGFR-2 fused with IgGl Fc	Recombinant humanized monoclonal IgG antibody, full sized, developed for oncology	PEGylated oli-gonucleotide aptamer
FDA approval	AMD (2006) RVO edema (2010) DME (2012) Diabetic retinopathy (2017)	AMD (2011) RVO edema (2012) DME (2014)	Off-label use in ophthal-mology (2005), approved as intravenous infusion for Oncology (2004)	AMD (2004)

AMD, age-related macular degeneration; *DME*, diabetic macular edema; *FDA*, US Food and Drug Administration; *PlGF*, placental growth factor; *RVO*, retinal vein occlusion; *VEGF*, vascular endothelial growth factor; *VEGFR*, vascular endothelial growth factor receptor.
Zhang Y, Han Q, Ru Y, Bo Q, Wei RH. Anti-VEGF treatment for myopic choroid neovascularization: from molecular characterization to update on clinical application. *Drug Design Dev Ther*. 2015;9:3413–3421 and Lu XM, Sun XD. Profile of conbercept in the treatment of neovascular age-related macular degeneration. *Drug Design Dev Ther*. 2015;9:2311–2320.

Aflibercept (Eylea; Regeneron, Tarrytown, New York, USA), approved by the FDA in 2011, consists of a fusion protein comprising the second immuno-globulin domain of VEGF receptor 1, the third immu-noglobulin domain of VEGF receptor 2, and the Fc portion of human IgG1. Also known as VEGF trap, it functions as a decoy receptor and sequesters VEGF. Aflibercept has a 100-fold increase in binding affinity compared with ranibizumab or bevacizumab. In addi-tion, the intravitreal half-life of aflibercept is 4.8 days in comparison with 3.2 and 5.6 days for ranibizumab and bevacizumab, respectively. These aspects of afliber-cept are thought to allow fewer overall injections, with a similar treatment efficacy as compared with the other anti-VEGF agents.[1]

Early use and approval of anti-VEGF agents was focused on neovascular AMD. However, VEGF also plays a crucial role in other ocular disorders, including NV in proliferative diabetic retinopathy (PDR), macu-lar edema from retinal vein occlusion (RVO), and dia-betic macular edema (DME), among others. The use of anti-VEGF agents for diabetic ocular disease is the focus for the remainder of this chapter.

ANTI-VEGF AGENTS IN DME

DME, the leading cause of central vision loss in patients with diabetes, is characterized by retinal edema and thick-ening in the macula, often with lipid exudate and micro-aneurysms.[4] Chronic elevation of blood glucose along with accumulation of glycosylated products and oxygen free radicals is hypothesized to lead to increased levels of VEGF-A,[5] which then contributes to the breakdown of the blood-retinal barrier via several mechanisms. VEGF-A induces phosphorylation of tight junction–associ-ated proteins, such as occludin, B-catenin, and zonula occludens-1, which facilitate opening of intercellular junctions and increase paracellular and transcellular per-meability. Furthermore, VEGF-A induces pericyte degen-eration and depletion in the retinal vascular wall as well as apoptosis of astrocytes and neurons.[6] This leads to vascular incompetence, followed by the development of macular edema and associated loss of visual acuity.

From the 1980s until recently, macular laser photoco-agulation, as demonstrated by the Early Treatment Dia-betic Retinopathy Study (ETDRS), was the gold standard treatment for DME and the standard with which newer therapies were compared.[5] Laser typically stabilized vision and reduced the degree of visual loss that patients had compared with the natural history of DME. The more recently developed anti-VEGF agents have the ability to improve visual acuity, which has revolutionized the management of diabetic retinopathy and shifted the treatment paradigm away from predominantly laser therapy.[7] In 2013, 90% of retinal specialists in the United States reported using anti-VEGF agents for the initial treatment of DME.[8] There is considerable variation however, in the choice of anti-VEGF agent, the use of other options such as corticosteroid, laser, or surgery, and treatment patterns. Table 7.2 outlines some of the studies that led to anti-VEGF agent approval as well as comparative studies between anti-VEGF agents. Further clinical research and drug development will help clinicians choose the most effective therapy individualized to the patient's needs.

Pegaptanib

In 2005, a Phase II randomized trial compared multiple concentrations of pegaptanib with sham in 172 patients with DME. Subjects treated with 0.3 mg intravitreal pegaptanib every 6 weeks for 3 months were found to have better visual outcomes compared with sham and more likely to have a reduction in central retinal thickness (CRT). Also, the pegaptanib group was less likely to need supplemental treatment with laser at follow-up.[9] These findings were confirmed in a subsequent Phase II/III trial in 2011, and at 102 weeks, pegaptanib-treated eyes gained 6.1 letters in mean best corrected visual acuity (BCVA) compared with a 1.3-letter gain in sham eyes ($P<.01$). Pegaptanib was well tolerated, and frequencies of treatment-related and serious adverse events were comparable in the pegaptanib and sham groups.[10] Today, pegaptanib is rarely used as its comparative efficacy is lower than that of the other available treatment options.

Ranibizumab

Ranibizumab was the first FDA-approved anti-VEGF agent for the treatment of DME.[11-12] The RESOLVE study (Safety and Efficacy of Ranibizumab in Diabetic Macular Edema With Center Involvement) was a Phase II randomized clinical trial that evaluated the efficacy and safety of ranibizumab compared with sham over 12 months. Subjects received either IVR 0.3 or 0.5 mg or sham injection. All patients had baseline visual acuities between 20/40 and 20/160 and CRT ≥300 μm. Rescue laser photocoagulation and dose doubling were allowed during the study based on specific protocol-defined criteria. At 12 months, BCVA improved 10.2 letters in the ranibizumab group and declined 1.4 letters in the sham group ($P<.0001$). There was also a

significant mean reduction in CRT in the ranibizumab group compared with sham (194 ± 135 μm in ranibizumab vs. 48.4 ± 153 μm in sham, $P<.0001$). [13]

The READ-2 (Ranibizumab for Edema of the mAcula in Diabetes-2) study provided early evidence that ranibizumab is effective for DME and that its combination with laser treatment may reduce the frequency of injections needed to control DME. Patients were randomized to one of three groups: 0.5 mg ranibizumab injection at baseline and at months 1, 3, and 5 (Group 1), laser treatment at baseline and then at month 3 as needed (Group 2), or ranibizumab injections and laser treatment at baseline and at month 3 (Group 3). All patients had baseline acuity between 20/40 and 20/320 and CRT ≥250 μm. The mean BCVA change from baseline to month 24 was +7.7 letters in Group 1, +5.1 letters in Group 2, and +6.8 letters in Group 3, although mean differences were not significantly different between the groups. The percentage of patients who gained three lines or more of BCVA was 24%, 18%, and 26% at month 24 and the percentage of patients with 20/40 or better Snellen equivalent at month 24 was 45%, 44%, and 35%, respectively. In addition, the mean foveal thickness at month 24 was 340, 286, and 258 μm for Groups 1, 2, and 3, respectively. Patients in Groups 2 and 3 who were treated with laser required fewer injections than those receiving ranibizumab alone (Group 1).[14] The READ-3 studies compared ranibizumab 0.5 and 2 mg doses and showed that the higher 2 mg ranibizumab dose did not have significant benefit over the lower dose over a 6-month period.[15]

RISE (A Study of Ranibizumab Injection in Subjects with Clinically Significant Macular Edema With Center Involvement Secondary to Diabetes Mellitus) and RIDE (A Study of Ranibizumab Injection in Subjects with Clinically Significant Macular Edema With Center Involvement Secondary to Diabetes Mellitus) were two parallel, Phase III, double-masked, sham-controlled randomized clinical trials that compared the efficacy and safety of two doses of IVR (0.3 vs. 0.5 mg) over 24 months. In both studies, the proportion of patients who gained 15 or more letters in the ranibizumab treatment groups was twice that of patients who received sham injections. There was a mean gain of 8.5–9.9 letters from baseline at month 24 in all ranibizumab-treated eyes compared with sham. Significant improvements in macular edema were noted on optical coherence tomography (OCT), and the level of diabetic retinopathy was also less likely to worsen and more likely to improve in ranibizumab-treated eyes. Improvements were noted in both the 0.3 and 0.5 mg ranibizumab groups, with less adverse effects in

TABLE 7.2
Clinical Studies of Anti-VEGF Agents in Diabetic Retinopathy

ANTI-VEGF AND DME

Author, Study	No. (Eyes)	Inclusion Criteria	Intervention (Study Groups)	Control Group	Study Duration	Primary Outcome	Secondary Outcome(s)	Results
Cunning-ham[9]	172	DME	IVP (either 0.3, 1, or 3 mg dose) at study entry, week 6 & week 12 with additional IVP/focal laser PRN for 18 weeks	Sham injection	36 weeks	VA, OCT, CRT, additional photocoagulation between weeks 12–36	NA	IVP group had better VA outcomes, more likely to have reduced CRT, and less need for additional focal laser at 36 weeks
Sultan[10]	317	DME	IVP 0.3 mg every 6 weeks in year 1 and as often as every 6 weeks in year 2 per prespecified criteria	Sham injection	102 weeks	≥10-letter gain	Mean VA change, ≥15-letter gain, degree of DR, CRT, requirement for laser, visual function	Greater proportion in IVP group had ≥10-letter gain at week 54 & VA increase at week 102. IVP had less retinopathy at week 54, received less focal/grid laser & higher visual functioning on NEI-VFQ-25. CRT and frequencies of adverse events were comparable
Massin, RESOLVE[13]	151	DME	IVR 0.3 mg or IVR 0.5 mg, monthly ×3 injections, then PRN with rescue laser	Sham	12 months	BCVA, CRT	Safety	BCVA improvement & CRT reduction significantly more in IVR group IVR was well tolerated without new safety concerns
Nguyen, READ-2[14]	126	DME	3 groups: IVR 0.5 mg at baseline, months 1, 3, 5 (Group 1), focal or grid laser at baseline and month 3 if needed (Group 2), or combined IVR 0.5 mg & focal/grid laser at baseline and month 3 (Group 3)	NA	24 months	Mean change BCVA	CRT, frequency of injections	IVR eyes had reduced residual edema and decreased frequency of injections for at least 24 months when combined with focal or grid laser
Do, READ-3[15]	152	DME	IVR 2.0 mg or IVR 0.5 mg, each monthly ×6 injections	NA	6 months	Mean change in BCVA at month 6	Incidence/ severity of systemic/ ocular adverse events, mean change in CRT	No statistically significant difference in mean number of letters gained or CRT between groups. One death in the 0.5-mg group & 3 deaths in the 2.0-mg group all due to MI in patients with preexisting heart disease

Study	N	Disease	Intervention	Comparator	Duration	Primary outcome	Secondary outcome	Results
Nguyen, RISE/RIDE, 24 months[16]	759	DME	IVR 0.5 mg or IVR 0.3 mg monthly for 2 years	Sham injection	24 months	Proportion gaining ≥15 ETDRS letters	CRT, DR severity level	Greater proportion eyes gained ≥15 letters, improved CRT, reduced DR severity score in IVR groups
Ip, RISE/RIDE, secondary analyses[17]	759	DME	IVR 0.5 mg or IVR 0.3 mg monthly	Sham injection	24 months	Diabetic retinopathy severity score and DR progression	NA	IVR reduced risk of DR progression, many IVR-treated eyes had improvement in DR severity score
Brown, RISE/RIDE, 36 months[18]	594	DME	1 eye per patient randomized to IVR 0.5 or 0.3 mg monthly	Sham injection with cross-over to monthly 0.5 mg IVR after 24 months	36 months	Proportion gaining ≥15 ETDRS letters at month 24	Proportion gaining ≥15 ETDRS letters at month 36, mean change in BCVA, proportion lost >15 letters, proportion with 20/40 VA or better, CRT	IVR groups had greater proportion who gained ≥15 ETDRS letters, greater average change in BCVA, fewer lost >15 letters, and more patients with BCVA 20/40 or better. Greater reductions in CRT in IVR groups. Delayed treatment in patients receiving sham did not result in the same extent of VA improvement observed in patients originally randomized to IVR
Mitchell, RESTORE[19]	345	DME	3 groups: IVR + sham laser, IVR + laser, sham injection + laser	NA	12 months	BCVA, safety	CRT, visual function scores (NEI-VFQ-25)	IVR alone and IVR+laser superior to laser alone in improving BCVA & reducing CRT. IVR groups had greater visual function scores. At 1 year, no difference between IVR and IVR+laser groups. IVR groups had safety profiles in DME similar to that in AMD
Schmidt-Erfurth, RESTORE extension study[20]	208	DME	Individualized IVR as of month 12 in RESTORE study guided by BCVA & disease progression criteria	NA	36 months	BCVA, safety	CRT	Consecutive individualized IVR treatment during extension study led to maintenance of BCVA and CRT observed at month 12 over 2-year extension study. IVR was well tolerated with no new safety concerns

Continued

TABLE 7.2
Clinical Studies of Anti-VEGF Agents in Diabetic Retinopathy—cont'd

Author, Study	No. (Eyes)	Inclusion Criteria	Intervention (Study Groups)	Control Group	Study Duration	Primary Outcome	Secondary Outcome(s)	Results
Mitchell, RESTORE extension study[21]	240	DME	IVR 0.5 mg	NA	36 months	Visual function scores (NEI-VFQ-25)	NA	Gains in visual function at month 12 in IVR groups decreased slightly by 36 months. Eyes originally receiving laser alone for 12 months then IVR for 24 months achieved similar gains by 36 months to groups receiving IVR for 36 months
Ishibashi, REVEAL[22]	396	DME in Asian patients	3 groups: IVR 0.5 mg, IVR 0.5 mg + laser, laser monotherapy	NA	12 months	BCVA, safety	CRT	IVR alone or combined with laser was superior to laser in improved mean change BCVA, gain of ≥15 letters, reduction in CRT. No new ocular or nonocular safety findings
DRCR.net Protocol I, 1 year[23]	854	DME	4 groups: IVR 0.5 mg + deferred laser, IVR 0.5 mg + prompt laser, triamcinolone 4 mg + prompt laser, sham injection + prompt laser	Sham injection + focal/grid laser	1 year	BCVA, safety	CRT	Mean change in VA letter score significantly greater in IVR groups. In pseudophakic eyes, intravitreal triamcinolone + prompt laser more effective than prompt laser alone but some increases in IOP. No systemic events attributable to study treatment
DRCR.net Protocol I,2-year[24]	854	DME	4 groups: IVR 0.5 mg + deferred laser, IVR 0.5 mg + prompt laser, triamcinolone 4 mg + prompt laser, sham injection + prompt laser	Sham injection + focal/grid laser	2 years	BCVA, safety	CRT	Mean change in VA greater in IVR groups compared with sham + prompt laser group at 2 years. No systemic events attributable to study treatment

Study	N	Condition	Intervention		Duration	Outcomes		Results
DRCR.net Protocol I, 3-year[25]	361	DME	IVR 0.5 mg every 4 weeks for at least 4 doses; additional dose at week 16 and 20 unless met success criteria (Snellen 20/20 or better or OCT CRT ≤250 μm). Then given Q4 weeks if eye improved (defined by OCT CRT decreased by ≥10% or VA increase by ≥5 letters compared with prior) and did not yet meet success criteria. Focal/grid laser applied either promptly (7–10 days post first IVR) or deferred for at least 24 weeks	NA	3 years	BCVA, safety	CRT	Mean change in VA significantly greater in deferred laser group compared with prompt laser Focal/grid laser at initiation of IVR is no better, and possibly worse, for VA than deferring laser for 24 weeks or more
DRCR.net Protocol I, 5-year[26]	235	DME	As above	NA	5 years	BCVA		Focal/grid laser at IVR initiation is no better than deferring laser for ≥24 weeks. Most eyes treated with IVR and either prompt or deferred laser maintain vision gains
DRCR.net Protocol H[27]	121	DME	5 groups: focal laser (A), IVB (1.25 mg) at baseline and 6 weeks (B), IVB (2.5 mg) at baseline and 6 weeks (C), IVB (1.25 mg) at baseline and sham at 6 weeks (D), IVB (1.25 mg) at baseline and 6 weeks with laser at 3 weeks (E)	NA	24 weeks	CRT, BCVA	NA	Compared with focal laser alone, groups treated with IVB had greater reduction in CRT at 3 weeks but not after. Both IVB doses had about one line better mean VA over 12 weeks compared with laser Comparisons of 2.5 mg and 1.25 mg doses suggested that there is likely no difference between the two
Arevalo, PACORES 12 months[28]	101	DME	IVB 1.25 or IVB 2.5 mg	NA	12 months	BCVA, CRT	FA	IVB 1.25 and 2.5 mg provided stability or improved BCVA, OCT, and FA at 12 months. No difference in results between 1.25 and 2.5 mg doses. At least 3 injections needed over 12 months to maintain BCVA results

Continued

TABLE 7.2
Clinical Studies of Anti-VEGF Agents in Diabetic Retinopathy—cont'd

Author, Study	No. (Eyes)	Inclusion Criteria	Intervention (Study Groups)	Control Group	Study Duration	Primary Outcome	Secondary Outcome(s)	Results
Arevalo, PACORES 24 months[29]	139	DME	IVB 1.25 or IVB 2.5 mg	NA	24 months	BCVA, CRT	FA	IVB at doses of 1.25 or 2.5 mg provided stability or improvement in BCVA, OCT, FA at 24 months. No difference in results between 1.25 and 2.5 mg doses
Rajendram, BOLT[30]	80	DME	IVB 1.25 mg	Macular laser therapy (MLT)	24 months	Difference in ETDRS BCVA	Mean change BCVA, ETDRS letters gained or lost, change in CRT, retinopathy severity, safety	At 2 years, ETDRS BCVA was better in the IVB than in the MLT group. IVB group had greater mean improved BCVA, gained more ETDRS letters, & lost fewer letters than the MLT arm. No significant difference in change in CRT between arms
Do, DA-VINCI[31]	221	DME	5 groups: IAI (0.5 mg every 4 weeks), IAI (2 mg every 4 weeks), IAI (2 mg for 3 monthly doses then every 8 weeks), IAI (2 mg for 3 monthly doses then PRN), macular laser	NA	24 weeks	Mean change in VA & CRT	NA	Patients in the 4 IAI groups had mean VA benefits ranging from +8.5 to 11.4 ETDRS letters compared with +2.5 letters in laser group. Mean reductions in CRT in 4 IAI groups ranged from −127.3 to 194.5 μm compared with −67.9 μm in laser group. IAI doses were well tolerated
Do, DAVINCI 12 months[32]	221	DME	5 groups: IAI (0.5 mg every 4 weeks), IAI (2 mg every 4 weeks), IAI (2 mg for 3 monthly doses then every 8 weeks), IAI (2 mg for 3 monthly doses then PRN), macular laser		52 weeks	Mean change in VA and CRT	NA	Significant gains in BCVA from baseline achieved at week 24 were maintained or improved at week 52 in all IAI groups. IAI continued to be well tolerated

Study	N	Condition	Intervention	Comparator	Duration	Primary Outcome	Secondary Outcome	Results
Brown, VISTA AND VIVID 100 weeks[33]	872	DME	IAI (2 mg) every 4 weeks, IAI (2 mg) every 8 weeks after 5 monthly doses	Macular laser photocoagulation	100 weeks	Mean change in BCVA	Diabetic retinopathy severity	Mean BCVA gain was greater in the IAI groups compared with laser. Significantly more eyes in the IAI groups gained ≥15 letters and lost ≤15 letters compared with laser. Significantly more eyes in IAI groups had ≥2 step improvement in diabetic retinopathy severity score. Safety was consistent with known safety profile. Similar efficacy when IAI was given every 4 or 8 weeks
DRCR.net Protocol T[34]	660	DME	IAI 2.0 mg, IVB 1.25 mg, IVR 0.3 mg as often as every 4 weeks according to protocol-specified algorithm	NA	1 year	Mean change in VA	NA	IAI, IVB, and IVR improved VA but the relative effect depended on baseline VA. When the initial VA loss was mild (20/40 or better), there was no statistically significant difference between the three agents, but when initial VA was more severe (20/50 or worse), IAI was more effective at improving vision

ANTI-VEGF AND PDR

Study	N	Condition	Intervention	Comparator	Duration	Primary Outcome	Secondary Outcome	Results
Adamis[40]	16	PDR, no PRP within 6 months before enrollment	IVP (0.3, 1, 3 mg) at study entry, week 6 and 12 with additional injections and/or focal laser as needed during ensuing 18 weeks	Sham injection	36 weeks	Regression of NV on fundus photographs and FA	NA	8 of 13 in IVP group, 0 of 3 in the sham group, and 0 of 4 in the fellow (nonstudy) eyes had regression of NV at 36 weeks
Bhavsar[41]	261	VH precluding PRP	IVB 0.5 mg at baseline, 4, and 8 weeks	Saline at baseline, 4, and 8 weeks	52 weeks	Cumulative probability of PPV at 16 weeks	Mean VA	No difference in PPV rates or mean VA at 52 weeks
Gonzalez[43]	20	Active PDR	IVP 0.3 mg every 6 weeks	PRP	36 weeks	Regression of NV	Change in BCVA; Change in CMT	IVP resulted in regression of NV by 12 weeks and improved CMT at 36 weeks

Continued

TABLE 7.2
Clinical Studies of Anti-VEGF Agents in Diabetic Retinopathy—cont'd

Author, Study	No. (Eyes)	Inclusion Criteria	Intervention (Study Groups)	Control Group	Study Duration	Primary Outcome	Secondary Outcome(s)	Results
Ernst[44]	30	PDR or severe NPDR & no prior PRP	IVB (2.5 mg) every 2 months	PRP	1 year	CMT	BCVA	CMT significantly less after IVB; no difference in BCVA
DRCR.net Protocol S[42]	394	PDR	IVR 0.5 mg at baseline and as frequently as every 4 weeks based on retreatment protocol	PRP completed in 1–3 visits	2 years	Mean VA change	Peripheral VF, vitrectomy rate, DME development, retinal neovascularization	In eyes with PDR, treatment with IVR resulted in visual acuity that was noninferior to PRP treatment at 2 years. Mean peripheral VF sensitivity loss was worse, vitrectomy was more frequent, and DME development was more frequent in the PRP group versus IVR group. There was no significant difference in retinal neovascularization
Mirshahi[45]	80	High-risk PDR & no prior PRP	IVB (1.25 mg) + PRP	PRP	16 weeks	FA leakage	NA	Significantly greater regression of NV at 6 weeks in IVB/PRP but not at 16 weeks
Tonello[46]	30	High-risk PDR & no prior PRP	IVB 1.5 mg at 1 and 3 weeks + PRP	PRP	16 weeks	BCVA	Area of FA leakage	No difference in BCVA; Decreased FA leakage in IVB/PRP group
Cho[47]	41	High-risk PDR & no prior PRP	IVB 1.25 mg + PRP	PRP	3 months	Change in BCVA; change in CMT	Proportion of vision loss ≥ 0.1 logMAR; Increase in CMT ≥ 50 μm; VH; Progression of PDR	Superior BCVA and CMT outcomes in combined IVB/PRP; significantly less VH/PDR progression in combined IVB/PRP
Filho[48]	29	High-risk PDR and no previous PRP	IVR 0.5 mg + PRP	PRP	48 weeks	BCVA	CMT; FA leakage area	No difference in BCVA or CMT; less FA leak in IVR/PRP

Study	N	Condition	Intervention	Procedure	Follow-up	Primary outcome	Secondary outcome	Results
Messias[49]	20	High-risk PDR & no prior PRP	IVR 0.5 mg + PRP	PRP	48 weeks	ERG parameters	Number of laser spots	Improved scotopic postreceptoral responses in IVR/PRP; fewer laser spots in IVR/PRP
Preti[50]	84	High-risk PDR with and without DME	IVB 1.25 mg given 1 week before PRP/macular laser and again at completion	PRP ± macular laser	6 months	Between-group analysis of BCVA and CMT	Within-group analysis of BCVA and CMT	Addition of IVB prevented decline in BCVA and increase in CMT associated with PRP
Preti[51]	84	High-risk PDR & no previous PRP	IVB 1.25 mg with PRP	PRP	6 months	Change in contrast sensitivity (CS)	NA	Combined IVB/PRP prevented some deterioration in CS function observed in PRP
Jorge[52]	15	PDR refractory to laser treatment	IVB 1.5 mg at baseline	NA	12 weeks	Total area FA leakage	Mean BCVA	Significant decrease in active area of FA leakage and significant increase in mean BCVA post IVB
Moradian[53]	30	PDR	IVB 1.25 mg, 1 to 3 injections at intervals of either 6 or 12 weeks	NA	20 weeks	Clearing of VH & regression of FVT	Change in BCVA and incidence of adverse events	VH resolved significantly after 1, 12, and 20 weeks. Vascular component of FVT regressed, although FVT area did not change. Mean BCVA improved significantly compared with baseline at all follow-up examinations. Two patents developed TRD
ANTI-VEGF AND PPV								
Lucena[56]	20	PDR with macular involved TRD	IVB 1.5 mg at 3 weeks before PPV	PPV	3 weeks	RBC count in vitrectomy cassette	NA	Significantly fewer RBC in the IVB/PPV group
Rizzo[57]	22	Severe PDR	IVB (1.25 mg) 5–7 days before PPV	PPV	6 months	Mean surgical time	Mean surgical instrument changes, bleeding, endodiathermy, BCVA	Combined IVB/PPV resulted in shorter surgery time and superior BCVA at 6 months

Continued

TABLE 7.2
Clinical Studies of Anti-VEGF Agents in Diabetic Retinopathy—cont'd

Author, Study	No. (Eyes)	Inclusion Criteria	Intervention (Study Groups)	Control Group	Study Duration	Primary Outcome	Secondary Outcome(s)	Results
Modarres[58]	40	PDR with a surgical complexity score of ≥4	IVB 2.5 mg at 3–5 days before PPV	PPV	7 months	Facilitation of surgery	Anatomic and visual outcomes	Combined IVB/PPV resulted in shorter surgery time and superior BCVA at final visit
Farahvash[59]	35	PDR with dense VH	IVB 1.25 mg at 7 days before PPV	PPV	8.1 months	Intraoperative bleeding score and number of breaks	BCVA	No difference in primary or secondary outcomes
Hernandez-Da Mota[60]	40	PDR with TRD threatening macula	IVB 1.25 mg at 2 days before PPV	PPV	6 months	Duration of surgery	BCVA; bleeding	Combined IVB/PPV resulted in shorter surgery time, superior BCVA, and less bleeding
di Lauro[61]	72	PDR with TRD and VH	IVB 1.25 mg at 7 or 20 days before PPV	Sham & PPV	6 months	BCVA	Duration of surgery and intraoperative complications	IVB at 7 and 20 days before PPV resulted in significant improvement in BCVA and a shorter duration of surgery with fewer complications
Ahmadieh[62]	68	PDR with VH, TRD, or active & progressing PDR	IVB 1.25 mg at 7 days before PPV	Sham & PPV	1 month	Incidence of early postoperative VH	BCVA and adverse events	IVB/PRP resulted in fewer incidences of postoperative VH and better BCVA
Ahn[63]	107	PDR with VH, TRD, or vitreoretinal adhesions	IVB 1.25 mg at 1–14 days before PPV or at time of PPV	PPV	6 months	Incidence of early (≤4 weeks) and late (>4 weeks) VH	Initial time to vitreous clearing; BCVA	Decreased incidence of early VH & shorter clearing time with intraoperative IVB; no difference in late VH or BCVA

Study	N	Condition	Intervention	Comparison	Follow-up	Outcome measure	Outcome measure	Results
Sohn[64]	20	PDR with macula involving TRD, TRD/RRD, TRD/VH	IVB 1.25 mg at 3–7 days before PPV	Sham & PPV	3 months	Levels of VEGF and CTGF (connective tissue growth factor) in ocular fluid	BCVA, adverse events	Significant decrease in VEGF with IVB, no difference in other outcomes
Han[65]	24	Active PDR with VH, TRD, or DME	IVB 1.25 mg at 6 days before PPV	Sham & PPV	NK	Endothelial cell counts in neovascular membranes	Expression of VEGF and HIF-1α in NVMs	IVB resulted in decreased cell counts, VEGF, and HIF-1α in neovascular membranes
El-Batarny[66]	30	PDR with macula involving or threatening TRD, TRD/VH	IVB 1.25 mg at 5–7 days before PPV	PPV	≥6 months	Feasibility of surgery	Postoperative complications	Shorter duration of surgery with less bleeding & fewer diathermy applications. No difference in final BCVA
ANTI-VEGF AND NVI/NVG								
Chalam[67]	16	NVI with or without NVG secondary to proliferative retinal vasculopathy	Intracameral bevacizumab 1.25 mg	NA	6 to 36 weeks	Change in degree of NVI	Iris FA leakage, IOP control, VA	All patients with NVI had complete or partial reduction in leakage of NVI within 3 weeks post injection. IVB facilitated IOP control in patients with associated glaucoma and improved VA
Costagliola[68]	26	NVG secondary to proliferative retinal vasculopathy	IVB 1.25 mg given at 4 week intervals ×3 injections	NA	12 months	Regression of NVI (reduced IFA leakage)	IOP, VA	After the first IVB, all patients had reduction in corneal edema, significant pain reduction, and partial regression of leakage from iris vessels. After 3 IVB, regression of NVI and improved VA was noted in all patients. IOP reduction from baseline ranged from 30 to 0 mm Hg

Continued

TABLE 7.2
Clinical Studies of Anti-VEGF Agents in Diabetic Retinopathy—cont'd

Author, Study	No. (Eyes)	Inclusion Criteria	Intervention (Study Groups)	Control Group	Study Duration	Primary Outcome	Secondary Outcome(s)	Results
Lim[69]	5	NVG	Intracameral bevacizumab 1.25 mg	NA	2 weeks	VEGF concentration in aqueous humor	Regression of NVI, IOP, corneal endothelial cells	After IVB, all patients had substantial regression of NVI or iris FA leakage. Two weeks after IVB, anti-VEGF concentrations in aqueous humor decreased significantly. There were no significant changes in IOP or corneal endothelial cells
Eid[70]	20	Intractable NVG	IVB 1.25 mg and Ahmed valve	Historical group of 10 NVG eyes treated with PRP + aqueous shunt surgery without IVB	12 months	Success rate of surgery	IOP, number of glaucoma medications, VA, postsurgical complications	Success rate was higher in IVB group compared with historical group. No statistically significant difference in final IOP, number of glaucoma medications, postoperative VA, or postsurgical complications between groups
Yazdani[71]	26	NVG	IVB 2.5 mg at 3 week intervals ×3	Subconjunctival normal saline	5.9 ± 1.4 months	NVI, IOP	VA	IVB group had significantly greater reduction in IOP and NVI compared with baseline. Control group IOP and NVI were unchanged or increased at follow-up. No significant difference in VA within the study groups at any time
Vasudev[72]	14	NVG	IVB 1.25 mg + PRP post	PRP only	1 year	Long-term angle anatomy	IOP, VA, patient compliance, control of systemic diseases	Better long-term preservation of open angle & IOP control in eyes treated with IVB + PRP
Ehlers[73]	23	NVG	IVB 1.25 mg + PRP	PRP only	Mean 143 days IVB group, 118 days PRP group	IOP, rate of NV regression	VA	Significant reduction in IOP, regression of NV in IVB group. No significant difference in VA between groups

AMD, age-related macular degeneration; BCVA, best corrected visual acuity; CMT, central macular thickness; CRT, central retinal thickness; CS, contrast sensitivity; DME, diabetic macular edema; DR, diabetic retinopathy; ERG, electroretinogram; ETDRS, Early Treatment Diabetic Retinopathy Study; FA, fluorescein angiography; FVT, fibrovascular tissue; HIF-1alpha, hypoxia inducible factor-1alpha; IAI, intravitreal aflibercept; IOP, intraocular pressure; IVB, intravitreal bevacizumab; IVP, intravitreal pegaptanib; IVR, intravitreal ranibizumab; MI, myocardial infarction; MLT, macular laser therapy; NA, not applicable; NEI-VFQ, National Eye Institute Visual Function Questionnaire; NPDR, nonproliferative diabetic retinopathy; NV, neovascularization; NVG, neovascular glaucoma; NVM, neovascular membrane; OCT, optical coherence tomography; PDR, proliferative diabetic retinopathy; PRN, pro re nata; PRP, panretinal laser photocoagulation; RBC, red blood cell; RRD, rhegmatogenous retinal detachment; TRD, tractional retinal detachment; VA, visual acuity; VEGF, vascular endothelial growth factor; VF, visual field; VH, vitreous hemorrhage.

the 0.3 mg group, driving the decision to seek approval of the 0.3 mg dose for DME. An extension study found that the strong vision gains and improvement in retinal anatomy achieved with ranibizumab at month 24 were sustained through month 36. In addition, delayed ranibizumab treatment in eyes initially randomized to sham did not seem to result in the same extent of visual acuity improvement observed in patients who were originally randomized to ranibizumab.[16-18]

RESTORE (A 12 Month Core Study to Assess the Efficacy and Safety of Ranibizumab in Patients With Visual Impairment Due to Diabetic Macular Edema and a 24 Month Open-label Extension Study) and REVEAL (Efficacy and Safety of Ranibizumab in Patients With Visual Impairment Due to Diabetic Macular Edema) were Phase III trials that demonstrated the superiority of IVR compared with laser therapy alone. RESTORE examined the efficacy of ranibizumab 0.5 mg as monotherapy or combined with laser therapy versus laser treatment alone. A significant improvement in BCVA was seen in eyes treated with ranibizumab alone (+6.1 letters) and ranibizumab combined with laser (+5.9 letters) compared with laser monotherapy (+0.8 letters) at 12 months. The proportion of eyes that gained 10 or more letters and 15 or more letters were two to three times greater in the ranibizumab groups compared with the laser group.[19-21] The REVEAL study randomized Asian patients to receive ranibizumab plus sham laser, ranibizumab plus active laser, or sham injection plus active laser. Ranibizumab monotherapy or combined therapy with laser was superior to laser alone in improving the mean average change in BCVA from baseline to months 1 through 12. At month 12, a greater proportion of patients gained 15 or more letters in the ranibizumab groups compared with laser monotherapy. Furthermore, mean CRT was reduced significantly from baseline to month 12 in ranibizumab groups compared with laser alone. There were no new ocular or nonocular safety findings, and the treatment was well tolerated over the 12-month period.[22]

In 2010, DRCR.net released the 1-year results of Protocol I, a 5-year, independent, multicenter, prospective randomized trial evaluating the role of IVR with either prompt or deferred laser for DME. Patients with center-involving DME and associated vision impairment were randomly assigned to one of four treatment groups: ranibizumab (0.5 mg) with prompt focal/grid laser, ranibizumab (0.5 mg) with deferred laser, intravitreal triamcinolone (4 mg) with prompt laser, or sham injection with prompt laser. In the ranibizumab plus deferred laser group, laser was deferred for at least 24 weeks and only added if DME persisted and was not improved despite IVR every 4 weeks. Results at 3 years

of follow-up suggested that focal/grid laser treatment at initiation of ranibizumab treatment was no better and possibly worse than deferring laser treatment with respect to visual acuity outcomes. At the end of year three, a subset of patients in the ranibizumab groups were enrolled in a 2-year extension, with results published in 2015. The 5-year results echoed these findings regarding prompt versus deferred laser and demonstrated treatment with IVR in any arm maintained visual gains through 5 years, with little additional treatment after 3 years. Previous to this study, focal/grid laser had been the gold standard treatment for DME since 1985. The 5-year follow-up of Protocol I confirmed superior visual acuity (VA) outcomes with anti-VEGF (ranibizumab) treatment and showed that maintenance of this visual improvement required few additional treatments 4 to 5 years after initiation of therapy.[23–26]

Bevacizumab

Intravitreal bevacizumab (IVB) has been widely used off-label for the treatment of neovascular AMD, macular edema due to RVO, DME, and PDR because of its low cost and wide availability.[4] Various trials have demonstrated the benefit of IVB over macular laser for DME. Protocol H of the DRCR.net was a short-term pilot study that randomized eyes with DME to two different doses of IVB (1.25 or 2.5 mg) or focal laser. Compared with focal laser alone, bevacizumab-treated eyes had a greater reduction in CRT at 3 weeks and about one line greater mean visual acuity at 12 weeks. Comparisons of the 1.25 and 2.5 mg doses suggested there was not likely a difference in short-term effects between the two. Data from this study provided limited early evidence that IVB treatment may benefit eyes with DME.[27]

The study conducted by the Pan-American Collaborate Retina Study Group (PACORES) reviewed clinical data of 139 eyes with DME treated with bevacizumab at 11 centers in eight countries. Patients treated with IVB 1.25 or 2.5 mg demonstrated a significantly improved mean BCVA and CRT at 1 month after the first injection, with outcomes sustained at 24 months. Results showed that 51.8% of eyes improved by two or more ETDRS lines, 44.6% of eyes remained stable, and 3.6% decreased by two or more lines. At 24 months, CRT decreased from 446.4 ± 154.4 to $279.7 \pm 80\,\mu m$. The mean number of injections per eye was 5.8, and there was no significant difference in effect between the 1.25 and 2.5 mg dose.[28–29]

The 2-year outcomes of the bevacizumab or laser therapy (BOLT) study, a randomized controlled trial comparing IVB to macular laser therapy in patients with prior history of macular laser, also showed improved

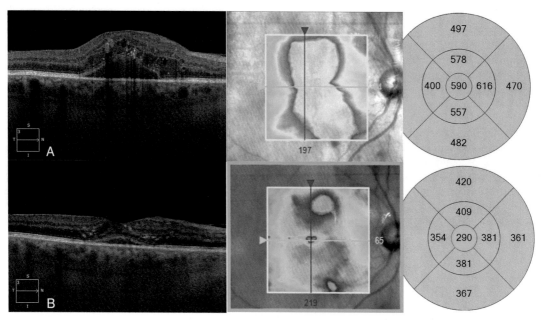

FIG. 7.1 Intravitreal bevacizumab for diabetic macular edema (DME). A 70-year-old man with a 10-year history of poorly controlled non-insulin-dependent diabetes mellitus and severe nonproliferative diabetic retinopathy presented with progression of DME despite focal laser 3 months earlier. His best corrected visual acuity (BCVA) was 20/400 and optical coherence tomography (OCT) **(A)** revealed subfoveal subretinal fluid, intraretinal cysts, and exudate with central foveal thickness (CFT) 590 μm. Four weeks status post a single intravitreal bevacizumab injection, OCT **(B)** demonstrated decreased intraretinal and subretinal fluid, improved CFT to 290 μm, and BCVA of 20/60.

BCVA in the bevacizumab group compared with laser-treated eyes (mean gain of 8.6 letters vs. 0.5 letters lost, respectively). About 32% of patients in the bevacizumab group gained 15 letters or more compared with 4% in the laser group. No patient in the bevacizumab group lost 15 or more letters compared with 14% in the laser-treated group. This prospective study reported no serious adverse events over 12 months and supported the use of IVB for the treatment of DME.[30] Fig. 7.1 features the type of patient included in the BOLT study. Despite focal laser treatment 3 months previously, DME progressed in this 70-year-old man with poorly controlled non-insulin-dependent diabetes mellitus and severe nonproliferative diabetic retinopathy (NPDR). Four weeks after a single injection of 1.25 mg bevacizumab (1B), BCVA improved from 20/400 to 20/60, with a reduction of central foveal thickness (CFT) from 590 to 290 μm.

Aflibercept

In July 2014, the FDA approved aflibercept for the treatment of DME.[4] A key randomized controlled study demonstrating the efficacy of aflibercept for DME was the Phase II DA VINCI (DME And VEGF Trap-Eye INvestigation of Clinical Impact) study. DA VINCI randomized 221 subjects with center-involving DME with CRT ≥250 μm to receive intravitreal aflibercept at different dosages and schedules (four groups) or laser treatment. The groups receiving aflibercept had a mean change in BCVA from 8.5 to 11.4 letters compared with 2.5 letters in the laser group at week 24. CRT was also significantly decreased after aflibercept administration compared with the laser group. No significant differences were seen between the aflibercept groups, supporting the dosing regimen of every 8 versus 4 weeks. At 1 year, the change in mean BCVA ranged from 9.7 to 13.1 letters gained in the aflibercept groups versus loss of 1.3 letters in the laser group.[31–32]

The Phase III VIVID (Intravitreal Aflibercept Injection in Vision Impairment Due to DME) and VISTA (Study of Intravitreal Aflibercept Injection in Patients with Diabetic Macular Edema) trials compared the efficacy and safety of two dosing regimens of intravitreal

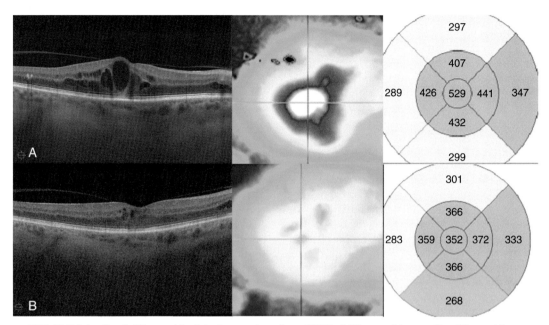

FIG. 7.2 Intravitreal aflibercept in diabetic macular edema (DME). A 60-year-old man with a 20-year history of non-insulin-dependent diabetes mellitus presented with worsening of vision in the right eye. The best corrected visual acuity (BCVA) was 20/70, and he had persistent DME after two intravitreal bevacizumab injections and focal laser. Optical coherence tomography (OCT) **(A)** showed cystic intraretinal fluid with central foveal thickness (CFT) 529 μm and vitreomacular adhesion. One month after a single aflibercept injection, OCT **(B)** demonstrated return of the foveal depression, reduced intraretinal cysts, and improved CFT to 352. BCVA remained stable at 20/70.

aflibercept with macular laser photocoagulation for DME and were vital for FDA approval. The mean BCVA gain from baseline to week 100 in the aflibercept groups (2 mg Q4 weeks or 2 mg Q8 weeks, each after five monthly loading doses) and laser control group was 11.5, 11.1, and 0.9 letters in VISTA and 11.4, 9.4, and 0.7 letters in VIVID, respectively. The proportion of eyes that gained 15 or more letters from baseline at week 100 was 38.3%, 33.1%, and 13.0% in VISTA and 38.2%, 31.1% and 12.1% in VIVID. Similarly, significantly fewer eyes lost 15 or more letters at week 100 in the aflibercept groups than in the laser control group and significantly more aflibercept-treated eyes had a ≥ 2-step improvement in the diabetic retinopathy severity score (DRSS).[33] An example response to aflibercept is demonstrated in Fig. 7.2. Center-involving DME persisted despite prior focal laser and two recent monthly IVB injections (2A). Four weeks after aflibercept administration (2B), OCT demonstrated improvement of CFT, although BCVA remained stable at 20/70 before and after aflibercept administration.

Conclusion

Numerous clinical trials have demonstrated the BCVA and OCT benefits of each of these anti-VEGF agents for the treatment of DME. Monthly injections seem to produce the best visual gain in clinical trials; however, this intensive treatment regimen can be difficult to mimic in real-world scenarios. Thus, treat-and-extend and pro re nata (PRN) regimens have been utilized by some to help maximize patient visual acuity and limit the injection burden. Although most physicians now chose anti-VEGF agents over laser for first-line therapy, which agent to use first is not universally agreed upon. Some may choose to use bevacizumab initially, as it is much less costly and more widely available, whereas others limit use to the more expensive FDA-approved medications, ranibizumab and aflibercept. In addition, changing between any of the anti-VEGF agents is also possible if a suboptimal response is obtained with the initial treatment choice.

Only one trial thus far has directly compared the efficacy of the three commonly used anti-VEGF medications for DME. In March 2015, Protocol T of the

DRCR.net published their 1-year results. In this study, patients were randomized to intravitreal treatment for center-involving DME with one of the aforementioned anti-VEGF agents on a monthly basis. Treatment was continued until there was no further improvement after two consecutive injections or there was treatment success defined as 20/20 visual acuity or <250 μm CRT on OCT. The study found that all three anti-VEGF treatments improved vision in eyes with center-involving DME, with the relative efficacy depending on baseline vision. In cases of mild vision loss (20/40 EDTRS vision or better, equivalent to a Snellen vision that is approximately one to two lines fewer), there was no significant difference between the three treatment option groups. In eyes with poorer baseline visual acuity (20/50 EDTRS vision or worse), aflibercept was more effective than both ranibizumab and bevacizumab in improving vision in the 12-month data, although ranibizumab caught up to aflibercept in the 2-year results. Anatomic results showed that the overall change in macular thickness was less with bevacizumab and a greater percentage of eyes had persistent macular thickening with bevacizumab compared with aflibercept and ranibizumab regardless of baseline visual acuity.[34]

In summary, all three agents have demonstrated efficacy in the treatment of DME and this finding has revolutionized current management. Further research on DME and its response to new emerging therapies will allow individualized patient care to optimize visual potential.

ANTI-VEGF AGENTS IN PDR

PDR is responsible for a substantial amount of visual morbidity worldwide. Retinal ischemia and NV, the hallmarks of PDR, can lead to severe visual loss, even with timely panretinal laser treatment (Fig. 7.3). Complications of PDR (Fig. 7.4) include vitreous hemorrhage, traction retinal detachment (TRD), and NVG.[35] Fig. 7.3 shows a 24-year-old woman with poorly controlled insulin-dependent diabetes mellitus (IDDM) who presented with reduced BCVA of 20/60 and bilateral high-risk PDR with extensive retinal and optic disc NV and preretinal hemorrhage (3A, 3B). One month after IVB administration in both eyes and panretinal photocoagulation (PRP) in the right eye, she progressed to an extrafoveal TRD in the right eye with 20/100 visual acuity (4A) and an extensive macula-involving TRD with light perception vision (4B) in the left eye.

In 1981, the Diabetic Retinopathy Study showed treatment with scatter photocoagulation reduced the risk of severe visual loss by 50% or more when compared with the natural history of PDR in patients with high-risk characteristics (preretinal or vitreous hemorrhage with retinal NV or mild disc NV; moderate or severe new vessels on or within one disc diameter of the optic disc).[35] Subsequently, the ETDRS recommended prompt PRP for eyes with high-risk PDR and consideration of PRP for those approaching the high-risk stage, including severe NPDR and moderate PDR.[36]

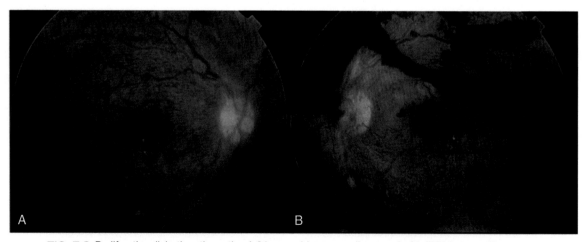

FIG. 7.3 Proliferative diabetic retinopathy. A 24-year-old woman, diagnosed with IDDM at age 10 years, was referred for rapidly progressive proliferative diabetic retinopathy. She had no prior history of treatment. The right eye **(A)** had extensive neovascularization of the disc and retina with preretinal hemorrhage along the inferior arcade. The left eye **(B)** also shows extensive neovascularization and preretinal hemorrhage superior to the disc, extending into the superior macula. The best corrected visual acuity was 20/60 in both eyes.

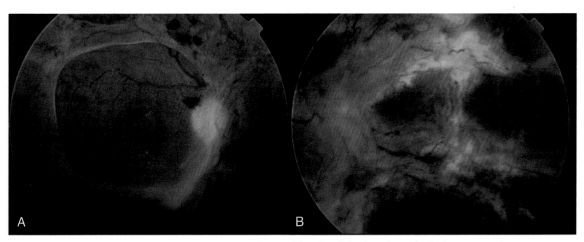

FIG. 7.4 Traction retinal detachments caused by proliferative diabetic retinopathy in the same patient as in Fig. 7.3. One month after treatment with intravitreal bevacizumab and panretinal laser photocoagulation, her best corrected visual acuity worsened to 20/100 with persistent neovascularization and new preretinal traction extending between the vascular arcades **(A)**. She received another intravitreal bevacizumab but subsequently developed a macula-off traction detachment in the right eye with 20/400 vision. She underwent vitrectomy with retinal detachment repair shortly thereafter. Postoperatively, her vision improved to 20/80 and the macula was attached. Despite treatment of the left eye with intravitreal bevacizumab, she quickly progressed to an extensive macula-involving traction detachment of the posterior pole **(B)** with light perception vision. She underwent surgery with vitrectomy for retinal detachment repair with panretinal photocoagulation and placement of silicone oil. Her vision is now stable at hand motion.

These studies established PRP as the gold standard for the treatment of PDR for years to come.[35–36]

The mechanism by which PRP exerts its beneficial effects is not fully understood but is believed to involve obliteration of ischemic retina, with a reduction of angiogenic stimuli and improved oxygenation from the choroid to the inner retina.[37] PRP, although effective and successful at reducing vision loss in PDR, is inherently destructive and associated with laser-related side effects, such as induction or worsening of DME, contraction of preretinal membranes, and peripheral visual field loss. Other reported adverse effects include decreased vision, pain, damage to posterior ocular structures, loss of accommodation, nyctalopia, choroidal effusion, and acute intraocular pressure (IOP) elevation, among others.[35–36,38]

Given the side effects of PRP, nondestructive approaches to PDR treatment, such as VEGF inhibition via intravitreal injection, have been sought. High VEGF levels are found in the vitreous of eyes with PDR, and VEGF has been shown to be a major mediator of preretinal angiogenesis in hyperglycemia-induced retinal ischemia.[39] It has been shown that vascular endothelial cells, RPE cells, Müller cells, astrocytes, and retinal neurons express VEGF-A in response to hypoxia, oxidative stress, and hyperglycemic states.[5] In PDR, VEGF-A promotes the proliferation and migration of vascular endothelial cells, induces tube formation, and maintains and stabilizes newly formed vessels.[39]

Anti-VEGF Agents Versus Sham or Saline

The effect of anti-VEGF agents in eyes with PDR has been studied in various trials and showed benefit over sham injection. In 2006, a retrospective analysis of a randomized clinical trial evaluating DME was performed to study the effects of IVP on retinal NV. At 36 weeks, 8 of 13 (62%) in the IVP-treated group, 0 of 3 in the sham group, and 0 of 4 fellow (nonstudy) eyes showed regression of NV on fundus photographs or regression or absence of leakage on fluorescein angiography (FA).[40]

In 2013, DRCR.net Protocol N examined the rates of pars plana vitrectomy (PPV) and PRP in patients with vitreous hemorrhage secondary to PDR treated with a series of three intravitreal injections of ranibizumab (IVR) versus saline. The primary outcome measure was the cumulative probability of PPV at 16 weeks, and secondary outcomes included improvement in visual acuity, rate of completion of PRP without PPV, and rate of recurrent diabetic vitreous hemorrhage by 16 weeks. There was no significant difference in the probability of vitrectomy between the two groups, although IVR offered superior outcomes in regards to the secondary outcomes, including an increased likelihood of completion of PRP, a greater gain in visual acuity, and a decreased incidence of recurrent diabetic vitreous hemorrhage. At 1 year, there was still a nonsignificant change in the rate of vitrectomy and visual acuity was similar between the two groups.[41]

Anti-VEGF Agents Versus PRP

Anti-VEGF agents have also been evaluated as an alternative to standard PRP therapy for PDR in multiple studies. In 2015, DRCR.net published the 2-year results of Protocol S, comparing IVR with PRP for the treatment of PDR. The primary study end point was noninferiority of visual acuity between the PRP and the IVR treatment groups at 2 years. Secondary end points included the development of DME, visual field changes, and safety, including adverse systemic events, injection-related complications, and the need for vitrectomy. Individual eyes were randomly assigned to receive PRP treatment completed in one to three visits (n = 203 eyes) or ranibizumab 0.5 mg injection at baseline and as frequently as every 4 weeks based on a structured retreatment protocol. Initial or additional PRP was allowed if there was "treatment failure," and eyes in both treatment arms could receive ranibizumab for DME or vitrectomy for retinal detachment or vitreous hemorrhage at the investigator's discretion.[42]

The ranibizumab group received a median of 10 injections in the absence of DME and 14 injections in the presence of DME over 2 years. DME was defined as a thickened central subfield OCT of at least two standard deviations beyond gender-specific and instrument-specific normal values for the population and a visual acuity letter score of 78 or lower (approximate Snellen equivalent of 20/32 or worse). Supplemental PRP was needed in 45% of eyes randomized to the PRP group, and 53% of PRP-treated eyes also received IVR for concurrent DME. At 2 years, visual outcomes in the ranibizumab group were noninferior to visual outcomes in the PRP-treated eyes, with a mean visual acuity difference of +2.2 letters favoring the ranibizumab group. The mean peripheral visual field sensitivity loss was worse, vitrectomy was more frequent (15% vs. 4%), and the development of DME was more frequent (28% vs. 9%) in the PRP group compared with the ranibizumab group.[42] There was no significant difference in rates of

systemic adverse events between the two groups. These results suggest that among eyes with PDR, treatment with IVR as per Protocol S may be a safe and effective alternative to PRP, with visual acuity results noninferior to PRP at 2 years.[42]

Other anti-VEGF agents have shown similar results when compared with PRP in PDR. In 2009, one study demonstrated that IVP every 6 weeks led to regression of retinal NV in 90% of eyes by week 3 and 100% by week 12. PRP-treated eyes, in comparison, were more likely to have only partial regression or persistent active PDR at 36 weeks. These findings suggested IVP produces a marked and rapid short-term regression of diabetic NV.[43]

In 2012, a prospective randomized study evaluated 20 eyes of 10 patients with severe NPDR or PDR and compared PRP with IVB injections. Eyes randomized to bevacizumab were injected every 2 months for 12 months (six injections). In eyes with PDR, leakage from NV completely resolved in 80% of bevacizumab-treated eyes compared with 20% of PRP-treated eyes as assessed by FA and clinical examination. In addition, the final central macular thickness (CMT) was significantly less in eyes treated with bevacizumab compared with PRP-treated eyes. There were no complications in bevacizumab-treated eyes, whereas two PRP-treated eyes developed vitreous hemorrhage and three PRP-treated eyes developed DME. Despite these findings, there was no significant difference in the final BCVA between groups at 12 months.[44]

Anti-VEGF Agents Plus PRP Versus PRP Alone

Although studies have shown some benefit of using anti-VEGF therapy alone for the treatment of PDR, others have evaluated its use as an adjunctive treatment to PRP. In 2008, a prospective, fellow-eye sham-controlled clinical trial was conducted to evaluate the therapeutic effect of a single IVB injection on standard laser treatment in the management of high-risk PDR. All cases received standard laser treatment according to the ETDRS protocol. The bevacizumab-assigned eyes received one injection (1.25 mg) on the first session of laser treatment FA was obtained at baseline and at weeks 6 and 16. At week 6, 87.5% of bevacizumab eyes showed complete regression of NV compared with only 25% of eyes given laser treatment. However, by week 16, PDR recurred in a majority of bevacizumab-treated eyes and the complete regression rate between the two groups became identical. The authors concluded that although bevacizumab augmented the short-term response to PRP in high-risk PDR, the effect was short lived.[45]

That same year, another prospective trial evaluated the effect of PRP compared with PRP plus a single bevacizumab injection on BCVA and total area of fluorescein leakage from active new vessels in high-risk PDR eyes. In all patients, PRP was administered at two time points (weeks 1 and 3), with the bevacizumab (1.5 mg) delivered at the end of the second laser session in the PRP-plus group. Standardized ophthalmic evaluation, including ETDRS BCVA, stereoscopic fundus photography, and FA, was performed at baseline and at weeks 4, 9, and 16. Twenty-two (n = 30 eyes) patients completed the 16-week follow-up. No significant difference in BCVA was observed between the groups throughout the study period; however, the total area of actively leaking NV was significantly reduced in the PRP-plus bevacizumab group compared with PRP alone at each time point. The authors concluded that, in the short term, the combination of bevacizumab plus PRP was associated with a higher rate of regression of actively leaking NV than PRP alone in high-risk PDR.[46]

In 2009, a study of 41 eyes with high-risk PDR with or without clinically significant macular edema (CSME) received either bevacizumab (1.25 mg) before PRP (Plus group) or PRP alone (PRP group) to evaluate the effect on BCVA and CMT. Secondary outcomes were the proportion of visual loss ≥0.1 logMAR, increase in CMT ≥50 μm, and development of vitreous hemorrhage. At 3 months, in eyes both with and without CSME, BCVA was significantly worse in the PRP group, whereas there was no significant change in the plus group. In the subgroup of eyes with CSME, CMT decreased significantly at 1 and 3 months in the Plus group, whereas there was no significant change in the PRP only group. In the eyes without CSME, CMT was unchanged in the Plus group but significantly worse in the PRP group. In addition, the Plus group was less likely to lose ≥0.1 logMAR at 1 month or to develop vitreous hemorrhage.[47]

In another prospective study of patients with high-risk PDR and no prior laser treatment, eyes were randomly assigned to receive PRP alone or PRP plus IVR to evaluate the difference in BCVA, fluorescein leakage on FA, and CMT on OCT. There was a significant reduction in fluorescein leakage at all study visits in both groups, with a significantly larger reduction in the PRP plus ranibizumab group compared with PRP alone at 48 weeks. BCVA worsened in the PRP alone group and there was a significant increase in CMT. In comparison, there were no significant BCVA changes in the PRP plus ranibizumab group, and there was a significant

decrease in CMT at week 16, although this effect was lost by week 32 and 48. These findings suggest IVR after PRP is associated with a larger reduction in fluorescein leakage compared with PRP alone in high-risk PDR eyes at 48 weeks and seems to protect against visual acuity loss as well as the increased CMT associated with PRP.[48]

PRP compared with combined PRP and anti-VEGF therapy has also been evaluated in regards to electroretinogram (ERG) abnormalities and contrast sensitivity. In one study, the rod b-wave amplitude was reduced more in the PRP only group than in the PRP plus ranibizumab treatment group, whereas there were no differences in a-wave, oscillatory potential, cone single flash, or 30-Hz flicker responses between the two groups. The use of ranibizumab combined with PRP may allow the clinician to use less extensive PRP, which in turn induces less retinal functional loss as measured on rod-driven responses when compared with PRP alone.[49] Furthermore, PRP treatment in eyes with high-risk PDR was found to be associated with deterioration in contrast sensitivity and this was lessened with the use of supplemental bevacizumab. The authors hypothesized that IVB may have improved preexisting DME as well as inhibited the formation of DME secondary to PRP. This is in agreement with prior studies that showed improved visual acuity and decreased DME in eyes treated with PRP combined with IVB compared with PRP alone.[50–51]

Overall, these studies have demonstrated a beneficial effect on visual acuity, CMT, and visual function by combining an anti-VEGF agent with PRP to treat PDR. It may be possible to administer less aggressive PRP and induce more rapid regression of NV with the addition of an anti-VEGF agent, as well as treat or prevent the development of DME that can be induced by PRP. However, regression of NV is may not permanent with only short-term treatment and eventual reperfusion of abnormal vessels may be a factor limiting anti-VEGF agents.

Anti-VEGF in Eyes Unresponsive to PRP

The efficacy of anti-VEGF agents to induce further regression of persistent NV in eyes with incomplete response following extensive PRP has been mostly favorable. In 2006, Jorge and colleagues administered a single bevacizumab injection to 15 eyes with persistent PDR despite PRP and found that BCVA and the mean area of fluorescein leakage significantly improved from baseline at 1, 6, and 12 weeks, without significant adverse events.[52] Moradian et al. evaluated 38 eyes unresponsive to traditional PRP that received

IVB at baseline and after 6 or 12 weeks. They found a trend toward significance of clearance of vitreous hemorrhage at 6 weeks and regression of neovascular vessels but no significant change in the area of active fibrovascular tissue. This last study did, however, report the occurrence of tractional retinal detachments in 5.3% of study eyes.[53]

This concern of anti-VEGF "crunch" describes the situation in which existing fibrovascular membranes undergo rapid involution after anti-VEGF injection, leading to contraction of membranes and tractional retinal detachment. A case series by Arevalo et al. reported a 5.2% occurrence rate (11 eyes of 211), with patients developing or having progression of TRD status post anti-VEGF injection at a mean of 13 days post-injection (range, 3–31 days). All patients who developed TRD had poor glycemic control and refractory disease despite PRP, and none of the eyes were treatment-naïve.[54] In contrast, no patients were reported to experience anti-VEGF-induced "crunch" in the DRCR.net protocol S trial.[42] Future studies may help to identify risk factors for this complication. In the interim, anti-VEGF injection of PDR eyes with active preretinal fibrovascular tissue requires close monitoring and a plan for urgent surgery should membrane contraction with traction develop.

Combined Anti-VEGF Agents with PPV Versus PPV Alone

Another approach to treatment has included the use of anti-VEGF before or during PPV. A meta-analysis was performed on outcome measures for 11 controlled studies investigating the role of IVB as adjunctive treatment before PPV for PDR.[55–66] One of the studies also included an additional arm in which patients received intraoperative bevacizumab.[62] Most of the studies included estimates of surgical complexity (duration of surgery, intraoperative bleeding, endodiathermy use, intraoperative retinal breaks, etc.). The main postoperative outcomes were recurrent early (≤1 month) or late (>1 month) postoperative vitreous hemorrhage and BCVA. Benefits of IVB that were found included reduction in the duration of surgery, fewer intraoperative retinal breaks, a significant reduction in intraoperative bleeding, and a reduced requirement of intraoperative endodiathermy. Meta-analysis of the incidence of postoperative vitreous hemorrhage suggested that addition of IVB results in fewer occurrences of early postoperative vitreous hemorrhage but not late vitreous hemorrhage. Data available for analysis of visual acuity were limited, and meta-analysis on change in BCVA was not performed.[51,55–66]

Conclusion

As anti-VEGF agent use became more widespread for neovascular AMD and macular edema, it was also utilized for the treatment of PDR. Initially, off-label bevacizumab was used most often due to its wide availability and low cost. However, more recently, ranibizumab and then aflibercept were approved for the treatment of diabetic retinopathy in patients with DME and in 2017, ranibizumab was approved for the treatment of diabetic retinopathy without the presence of DME. Although all the studies to date show some benefit of anti-VEGF agents for PDR, the optimal treatment regimen or agent to manage PDR and its complications has yet to be determined.

ANTI-VEGF AGENTS: ROLE IN THE TREATMENT OF NVI AND NVG

Anti-VEGF agents have shown efficacy in the treatment of iris NV (NVI) and NVG from various etiologies. In a study of 16 eyes with NVI with or without NVG secondary to proliferative retinal vasculopathies including PDR, treatment with IVB led to partial to complete reduction in leakage from NVI within 3 weeks after injection. Leakage from NVI resolved in 75% of eyes, and IOP was controlled with maximum medical therapy in eight of nine eyes, reducing the need for a more definitive filtering procedure. Recurrent leakage, however, was seen in two cases by as early as 4 weeks.[67]

In another study of 26 eyes, IVB was used for the management of NVG in eyes that had already undergone standard retinal ablation. Three bevacizumab injections were given at 4-week intervals, and data including visual acuity, iris FA stage, and IOP were collected. Results demonstrated regression of corneal edema and reduction in pain in all eyes after the first bevacizumab injection without improvement in visual acuity. After the three injections, there was regression of NVI in all eyes in addition to improvement in visual acuity. IOP reduction from baseline ranged from 0 to 30 mm Hg.[68] Intracameral bevacizumab has also been investigated to treat NVG. Aqueous humor VEGF concentrations were decreased and there was substantial regression of NVI and fluorescein leakage in all treated eyes.[69]

IVB has also been used as an adjunct to aqueous shunting procedures. Twenty eyes with NVG were treated with IVB before aqueous shunting procedure and compared with a historical control group of NVG eyes treated with PRP followed by aqueous shunting procedure. The mean preoperative IOP was 46.5 mm Hg in the bevacizumab group and 49.2 mm Hg in the PRP group. Complete success in IOP control and number of glaucoma drops were similar in both groups (final IOP 18.8 and

15.9 mm Hg, respectively). Postsurgical complications were also comparable between the two groups. However, the success of aqueous shunting tube surgery in patients who received bevacizumab (85%) was better than that seen in eyes treated with PRP only (70%). Three eyes required repeated bevacizumab treatment.[70]

In a comparison of NVG treated with 4-week intervals of IVB or sham, the bevacizumab group demonstrated a significant reduction in IOP and NVI from baseline at 1, 3, and 6 months in contrast to the sham group in which IOP and NVI remained unchanged or increased at follow-up. There was no significant change in visual acuity at any time, and the two groups were comparable in terms of the need for PRP and cyclodestructive procedures. This showed that IVB can be a useful adjunct in reducing NVI and IOP but does not eliminate the need for more definitive surgical procedures for NVG.[71]

Overall, patients treated with IVB in addition to PRP had more open angle structures, improved control of IOP, an increased rate of neovascular regression, and a trend toward a decreased need for surgical intervention compared with those treated with PRP alone.[72,73] In the real world, no anti-VEGF agent is FDA approved to treat NVI or NVG. Thus, off-label use of IVB is the most common treatment used for this indication, often in conjunction with PRP and before more definitive aqueous shunting procedures if necessary to help with reducing IOP, hemorrhage, and pain and to help in the preservation of open angle structures.

ANTI-VEGF AGENTS: SAFETY

In addition to the potential complications associated with the injection of medication into the vitreous cavity, such as hemorrhage, infection, and retinal detachment, controversy remains regarding the systemic safety of anti-VEGF agents based on their mechanism of action. Despite systemic safety concerns of anti-VEGF agents when used intravenously for the treatment of malignancy, the much smaller intravitreal dose appears to be safe based on numerous clinical trials. However, many of these trials are not powered to evaluate infrequent adverse events and may have excluded high-risk patients such as those with prior cerebrovascular accident (CVA) or myocardial infarction (MI). Meta-analyses have demonstrated safety when the entire study population is examined; however, there is concern whether any particular subgroups may be at increased risk.

A systematic review and meta-analysis of the literature evaluated the systemic safety of intravitreal anti-VEGF injections in patients with DME. Patients with DME were chosen as a high-risk group given their increased risk of developing arteriothrombotic events (ATEs), such as impaired wound healing, CVA, and death. Furthermore, the analysis investigated the subgroup of these patients with the highest level of exposure to anti-VEGF agents, those who underwent monthly treatment for 2 years. Primary end points included CVA and all-cause mortality in the highest-dose arms. Secondary outcomes included MI, ATE, and vascular-related death. Four studies (representing 1328 patients) met the search criteria, two that used monthly aflibercept and two that used monthly ranibizumab (0.5 mg). The primary evaluation of 1078 patients demonstrated an increased risk of death compared with sham and laser treatment and an increased risk for CVA and vascular death. There was no increased risk for MI and ATEs seen. This meta-analysis suggested a possible increased risk for death and CVA in the highest-level exposure group.[74]

ANTI-VEGF AGENTS: CONCLUSIONS

Despite these potential systemic risks, the development of ocular anti-VEGF agents has been one of the most important advancements in ophthalmology. These agents have enabled improvement in visual acuity when the prior mainstay of treatment had a goal of reducing visual loss and have proved to serve numerous other benefits. This is especially important as individuals with diabetic disease may be younger at the onset of their disease and prompt treatment of retinopathy can reduce visual dysfunction and improve quality of life. VEGF is a key molecule in the pathogenesis of DME and PDR, and widespread use of anti-VEGF agents has revolutionized the way ophthalmologists treat diabetic-related ocular complications. Continued efforts are needed to improve cost effectiveness, prolong efficacy, and ultimately prevent or cure diabetic-related ocular morbidity.

REFERENCES

1. Kim LA, D'Amore PA. A brief history of anti-VEGF for the treatment of ocular angiogenesis. *Am J Pathol.* 2012;181(2):376–379.
2. Michels S, Rosenfeld PJ, Puliafito CA, Marcus EN, Venkatraman AS. Systemic bevacizumab (Avastin) therapy for neovascular age-related macular degeneration twelve-week results of an uncontrolled open-label clinical study. *Ophthalmology.* 2005;112:1035–1047.
3. Tremolada G, Del Turco C, Lattanzio R, et al. The role of angiogenesis in the development of proliferative diabetic retinopathy: impact of intravitreal anti-VEGF treatment. *Exp Diabetes Res.* 2012;2012:728325.

4. Mitchell P, Wong TY. Management paradigms for diabetic macular edema. *Am J Ophthalmol.* 2014;157(3):505–513.

5. Early Treatment Diabetic Retinopathy Study Research Group. Photocoagulation for diabetic macular edema. *Arch Ophthalmol.* 1985;103:1796–1806.

6. Zhang X, Bao S, Hambly BD, Gillies MC. Vascular endothelial growth factor-A: a multifunctional molecular player in diabetic retinopathy. *Int J Biochem Cell Biol.* 2009;41(12):2368–2371.

7. Stewart MW. Anti-VEGF therapy for diabetic macular edema. *Curr Diabetes Rep.* 2014;14(8):510.

8. Wells JA, Glassman AR, Ayala AR, et al. Aflibercept, bevacizumab, or ranibizumab for diabetic macular edema. *N Engl J Med.* 2015;372(13):1193–1203.

9. Cunningham ET Jr, Adamis AP, Altaweel M, et al. A phase II randomized double-masked trial of pegaptanib, an anti-vascular endothelial growth factor aptamer, for diabetic macular edema. *Ophthalmology.* 2005;112:1747–1757.

10. Sultan MB, Zhou D, Loftus J, Dombi T, Ice KS. Macugen Study G. A phase 2/3, multicenter, randomized, double-masked, 2-year trial of pegaptanib sodium for the treatment of diabetic macular edema. *Ophthalmology.* 2011;118(6):1107–1118.

11. Ferrara N, Damico L, Shams N, Lowman H, Kim R. Development of ranibizumab, an anti-vascular endothelial growth factor antigen binding fragment, as therapy for neovascular age-related macular degeneration. *Retina.* 2006;26(8):859–870.

12. Chun DW, Heier JS, Topping TM, Duker JS, Bankert JM. A pilot study of multiple intravitreal injections of ranibizumab in patients with center-involving clinically significant diabetic macular edema. *Ophthalmology.* 2006;113(10):1706–1712.

13. Massin P, Bandello F, Garweg JG, et al. Safety and efficacy of ranibizumab in diabetic macular edema (RESOLVE Study): a 12-month, randomized, controlled, double-masked, multicenter phase II study. *Diabetes Care.* 2010;116(11):2146–2151.

14. Nguyen QD, Shah SM, Khwaja AA, et al. Two-year outcomes of the ranibizumab for edema of the mAcula in diabetes (READ-2) study. *Ophthalmology.* 2010;117(11):2146–2151.

15. Do DV, Sepah YJ, Boyer D, et al. Month-6 primary outcomes of the READ-3 study (Ranibizumab for Edema of the mAcula in diabetes-protocol 3 with high dose). *Eye.* 2015;29(12):1538–1544.

16. Nguyen QD, Brown DM, Marcus DM, et al. Ranibizumab for diabetic macular edema: results from 2 phase III randomized trials: RISE and RIDE. *Ophthalmology.* 2012;119(4):789–801.

17. Ip MS, Domalpally A, Hopkins JJ, Wong P, Ehrlich JS. Long-term effects of ranibizumab on diabetic retinopathy severity and progression. *Arch Ophthalmol.* 2012;130(9):1145–1152.

18. Brown DM, Nguyen QD, Marcus DM, et al. Long term outcomes of ranibizumab therapy for diabetic macular edema: the 36-month results from two phase III trials: RISE and RIDE. *Ophthalmology.* 2013;120(10):2013–2022.

19. Mitchell P, Bandello F, Schmidt-Erfurth U, et al. The RESTORE study: ranibizumab monotherapy or combined with laser versus laser monotherapy for diabetic macular edema. *Ophthalmology.* 2011;118(4):615–625.

20. Schmidt-Erfurth U, Lang GE, Holz FG, et al. Three-year outcomes of individualized ranibizumab treatment in patients with diabetic macular edema: the RESTORE extension study. *Ophthalmology.* 2014;121(5):1045–1053.

21. Mitchell P, Massin P, Bressler S, et al. Three-year patient-reported visual function outcomes in diabetic macular edema managed with ranibizumab: the RESTORE extension study. *Curr Med Res Opin.* 2015;31(11):1967–1975.

22. Ishibashi T, Li X, Koh A, et al. The REVEAL study: ranibizumab monotherapy or combined with laser versus laser monotherapy in Asian patients with diabetic macular edema. *Ophthalmology.* 2015;122(7):1402–1415.

23. Diabetic Retinopathy Clinical Research Network. Randomized trial evaluating ranibizumab plus prompt or deferred laser or triamcinolone plus prompt laser for diabetic macular edema. *Ophthalmology.* 2010;117:1064–1077.

24. Diabetic Retinopathy Clinical Research Network. Expanded 2-year follow-up of ranibizumab plus prompt or deferred laser or triamcinolone plus prompt laser for diabetic macular edema. *Ophthalmology.* 2011;118:609–614.

25. Diabetic Retinopathy Clinical Research Network. Intravitreal ranibizumab for diabetic macular edema with prompt vs deferred laser treatment: 3-year randomized trial results. *Ophthalmology.* 2012;119:2312–2318.

26. Diabetic Retinopathy Clinical Research Network. Intravitreal ranibizumab for diabetic & macular edema with prompt versus deferred laser treatment- 5-year randomized trial results. *Ophthalmology.* 2015;122:375–381.

27. Diabetic Retinopathy Clinical Research Network, Scott IU, Edwards AR, et al. A phase II randomized clinical trial of intravitreal bevacizumab for diabetic macular edema. *Ophthalmology.* 2007;114(10):1860–1867.

28. Arevalo JF, Sanchez JG, JFromow-Guerra J, et al. Pan-American Collaborative Retina Study Group (PACROES). Comparison of two doses of primary intravitreal bevacizumab (Avastin) for diffuse diabetic macular edema: results from the Pan-American Collaborative Retina StudyGroup (PACORES) at 12-month follow-up. *Graefes Arch Clin Exp Ophthalmol.* 2009;247(6):735–743.

29. Arevalo JF, Sanchez JG, Wu L, et al. Primary intravitreal bevacizumab for diffuse diabetic macular edema. The Pan-American Collaborative retina study group at 24 months. *Ophthalmology.* 2009;116(8):1488–1497.

30. Rajendram R, Fraser-Bell S, Kaines A, et al. A 2-year prospective randomized controlled trial of intravitreal bevacizumab or laser therapy (BOLT) in the management of diabetic macular edema: 24-month data: report 3. *Arch Ophthalmol.* 2012;130(8):972–979.

31. Do DV, Schmidt-Erfurth U, Gonzalez VH, et al. The DA VINCI Study: phase 2 primary results of VEGF Trap-Eye in patients with diabetic macular edema. *Ophthalmology.* 2011;118(9):1819–1826.

32. Do DV, Nguyen QD, Boyer D, et al. One-year outcomes of the DAVINCI Study of VEGF Trap-Eye in eyes with diabetic macular edema. *Ophthalmology*. 2012;119(8):1658–1665.

33. Brown DM, Schmidt-Erfurth U, Do DV, et al. Intravitreal aflibercept for diabetic macular edema: 100-week results from the VISTA and VIVID studies. *Ophthalmology*. 2015;122(10):2044–2052.

34. Diabetic Retinopathy Clinical Research Network, Wells JA, Glassman AR, et al. Aflibercept, bevacizumab, or ranibizumab for diabetic macular edema. *N Engl J Med*. 2015;372:1193–1203.

35. The Diabetic Retinopathy Study Research Group. Photocoagulation treatment of proliferative diabetic retinopathy. Clinical application of Diabetic Retinopathy Study (DRS) findings, DRS Report Number 8. *Ophthalmology*. 1981;88(7):583–600.

36. Early Treatment Diabetic Retinopathy Study Research Group. Early photocoagulation for diabetic retinopathy. ETDRS report number 9. *Ophthalmology*. 1991;98(5):766–785.

37. Stefansson E. Oxygen and diabetic eye disease. *Graefes Arch Clin Exp Ophthalmol*. 1990;228(1):120–123.

38. Brucker AJ, Qin H, Antoszyk AN, et al. Observational study of the development of diabetic macular edema following panretinal (scatter) photocoagulation given in 1 or 4 sittings. *Arch Ophthalmol*. 2009;127(2):132–140.

39. Ma Y, Zhang Y, Zhao T, Jiang YR. Vascular endothelial growth factor in plasma and vitreous fluid of patients with proliferative diabetic retinopathy after intravitreal injection of bevacizumab. *Am J Ophthalmol*. 2012;153(2):307–312.

40. Adamis AP, Altaweel M, Bressler NM, et al. Changes in retinal neovascularization after pegaptanib (Macugen) therapy in diabetic individuals. *Ophthalmology*. 2006;113(1):23–28.

41. Bhavsar A, Torres K, Glassman A, et al. Evaluation of results 1 year following short-term use of ranibizumab for vitreous hemorrhage due to proliferative diabetic retinopathy. *JAMA Ophthalmol*. 2014;132:889–890.

42. Writing Committee for the Diabetic Retinopathy Clinical Research Network. Panretinal photocoagulation vs intravitreous ranibizumab for proliferative diabetic RetinopathyA randomized clinical trial. *JAMA*. 2015;314(20):2137–2146. http://dx.doi.org/10.1001/jama.2015.15217.

43. Gonzalez VH, Giuliari GP, Banda RM, Guel DA. Intravitreal injection of pegaptanib sodium for proliferative diabetic retinopathy. *Br J Ophthalmol*. 2009;93:1474–1478.

44. Ernst BJ, Garcia-Aguirre G, Oliver SC, et al. Intravitreal bevacizumab versus panretinal photocoagulation for treatment-naive proliferative and severe nonproliferative diabetic retinopathy. *Acta Ophthalmol*. 2012;90:e573–e574.

45. Mirshahi A, Roohipoor R, Lashay A, et al. Bevacizumab-augmented retinal laser photocoagulation in proliferative diabetic retinopathy: a randomized double-masked clinical trial. *Eur J Ophthalmol*. 2008;18:263–269.

46. Tonello M, Costa RA, Almeida FP, et al. Panretinal photocoagulation versus PRP plus intravitreal bevacizumab for high-risk proliferative diabetic retinopathy (IBeHi study). *Acta Ophthalmol*. 2008;86:385–389.

47. Cho WB, Oh SB, Moon JW, Kim HC. Panretinal photocoagulation combined with intravitreal bevacizumab in high-risk proliferative diabetic retinopathy. *Retina*. 2009;29:516–522.

48. Filho JA, Messias A, Almeida FP, et al. Panretinal photocoagulation (PRP) versus PRP plus intravitreal ranibizumab for high-risk proliferative diabetic retinopathy. *Acta Ophthalmol*. 2011;89:e567–e572.

49. Messias A, Ramos Filho JA, Messias K, et al. Electroretinographic findings associated with panretinal photocoagulation (PRP) versus PRP plus intravitreal ranibizumab treatment for high-risk proliferative diabetic retinopathy. *Doc Ophthalmol*. 2012;124:225–236.

50. Preti RC, Ramirez LM, Monteiro ML, et al. Contrast sensitivity evaluation in high risk proliferative diabetic retinopathy treated with panretinal photocoagulation associated or not with intravitreal bevacizumab injections: a randomised clinical trial. *Br J Ophthalmol*. 2013;97:885–889.

51. Preti RC, Vasquez Ramirez LM, Ribeiro Monteiro ML, et al. Structural and functional assessment of macula in patients with high-risk proliferative diabetic retinopathy submitted to panretinal photocoagulation and associated intravitreal bevacizumab injections: a comparative, randomised, controlled trial. *Ophthalmologica*. 2013;230:1–8.

52. Jorge R, Costa RA, Calucci D, Cintra LP, Scott IU. Intravitreal bevacizumab (Avastin) for persistent new vessels in diabetic retinopathy (Ibepe study). *Retina*. 2006;26(9):1006–1013.

53. Moradian S, Ahmadieh H, Malihi M, Soheilian M, Dehghan MH, Azarmina M. Intravitreal bevacizumab in active progressive proliferative diabetic retinopathy. *Graefes Arch Clin Exp Ophthalmol*. 2008;246(12):1699–1705.

54. Arevalo JF, Maia M, Flynn HW, et al. Tractional retinal detachment following intravitreal bevacizumab (Avastin) in patients with severe proliferative diabetic retinopathy. *Br J Ophthalmol*. 2008;92:213–216.

55. Simunovic MP, Maberley DA. Anti-vascular endothelial growth factor therapy for proliferative diabetic retinopathy: a systematic review and meta-analysis. *Retina*. 2015;35(10):1931–1942.

56. Lucena da R D, Ribeiro JA, Costa RA, et al. Intraoperative bleeding during vitrectomy for diabetic tractional retinal detachment with versus without preoperative intravitreal bevacizumab (IBeTra study). *Br J Ophthalmol*. 2009;93:688–691.

57. Rizzo S, Genovesi-Ebert F, Di Bartolo E, et al. Injection of intravitreal bevacizumab (Avastin) as a preoperative adjunct before vitrectomy surgery in the treatment of severe proliferative diabetic retinopathy (PDR). *Graefes Arch Clin Exp Ophthalmol*. 2008;246:837–842.

58. Modarres M, Nazari H, Falavarjani KG, et al. Intravitreal injection of bevacizumab before vitrectomy for proliferative diabetic retinopathy. *Eur J Ophthalmol*. 2009;19:848–852.

59. Farahvash MS, Majidi AR, Roohipoor R, Ghassemi F. Pre-operative injection of intravitreal bevacizumab in dense diabetic vitreous hemorrhage. *Retina*. 2011;31:1254–1260.

60. Hernandez-Da Mota SE, Nunez-Solorio SM. Experience with intravitreal bevacizumab as a preoperative adjunct in 23-G vitrectomy for advanced proliferative diabetic retinopathy. *Eur J Ophthalmol.* 2010;20:1047–1052.

61. di Lauro R, De Ruggiero P, di Lauro MT, Romano MR. Intravitreal bevacizumab for surgical treatment of severe proliferative diabetic retinopathy. *Graefes Arch Clin Exp Ophthalmol.* 2010;248:785–791.

62. Ahmadieh H, Shoeibi N, Entezari M, Monshizadeh R. Intravitreal bevacizumab for prevention of early postvitrectomy hemorrhage in diabetic patients: a randomized clinical trial. *Ophthalmology.* 2009;116:1943–1948.

63. Ahn J, Woo SJ, Chung H, Park KH. The effect of adjunctive intravitreal bevacizumab for preventing postvitrectomy hemorrhage in proliferative diabetic retinopathy. *Ophthalmology.* 2011;118:2218–2226.

64. Sohn EH, He S, Kim LA, et al. Angiofibrotic response to vascular endothelial growth factor inhibition in diabetic retinal detachment: report no. 1. *Arch Ophthalmol.* 2012;130:1127–1134.

65. Han XX, Guo CM, Li Y, Hui YN. Effects of bevacizumab on the neovascular membrane of proliferative diabetic retinopa- thy: reduction of endothelial cells and expressions of VEGF and HIF-1alpha. *Mol Vis.* 2012;18:1–9.

66. El-Batarny AM. Intravitreal bevacizumab as an adjunctive therapy before diabetic vitrectomy. *Clin Ophthalmol.* 2008;2:709–716.

67. Chalam KV, Gupta SK, Grover S, Brar VS, Agarwal S. Intracameral Avastin dramatically resolves iris neovascularization and reverses neovascular glaucoma. *Eur J Ophthalmol.* 2008;18(2):255–262.

68. Costagliola C, Cipollone U, Rinaldi M, Della Corte M, Semeraro F, Romano MR. Intravitreal bevacizumab (Avastin) injection for neovascular glaucoma: a survey on 23 cases throughout 12-month follow-up. *Br J Clin Pharmacol.* 2008;66(5):667–750.

69. Lim TH, Bae SH, Cho YJ, Lee JH, Kim HK, Sohn YH. Concentration of vascular endothelial growth factor after intracameral bevacizumab injection in eyes with neovascular glaucoma. *Korean J Ophthalmol.* 2009;23(3):188–192.

70. Eid TM, Radwan A, El-Manawy W, El-Hawary I. Intravitreal bevacizumab and aqueous shunting surgery for neovascular glaucoma: safety and efficacy. *Can J Ophthalmol.* 2009;44(4):451–456.

71. Yazdani S, Hendi K, Pakravan M, Mahdavi M, Yaseri M. Intravitreal bevacizumab for neovascular glaucoma: a randomized controlled trial. *J Glaucoma.* 2009;18(8):632–637.

72. Vasudev D, Blair MP, Galasso J, Kapur R, Vajaranant T. Intravitreal bevacizumab for neovascular glaucoma. *J Ocul Pharmacol Ther.* 2009;25(5):453–458.

73. Ehlers JP, Spirn MJ, Lam A, Sivalingam A, Samuel MA, Tasman W. Combination intravitreal bevacizumab/panretinal photocoagulation versus panretinal photocoagulation alone in the treatment of neovascular glaucoma. *Retina.* 2008;28(5):696–702.

74. Avery RL, Gordon GM. Systemic safety of prolonged monthly anti-vascular endothelial growth factor therapy for diabetic macular edema: a systemic review and meta-analysis. *JAMA Ophthalmol.* 2016;124(1):21–29.

CHAPTER 8

Corticosteroid Therapy for Diabetic Retinopathy

ELAD MOISSEIEV, MD • ANAT LOEWENSTEIN, MD

THE ROLE OF INFLAMMATION IN DIABETIC RETINOPATHY

Diabetes mellitus is a complex systemic disease, with multiple factors playing a part in its etiology and pathogenesis. The hallmark of the disease is hyperglycemia, which has been shown to result in the synthesis of advanced glycation end products and activation of the sorbitol and hexosamine pathways of glucose metabolism, causing an excessive production of free radicals and oxidative stress. These processes cause tissues to activate multiple pathways, especially those related to angiogenesis and inflammation. The same mechanisms also participate in the development of diabetic retinopathy (DR). A significant factor is oxidative stress induced by the metabolic changes of diabetes mellitus, which causes tissue hypoxia and results in the upregulation of hypoxia-inducible factor 1α. This in turn upregulates the production of vascular endothelial growth factor (VEGF), which is responsible for numerous aspects related to DR, such as increased retinal vascular permeability, vasodilation, attraction of mononuclear leukocytes to the retina, and pathologic retinal neovascularization.[1] VEGF has been recognized as a key factor in the pathogenesis of DR and especially of diabetic macular edema (DME) and is currently the target of the most commonly used therapeutic agents for patients with this pathology. The most commonly utilized anti-VEGF agents include ranibizumab, bevacizumab, and aflibercept.

Despite the proven relevance of VEGF to the pathogenesis of DR and DME, there are other factors at play. There are substantial experimental and clinical data demonstrating the role of inflammation in the pathologic process of DR. Multiple inflammatory cytokines have been shown to be upregulated in response to the oxidative stress and metabolic changes induced by diabetes mellitus. These include interleukin (IL)-6, IL-8, tumor necrosis factor α (TNFα), nuclear factor kappa-light-chain-enhancer of activated B cells (NF-κB), protein kinase C, monocyte chemotactic protein, and nitric oxide synthase. These cytokines induce inflammation and other parainflammatory processes, such as activation of the complement pathway, attraction of leukocytes and macrophages to the retina, leukostasis, and breakdown of the blood-retinal barrier.[2] Inflammation is so central to the pathogenesis of DR that it has been considered as a chronic low-grade inflammatory disease.

It is important to emphasize that the angiogenesis and inflammatory pathways are not distinct in the pathogenesis of DR and DME. As mentioned earlier, they are both activated by the same triggers induced by diabetes mellitus. There is considerable evidence of cross-talk between them, as they share several common mediators and signaling pathways, such as the cyclooxygenase and prostaglandin pathways. It has also been shown that inflammatory cytokines, such as IL-1, IL-6, and TNFα, are capable of inducing angiogenesis in endothelial cells and VEGF is capable of eliciting inflammatory responses in these cells.[3]

The role of inflammation in DR makes it an appealing target for therapeutic intervention. Although inhibition of VEGF by anti-VEGF agents yields excellent results in many patients, it requires frequent monitoring and repeated treatments, and some patients respond incompletely to anti-VEGF agents as first line of treatment. The use of steroids to reduce the inflammatory component of DR and DME has been of clinical interest for many years. Corticosteroids confer an antiinflammatory effect by inhibiting the enzyme phospholipase A2, which produces arachidonic acid, which is necessary for the production of leukotrienes, thromboxanes, and prostaglandins, all of which are upregulated by inflammation and play a part in the increased vascular permeability and vasodilation of DR. Corticosteroids have also been demonstrated to decrease the production of numerous inflammatory mediators, as well as that of VEGF. They also stabilize the blood-retinal barrier and improve retinal oxygenation.[2] The administration of corticosteroids offers several advantages, including influencing a wider array of pathologic processes and having a longer duration of action, which make them more suitable for long-term treatment of patients who may require multiple interventions. Their ability to affect multiple pathways also makes them a better choice for refractory patients with inadequate response to anti-VEGF therapy. This chapter reviews the evolution and options of corticosteroid therapy for DR and DME.

CORTICOSTEROIDS FOR THE TREATMENT OF DIABETIC MACULAR EDEMA

As the most common vision-threatening manifestation of DR, as well as the one most responsive to treatment, DME is the main indication for treatment of DR in general and for the administration of steroids in particular. As a result, the vast majority of studies on steroid therapy focus on DME. Some of the most clinically relevant studies on this subject are outlined in Table 8.1.

The most common ocular adverse effects of corticosteroid therapy are the progression of cataract and elevated intraocular pressure (IOP), which may lead to glaucoma. These are class effects, which can occur with any method of corticosteroid administration, whether systemic, local, or topical. The rates of these complications vary and are dependent on the specific type of corticosteroid used, dosage, and route of administration. Although these complications are significant and can lead to further vision loss, it should be remembered that cataract progression is also accelerated by diabetes mellitus itself and that in the vast majority of cases cataract extraction is a simple procedure that achieves considerable visual improvement. Elevated IOP does not occur in all patients and in the majority of cases can be controlled by topical IOP-lowering drops.

Systemic administration of corticosteroids is not suitable for the treatment of DR, as it would require long-term use of high doses to achieve therapeutic concentrations in the eye. This would be hazardous to these patients, as systemic corticosteroids increase glucose levels in patients with diabetes. The following sections discuss the utility of the different routes available for ocular steroid administration.

Topical

Topical administration of steroids is not commonly used for the treatment of DME, as penetration into the posterior segment is limited, and thus therapeutic efficacy has been inadequate. Some clinicians recommend a trial of dexamethasone drops before intravitreal injection of steroids, to determine whether the patient is likely to develop IOP elevation (known as

a "steroid response"). Nevertheless, the simplicity of topical administration makes it an attractive target for future research and two studies are worthy of mentioning in this context.

A small study evaluated 20 patients with refractory DME who were topically treated by 0.05% difluprednate ophthalmic emulsion three times a day for 3 months. This steroid has improved penetration into the posterior segment, and a mean improvement of two lines of vision along with a significant reduction in central macular thickness (CMT) was achieved. However, 20% of patients had a significant IOP elevation.[4] Another development in topical treatment is in the form of microparticles. One study investigated topical 1.5% dexamethasone γ-cyclodextrin nanoparticle eye drops and compared it with sub-Tenon injection of triamcinolone for DME. This novel nanoparticle formulation improves stability and intraocular penetration of the steroid. A small group of patients with DME received three drops a day for 4 weeks, then two drops a day for 4 weeks, and then one drop a day for 4 weeks. The study reported comparable improvement in visual acuity (VA) and a reduction in CMT to those achieved with a sub-Tenon injection of triamcinolone but with a higher rate of IOP elevation.[5] These findings demonstrate that topical steroid therapy may eventually prove efficacious for DME but at present is limited by a drug formulation and a relatively high rate of IOP elevation.

Sub-Tenon Injection

Steroids may be delivered into the sub-Tenon space via a periocular injection, where a relatively large volume can be accommodated to allow a long-lasting effect. This method avoids the potential risks of intraocular damage and endophthalmitis posed by an intravitreal injection, with minimal systemic drug exposure.

This method of steroid administration was in clinical use before the advent of anti-VEGF agents, and therefore its efficacy was compared with the standard of treatment at that time, which was focal photocoagulation treatment as per the historic Early Treatment of Diabetic Retinopathy Study (ETDRS) study results. In a prospective controlled comparative study, patients with DME were treated with either macular (focal/grid) laser alone or in combination with posterior sub-Tenon injection of 20 mg of triamcinolone acetonide and followed for 24 weeks. At the end of the study period, 87% of the patients who received sub-Tenon triamcinolone had maintained their baseline VA compared with 75% of those treated with laser only. More importantly, 40% of the patients who received sub-Tenon triamcinolone had improved by two or more lines of vision, compared

TABLE 8.1
Major Studies in the Evolution of Corticosteroid Therapy for Diabetic Retinopathy (DR) and Diabetic Macular Edema (DME)

Study	Steroid Type, Route of Administration	Eyes (No.)	Design	Main Results	Clinical Significance
Martidis et al.[9]	Intravitreal triamcinolone	16	One group; eyes with refractory DME	Mean VA gain of 2.4 lines, 57.5% reduction in CMT	First clinical evidence of steroid efficacy for DME
Verma et al.[6]	Sub-Tenon triamcinolone	31	Eyes with diffuse DME; laser versus PST triamcinolone+laser	2 line VA gain 40% in PST+laser group versus 19% in laser alone group, Better overall VA improvement in PST+laser group	First evidence to support PST triamcinolone role in DME therapy
DRCR.net[11,12,33] Protocol B	Intravitreal triamcinolone	840	Eyes with new DME; 3 groups: 1 mg IVT versus 4 mg IVT versus laser	At 4 months VA better in 4 mg IVT group, but all groups were equal by 1 year VA better in laser group during second year Higher rates of cataract in IVT groups Lower rate of DR progression in 4 mg IVT group	Large long-term study, concluded IVT not superior to macular laser for DME Evidence that 4 mg IVT may reduce DR progression
DRCR.net, Protocol I[15]	Intravitreal triamcinolone	854	Eyes with new DME Ranibizumab with prompt laser versus ranibizumab with deferred laser versus IVT+laser versus laser only	In subanalysis of pseudophakic eyes, VA gain in IVT+laser-treated eyes was comparable with ranibizumab groups	In pseudophakic eyes, IVT may be as effective as ranibizumab
Haller et al.[21]	Intravitreal dexamethasone (Ozurdex)	171	Eyes with persistent DME; 3 groups: Ozurdex 0.7 mg versus Ozurdex 0.35 mg versus laser only	≥10 letter gain at day 180 - 30% in Ozurdex 0.7 mg, 19% in Ozurdex 0.35 mg, 23% in laser group	First evidence for utility of Ozurdex in DME Supports 0.7-mg dose
Campochiaro et al. FAME[31]	Intravitreal fluocinolone (Iluvien)	953	Eyes with persistent DME; 3 groups: Iluvien 0.5 µg versus Iluvien 0.2 µg versus laser	≥15 letter VA gain at 2 years 28.6% in Iluvien 0.5 µg, 28.7% in Iluvien 0.2 µg, 16.2% in laser group	First study showing long-term sustainability & efficacy of Iluvien Risk-benefit ratio supported 0.2 µg as preferred dose
Pearson et al.[32]	Intravitreal fluocinolone (Retisert)	196	Eyes with refractory DME; 0.59 mg Retisert versus macular laser	≥15 letter gain at 3 years 31.1% in Retisert, but not significantly better than laser High complication rate with Retisert: 61.4% IOP elevation, 33.8% required surgery	Retisert is effective for long-term DME therapy, but may have unfavorable safety profile

Continued

TABLE 8.1
Major Studies in the Evolution of Corticosteroid Therapy for Diabetic Retinopathy (DR) and Diabetic Macular Edema (DME)—cont'd

Study	Steroid Type, Route of Administration	Eyes (No.)	Design	Main Results	Clinical Significance
Boyer et al.[24] (MEAD)	Intravitreal dexamethasone (Ozurdex)	1048	Eyes with new DME; 3 groups: Ozurdex 0.7 mg versus Ozurdex 0.35 mg versus laser	≥15 letter gain at 3 years - 22.2% in Ozurdex 0.7 mg, 18.5% in Ozurdex 0.35 mg, 12% in laser group	Evidence that Ozurdex is effective as first-line DME treatment
Gillies et al.[29] (BEVORDEX)	Intravitreal dexamethasone (Ozurdex)	88	Eyes with new DME; Ozurdex every 4 months versus monthly bevacizumab	≥10 letter gain - 45% in bevacizumab versus 43% in Ozurdex. Higher rate of cataract in Ozurdex. Fewer injections in Ozurdex (2.7) versus bevacizumab (8.6) in 1st year	Only head-to-head comparative study. Ozurdex as effective as bevacizumab with reduction in injection burden
Kaur et al.[4]	Topical difluprednate	20	One group; eyes with refractory DME	Improvement of VA 2 lines, reduction in CMT	Proof of concept that topical therapy may be effective for DME

CMT, central macular thickness; *FAME*, fluocinolone acetonide in diabetic macular edema; *IVT*, intravitreal triamcinolone; *PST*, posterior sub-Tenon injection; *VA*, visual acuity; *MEAD*, Macular Edema: Assessment of Implantable Dexamethasone in Diabetes study; *BEVORDEX*, Intravitreal Bevacizumab (Avastin) Versus Intravitreal Dexamethasone (Ozurdex for Persistent Diabetic Macular Edema) study with only 19% of those treated with laser alone. The improvement in vision was significantly better in the sub-Tenon triamcinolone group, with no difference in the rates of IOP elevation.[6]

Although sub-Tenon injection of triamcinolone is a valid option for the treatment of DME, it is not frequently used because of its potential complications of cataract progression and IOP elevation. In addition, several comparative studies have demonstrated that intravitreal administration of steroids is more effective than sub-Tenon injection for DME treatment.[7,8] When sub-Tenon injection of triamcinolone is employed, the common administered dose is 40 mg (in 1 mL), which is expected to last for about at least 3 months.

Intravitreal Injection

Intravitreal injection of triamcinolone was the first route by which corticosteroids were shown to be effective for the treatment of DME. This technique is simple to perform and achieves rapid, therapeutic drug concentrations in the eye. Despite the greater potency of dexamethasone as a steroid agent, it has a very short half-life in the eye. Triamcinolone has a longer half-life and is more suitable for intravitreal injection.[2] In a seminal pilot study of 16 eyes with refractory DME that had at least two previous macular laser sessions, an intravitreal injection of 4 mg triamcinolone acetonide led to improvement of VA by 2.4 lines and a reduction of CMT by 57.5% at 3 months. Three eyes (18.7%) had an IOP elevation over 21 mm Hg.[9] This study demonstrated that intravitreal injection of triamcinolone is effective and relatively safe for the treatment of refractory DME.

Subsequent larger-scale randomized controlled trials have established the efficacy of intravitreal triamcinolone injection for DME therapy. A comparative study of 63 eyes with refractory DME treated with either 4 mg intravitreal triamcinolone acetonide (IVT) injection or a sham subconjunctival saline injection reported improved VA and CMT in treated eyes, which was maintained for 2 years. An improvement of more than one line of vision was achieved in 56% of IVT-treated eyes compared with 26% of control eyes, and the IVT-treated group had a significantly larger improvement in VA overall. Although higher rates of IOP elevation were noted in the IVT group, this was managed by topical therapy in all eyes.[10]

The DRCR.net studies (see Appendix A) have contributed greatly to the understanding of the efficacy and safety profiles of intravitreal steroids and have helped establish their place in the medical management against DME. Protocol B from the DRCR.net group randomized 840 eyes with DME and baseline VA of 20/40 to 20/320 to one of three treatments: macular laser, 1 mg IVT, or 4 mg IVT. Although eyes treated with 4 mg IVT had better VA at 4 months, by 1 year there was no difference between the groups and at the end of the second year, VA was better in the laser-treated group with lower rates of complications. The results were also slightly in favor of the laser-treated group in a subanalysis of pseudophakic eyes.[11] With repeated injections over the 3 years of study follow-up, a large proportion of IVT-treated eyes had progression of cataract, requiring surgery.[12] These results are in contrast to a smaller study that had compared three types of treatments for DME: macular laser, IVT (4 mg), and a combination of both laser and IVT. At 6 months, eyes treated by laser alone had the worst results, whereas eyes treated with IVT and IVT combined with laser demonstrated similar improvements in VA and CMT.[13] However, owing to the larger sample size and design, the results of the DRCR.net studies indicated that IVT is not superior to macular laser, which remained the treatment of choice for DME at that time, against which novel therapeutic modalities had to be compared.

Another long-term comparative study by DRCR.net (Protocol I) evaluated eyes with DME treated with ranibizumab with or without focal laser and demonstrated that deferring laser treatment is preferable, as its performance was found to be worse in terms of final visual improvement.[14] As intravitreal anti-VEGF injections are presently the most commonly used treatment for DME, based on the results of the Ranibizumab for Diabetic Macular Edema (RISE/RIDE) study and other studies, the results of this study have markedly reduced the use of macular laser therapy for DME, and it is currently reserved for a minority of patients who have non-center-involving focal DME. However, it is important to note that the Protocol I study also included a group of patients who were treated with 4 mg IVT and macular laser. In a subset of pseudophakic eyes at baseline, VA improvement in the IVT group was comparable with that of the ranibizumab groups.[15] These results were reported for 6 months, indicating that at least for the short term, IVT may be equally effective as ranibizumab for DME. A small study that compared DME treatment with either IVT or bevacizumab reported comparable short-term results, but at 12 months VA was better in the bevacizumab group.[16] It should be noted that despite the obvious efficacy of intravitreal injection of triamcinolone acetonide for DME, it has not been formally approved by the US Food and Drug Administration (FDA) for this indication and its use is considered off-label.

Sterile endophthalmitis is an uncommon, noninfectious, inflammatory reaction status post intravitreal injections. Because infectious endophthalmitis is a dreaded complication of any intravitreal injection, any patient presenting shortly after an injection with signs and symptoms suggestive of endophthalmitis is very concerning. In contrast to infectious etiology, the clinical picture of sterile endophthalmitis is milder, without pain, hypopyon, or anterior chamber fibrin. As an infectious cause is lacking, sterile endophthalmitis does not require intravitreal antibiotics or surgical intervention and may be managed conservatively with topical antiinflammatory drops. It has been demonstrated that it is an inflammatory response incited by the relatively high particle load injected into the eye,[17] which eventually settles down and the inflammation decreases. The reported rate of this complication varies between 0% and 13% following IVT. Preservative-free formulations (Triescence, Alcon, Ft Worth, TX, USA) are associated with a lower risk for this complication, whereas patients with a prior history of uveitis are at increased risk.[17–20] Sterile endophthalmitis should be differentiated from pseudoendophthalmitis or pseudohypopyon, which is a result of dispersion of triamcinolone crystals into the anterior chamber after intravitreal injection. This occurs in 0.8% of eyes after IVT and is more common in eyes with a posterior capsule opening, with zonular disruption, or after vitrectomy but can occur in any eye. The crystals settle in the inferior angle, and the condition may occur immediately at the time of injection or be noted in the first 3 days after IVT. Diagnosis is made by the slit lamp appearance of crystals that may be mobile, and this usually resolves spontaneously without specific therapy.

Intravitreal Injection of Slow-Release Corticosteroid Implants

Intravitreal injection of steroids have been proved to be an effective treatment for DME but are limited primarily by ocular complications, including cataract progression, IOP elevation, and the need for repeated injections for effect (although less frequent that anti-VEGF agents). Therefore, research has been directed at creating a long-lasting, slow-release injectable corticosteroid implant that will be as efficacious and allow a longer duration of action with an improved safety profile. At present, there are two types of sustained-release steroid implants approved by the FDA for the treatment of DME: a degradable dexamethasone implant (Ozurdex, Allergan Inc., Irvine, CA, USA) and a nondegradable fluocinolone acetonide implant (Iluvien, Alimera Sciences Inc., Alpharetta, GA, USA).

Ozurdex is made of a biodegradable copolymer (polylactic-co-glycolic acid), which is loaded with 700 μg of dexamethasone. It is injected into the vitreous cavity using a 22-gauge specialized applicator, where it floats freely, usually sinking to the inferior part of the eye. For this reason, it is also recommended to inject it in the inferior part of the eye, so it does not come close to the visual axis. As the polylactic-co-glycolic acid slowly hydrolyzes to lactic and glycolic acids, dexamethasone is released in a slow and stable manner, allowing for up to 6 months' duration of action. The efficacy of Ozurdex in DME was first demonstrated in a Phase II study that included 171 eyes with persistent DME that were randomized to one of three treatment groups: a single injection of Ozurdex 700 μg, Ozurdex 350 μg, or sham therapy. Persistent DME was defined as that which was present for more than 90 days' duration before treatment initiation. After 6 months, 30% of eyes treated with Ozurdex 700 μg had improved by two or more lines of vision compared with 19% of eyes treated with Ozurdex 350 μg and 23% of sham eyes. The patients treated with Ozurdex 700 μg also had a significantly reduced CMT.[21] Ozurdex was subsequently evaluated in a study of 55 eyes with refractory DME defined as that which persisted after previous treatments including vitrectomy for this indication. After 8 weeks, which is the time of peak drug effect of the Ozurdex implant, 30.4% of patients had improved by two or more lines of vision. At 6 months, mean VA had significantly improved by six letters compared with baseline VA. Transient IOP elevation peaked at 8 weeks and was only noted in 9% of eyes, much less than the rates previously reported for IVT.[22] The more controlled slow release of corticosteroids from the implant is responsible for the reduced rate of IOP elevation.

The PLACID (Safety and Efficacy of a New Treatment in Combination With Laser for Diabetic Macular Edema) study compared Ozurdex combined with macular laser and macular laser alone in a large cohort of patients with DME. Although the 12-month VA results were similar in both groups, a significantly greater proportion of patients had gained two or more lines of vision up to 9 months. About 15% of the Ozurdex-treated patients had transient IOP elevations, but these were all managed by topical therapy.[23] The results of this study indicated Ozurdex may be a better treatment for DME than macular laser.

The highest-quality evidence supporting the efficacy of Ozurdex for the treatment of DME comes from the MEAD (Macular Edema: Assessment of Implantable Dexamethasone in Diabetes) study. In this multicenter randomized controlled trial, 1048 patients with DME

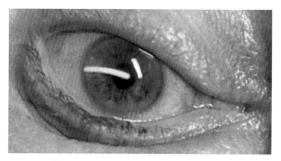

FIG. 8.1 Ozurdex migration into the anterior chamber in a pseudophakic eye with a large posterior capsule opening.

were randomized into one of three treatment groups (700 μg Ozurdex, 350 μg Ozurdex, or sham injection) and followed up for 3 years with retreatments possible at 6-month intervals. An improvement of three or more lines in VA was achieved in 22.2% of the patients treated with 700 μg Ozurdex, 18.5% of the patients treated with 350 μg Ozurdex, and only 12.0% of the patients in the sham group. The reduction in CMT was also significantly greater in the Ozurdex-treated groups than in the sham group. About a third of the Ozurdex-treated patients had an IOP elevation, but this were transient and only two patients in the entire study required trabeculectomy. Cataract progression was documented in 67.9% of the patients treated with 700 μg Ozurdex, 64.1% of the patients treated with 350 μg Ozurdex, and only 20.4% of the patients in the sham group.[24] Despite the increased rate of cataract progression and IOP elevations induced by repeated Ozurdex injections, this study demonstrated the efficacy of this therapeutic modality as a potential first-line treatment for DME. At present, it is recommended that IOP be monitored at 4–6 weeks following implantation to assess for IOP elevation in susceptible patients. It should also be noted that Ozurdex may migrate into the anterior chamber, where it can become trapped and require a surgical procedure for extraction (Fig. 8.1). For this reason, it is contraindicated in aphakic patients.

It is important to emphasize that the MEAD study design allowed reinjection with Ozurdex only at 6 months intervals, which is the length of effect the implant was originally designed to have. Subsequent data from smaller studies and real-world use of Ozurdex have shown that the response to this therapeutic modality is individual and that in many patients signs of decreasing efficacy (such as a decrease in VA, an increase in CMT, or recurrence of DME) that warrant retreatment occur after 3–4 months. For example, a multicenter, retrospective study reported the real-world

results achieved by administering multiple Ozurdex for DME therapy. Repeated Ozurdex injections were administered whenever intraretinal cysts were noted on OCT or VA had decreased. After 3 years, the mean improvement in VA was 9.5 letters, with 25.4% of eyes improving by 15 letters or more. The mean interval between injections was found to vary over time and was under 6 months during the first year.[25] Another large survey that assessed the real-life practice patterns of over 100 retina specialists in France reported that when used for the treatment of DME, Ozurdex was administered on average 2.4 times per year with a mean interval of 4.9 months between injections.[26] Additional smaller series that focused on Ozurdex for DME also reported that it is typically repeated before 6 months.[27,28] Therefore, using a patient-specific tailored approach to repeat Ozurdex DME may achieve better VA results than those reported in the MEAD study.

The BEVORDEX (Intravitreal Bevacizumab versus Intravitreal Dexamethasone/Ozurdex for Persistent Diabetic Macular Edema) study is unique because it is a comparative study, which was a head-to-head comparison of patients with DME treated with either 700 μg Ozurdex or intravitreal bevacizumab injections. The study included 88 eyes and patients were followed up for 12 months. At the final visit, 40% of the bevacizumab-treated eyes and 41% of the Ozurdex-treated eyes had improvement of two or more lines of vision. On the one hand, none of the bevacizumab-treated eyes lost more than two lines of vision, whereas 11% of those treated with Ozurdex lost vision as a result of cataract progression. On the other hand, patients in the bevacizumab group received a mean of 8.6 injections over 12 months, compared with only 2.7 injections in the Ozurdex group.[29] These results were subsequently reported to be maintained over 2 years of follow-up.[30] The BEVORDEX results imply that repeated Ozurdex injections may be as effective as bevacizumab for the treatment of DME by offering similar results with fewer injections but a higher rate of cataract progression.

The Iluvien implant contains 0.2 μg of fluocinolone acetonide, which is a very potent corticosteroid that lasts up to 3 years after injection into the eye. It is not biodegradable, and the drug is contained in a 3.5-mm inert polyimide tube that is injected into the vitreous in an office procedure. The Fluocinolone Acetonide in Diabetic Macular Edema (FAME) A and B studies were Phase III studies that evaluated the Iluvien implant for DME. These studies included 953 patients and evaluated two doses of fluocinolone (0.2 and 0.5 μg per day) compared with macular laser. The 2-year results demonstrated that 28.7% of subjects in the low-dose group and 28.6% of those receiving a high dose had a three-line improvement in VA compared with only 16.2% in the laser-treated group; 30.6% and 31.2% of subjects in the low- and high-dose group, respectively, had an increase in VA; the percentage of eyes with IOP greater than 30 mm Hg at any time point was 16.3% in the low-dose and 21.6% in the high-dose group; and surgical trabeculectomy was performed in 2.1% of low-dose patients and 5.1% of high-dose patients by 24 months.[31]

Retisert (Bausch and Lomb, Rochester, NY, USA) is another intraocular implant that contains fluocinolone acetonide. Unlike the injectable Iluvien implant, it is implanted into the eye via a surgical procedure entailing a 3.5-mm circumferential incision through the pars plana and sutured to the sclera. The implant is non-biodegradable and has been studied in a multicenter, randomized controlled clinical trial for the treatment of DME. Patients in the study were randomized 2:1 to receive either a 0.59-mg fluocinolone implant or macular laser. At 36 months, there was no evidence of edema in 58% of implanted eyes compared with 30% of eyes that received the standard-of-care laser treatment ($P<.001$). VA improvement of three lines or more occurred more frequently in Retisert-implanted versus laser-treated eyes (28% vs. 15%, respectively, $P<.05$). The most common serious adverse events in the Retisert-implanted eyes were those found in all studies employing intravitreal steroids, with cataract development requiring extraction and an increase in IOP. Of the phakic Retisert-implanted eyes, 95% required cataract surgery and 35% experienced increased IOP. A filtering procedure was necessary in 33.8% of implanted eyes, and explantation was required in 5% of eyes to manage IOP elevation.[32] Although this study indicated that the Retisert implant is effective for the long-term management of DME, the high rates of complications especially with regards to IOP prevent it from being recommended for use, and it was not approved by the FDA for the treatment of DME.

Injection Into the Suprachoroidal Space

A specialized microinjector to deliver medication into the suprachoroidal space is being evaluated. The hypothesis is that the suprachoroidal space allows access of therapeutic agents to the posterior segment while limiting potential anterior segment side effects. A Phase I/II trial is currently evaluating a proprietary suspension of triamcinolone acetonide (Zuprata, Clearside Biomedical) via suprachoroidal delivery as monotherapy or in combination with aflibercept for DME.

EFFECT OF CORTICOSTEROIDS ON THE PROGRESSION OF DIABETIC RETINOPATHY

The RISE/RIDE studies demonstrated that monthly intravitreal injections of ranibizumab not only were effective for the treatment of DME, but also resulted in considerable regression of DR severity staging score. One of the DRCR.net reports (Protocol B) has analyzed the effect of macular laser, 1 mg IVT, and 4 mg IVT on the progression of DR in patients who were treated for DME and followed up for 3 years. Progression of DR was defined as conversion from nonproliferative DR to proliferative DR, need for panretinal photocoagulation, occurrence of a vitreous hemorrhage, or worsening of two or more levels in the ETDRS DR severity scale. Along the entire study period, rates of DR progression were significantly lower in the 4 mg IVT group than in the 1 mg IVT or macular laser groups, with final 3-year progression rates of 21% versus 29% and 31%, respectively.[33] This suggests that 4 mg IVT may be efficacious to reduce the risk of DR progression; however, the use of corticosteroids to slow the progression of DR has not been approved by the FDA at any stage.

COMBINATION THERAPY

It is possible to combine corticosteroid therapy with anti-VEGF therapy, as both agents may be injected intravitreally to exert their effects simultaneously. This approach may offer some advantages in treating patients with refractory DME but at present has received relatively little research attention. One small randomized controlled study included 40 eyes with persistent DME after multiple anti-VEGF injections, which were followed up monthly for 12 months and randomized to receive monthly bevacizumab injections or monthly bevacizumab injections but Ozurdex on months 1, 5, and 9. Bevacizumab injections were administered if VA was less than 20/25 or the CMT was more than 250 μm. At 12 months, the mean improvement in VA was comparable in both groups (5.4 letters in the combination group; 4.9 letters in the bevacizumab group). However, the reduction in CMT was significantly greater in the combination group, and a larger proportion of patients had CMT of less than 250 μm. On average the eyes in the combination group received three fewer injections of bevacizumab during the study period, but the overall number of injections was similar when the Ozurdex injections were also included.[34]

A post hoc analysis of VA from the DRCR.net Protocol I data was performed to assess whether the long-term response to anti-VEGF treatment of DME could be predicted after three injections.[35] This Early Anti-VEGF Response and Long-term efficacY (EARLY) analysis may offer some insight into the management of patients with DME who do not respond adequately to anti-VEGF therapy, and further research in this direction may lead to more validated guidelines on switching anti-VEGF agents, switching to corticosteroid therapy, or considering a combination of treatments.

CONCLUSION

Corticosteroid therapy for DME is effective and safe, especially if administered by an intravitreally injected slow-release implant. Although anti-VEGF therapy is currently the primary choice of treatment for DME, it should be remembered that corticosteroid therapy is approved by the FDA as a first-line treatment for this indication as well. Intravitreal corticosteroids are a suitable option in refractory patients, especially if they are pseudophakic. Ozurdex and intravitreal triamcinolone are the most commonly utilized steroids for DME, and data support that their efficacy is similar to that of some of the anti-VEGF agents (bevacizumab). They offer the advantages of longer-lasting effect and a reduced injection burden compared with anti-VEGF agents; however, they are also associated with an increased rate of cataract progression and IOP elevation. There may be specific situations in which intravitreal steroid is preferable to anti-VEGF therapy, such as in pregnant women, children, patients with significant cardiovascular disease, and patients who cannot commit to monthly monitoring. Future research into reducing potential side effects especially IOP, longer-duration implants, or topical formulations with adequate penetrance may change current practice trends and increase steroid use in patients with diabetes. Also, studies to predict the response to anti-VEGF agents and of combination therapies may establish clearer guidelines for corticosteroid therapy.

REFERENCES

1. Ozaki H, Hayashi H, Vinores SA, Moromizato Y, Campochiaro PA, Oshima K. Intravitreal sustained release of VEGF causes retinal neovascularization in rabbits and breakdown of the blood-retinal barrier in rabbits and primates. *Exp Eye Res.* 1997;64:505–517.
2. Stewart MW. Corticosteroid use for diabetic macular edema: old fad or new trend? *Curr Diabetes Rep.* 2012;12:364–375.
3. Semeraro F, Cancarini A, dell'Omo R, Rezzola S, Romano MR, Costagliola C. Diabetic retinopathy: vascular and inflammatory disease. *J Diabetes Res.* 2015;2015:582060.
4. Kaur S, Yangzes S, Singh S, Sachdev N. Efficacy and safety of topical difluprednate in persistent diabetic macular edema. *Int Ophthalmol.* 2016;36:335–340.
5. Ohira A, Hara K, Jóhannesson G, et al. Topical dexamethasone γ-cyclodextrin nanoparticle eye drops increase visual acuity and decrease macular thickness in diabetic macular oedema. *Acta Ophthalmol.* 2015;93:610–615.
6. Verma LK, Vivek MB, Kumar A, Tewari HK, Venkatesh P. A prospective controlled trial to evaluate the adjunctive role of posterior subtenon triamcinolone in the treatment of diffuse diabetic macular edema. *J Ocul Pharmacol Ther.* 2004;20:277–284.
7. Cardillo JA, Melo Jr LA, Costa RA, et al. Comparison of intravitreal versus posterior sub-Tenon's capsule injection of triamcinolone acetonide for diffuse diabetic macular edema. *Ophthalmology.* 2005;112:1557–1563.
8. Bonini-Filho MA, Jorge R, Barbosa JC, Calucci D, Cardillo JA, Costa RA. Intravitreal injection versus sub-Tenon's infusion of triamcinolone acetonide for refractory diabetic macular edema: a randomized clinical trial. *Invest Ophthalmol Vis Sci.* 2005;46:3845–3849.
9. Martidis A, Duker JS, Greenberg PB, et al. Intravitreal triamcinolone for refractory diabetic macular edema. *Ophthalmology.* 2002;109:920–927.
10. Gillies MC, Sutter FK, Simpson JM, Larsson J, Ali H, Zhu M. Intravitreal triamcinolone for refractory diabetic macular edema: two-year results of a double-masked, placebo-controlled, randomized clinical trial. *Ophthalmology.* 2006;113:1533–1538.
11. Diabetic Retinopathy Clinical Research Network. A randomized trial comparing intravitreal triamcinolone acetonide and focal/grid photocoagulation for diabetic macular edema. *Ophthalmology.* 2008;115:1447–1449. 1449.e1-e10.
12. Diabetic Retinopathy Clinical Research Network (DRCR.net), Beck RW, Edwards AR, et al. Three-year follow-up of a randomized trial comparing focal/grid photocoagulation and intravitreal triamcinolone for diabetic macular edema. *Arch Ophthalmol.* 2009;127:245–251.
13. Lam DS, Chan CK, Mohamed S, et al. Intravitreal triamcinolone plus sequential grid laser versus triamcinolone or laser alone for treating diabetic macular edema: six-month outcomes. *Ophthalmology.* 2007;114: 2162–2167.
14. Elman MJ, Ayala A, Bressler NM, et al. Intravitreal Ranibizumab for diabetic macular edema with prompt versus deferred laser treatment: 5-year randomized trial results. *Ophthalmology.* 2015;122:375–381.
15. Diabetic Retinopathy Clinical Research Network, Elman MJ, Aiello LP, et al. Randomized trial evaluating ranibizumab plus prompt or deferred laser or triamcinolone plus prompt laser for diabetic macular edema. *Ophthalmology.* 2010;117:1064–1077.

16. Kriechbaum K, Prager S, Mylonas G, et al. Intravitreal bevacizumab (Avastin) versus triamcinolone (Volon A) for treatment of diabetic macular edema: one-year results. *Eye (London)*. 2014;28:9–15.

17. Otsuka H, Kawano H, Sonoda S, Nakamura M, Sakamoto T. Particle-induced endophthalmitis: possible mechanisms of sterile endophthalmitis after intravitreal triamcinolone. *Invest Ophthalmol Vis Sci*. 2013;54(3):1758–1766.

18. Dodwell DG, Krimmel DA, de Fiebre CM. Sterile endophthalmitis rates and particle size analyses of different formulations of triamcinolone acetonide. *Clin Ophthalmol*. 2015;9:1033–1040.

19. Stepien KE, Eaton AM, Jaffe GJ, Davis JL, Raja J, Feuer W. Increased incidence of sterile endophthalmitis after intravitreal triamcinolone acetonide in spring 2006. *Retina*. 2009;29(2):207–213.

20. Taban M, Singh RP, Chung JY, Lowder CY, Perez VL, Kaiser PK. Sterile endophthalmitis after intravitreal triamcinolone: a possible association with uveitis. *Am J Ophthalmol*. 2007;144(1):50–54.

21. Haller JA, Kuppermann BD, Blumenkranz MS, et al. Randomized controlled trial of an intravitreous dexamethasone drug delivery system in patients with diabetic macular edema. *Arch Ophthalmol*. 2010;128:289–296.

22. Boyer DS, Faber D, Gupta S, et al. Dexamethasone intravitreal implant for treatment of diabetic macular edema in vitrectomized patients. *Retina*. 2011;31:915–923.

23. Callanan DG, Gupta S, Boyer DS, et al. Dexamethasone intravitreal implant in combination with laser photocoagulation for the treatment of diffuse diabetic macular edema. *Ophthalmology*. 2013;120:1843–1851.

24. Boyer DS, Yoon YH, Belfort Jr R, et al. Three-year, randomized, sham-controlled trial of dexamethasone intravitreal implant in patients with diabetic macular edema. *Ophthalmology*. 2014;121:1904–1914.

25. Malclès A, Dot C, Voirin N, et al. Real-life study in diabetic macular edema treated with dexamethasone implant: The Reldex Study. *Retina*. 2017;37:753–760.

26. Querques G, Darvizeh F, Querques L, Capuano V, Bandello F, Souied EH. Assessment of the real-life usage of intravitreal dexamethasone implant in the treatment of chronic diabetic macular edema in France. *J Ocul Pharmacol Ther*. 2016;32:383–389.

27. Matonti F, Pommier S, Meyer F, et al. Long-term efficacy and safety of intravitreal dexamethasone implant for the treatment of diabetic macular edema. *Eur J Ophthalmol*. 2016. [ahead of print].

28. Aknin I, Melki L. Longitudinal study of sustained-release dexamethasone intravitreal implant in patients with diabetic macular edema. *Ophthalmologica*. 2016;235:187–188.

29. Gillies MC, Lim LL, Campain A, et al. A randomized clinical trial of intravitreal bevacizumab versus intravitreal dexamethasone for diabetic macular edema: the BEVORDEX study. *Ophthalmology*. 2014;121:2473–2481.

30. Fraser-Bell S, Lim LL, Campain A, et al. Bevacizumab or dexamethasone implants for DME: 2-year results (the BEVORDEX study). *Ophthalmology*. 2016;123:1399–1401.

31. Campochiaro PA, Brown DM, Pearson A, et al. Long-term benefit of sustained-delivery fluocinolone acetonide vitreous inserts for diabetic macular edema. *Ophthalmology*. 2011;118:626–635.

32. Pearson PA, Comstock TL, Ip M, et al. Fluocinolone acetonide intravitreal implant for diabetic macular edema: a 3-year multicenter, randomized, controlled clinical trial. *Ophthalmology*. 2011;118:1580–1587.

33. Bressler NM, Edwards AR, Beck RW, et al. Exploratory analysis of diabetic retinopathy progression through 3 years in a randomized clinical trial that compares intravitreal triamcinolone acetonide with focal/grid photocoagulation. *Arch Ophthalmol*. 2009;127:1566–1571.

34. Maturi RK, Bleau L, Saunders J, Mubasher M, Stewart MW. A 12-month, single-masked, randomized controlled study of eyes with persistent diabetic macular edema after multiple anti-vegf injections to assess the efficacy of the dexamethasone-delayed delivery system as an adjunct to bevacizumab compared with continued bevacizumab monotherapy. *Retina*. 2015;35:1604–1614.

35. Gonzalez VH, Campbell J, Holekamp NM, et al. To anti-vascular endothelial growth factor therapy in diabetic macular edema: analysis of Protocol I data. *Am J Ophthalmol*. 2016.

CHAPTER 9

Laser Treatment of Diabetic Retinopathy

SEAN PLATT, MD • SOPHIE BAKRI, MD

Diabetic retinopathy can be treated with a variety of methods, including corticosteroids, anti–vascular endothelial growth factor (VEGF) injections, corticosteroids, and laser photocoagulation. The therapies may be used solely, sequentially, or at times in combination to achieve the desired outcome. This chapter outlines the current role of laser photocoagulation for diabetic retinopathy in the anti-VEGF era and recent developments in laser treatment modalities.

HISTORY OF LASER TREATMENT

The photo effects of bright light have been known for centuries as noted by Socrates who warned against staring at a solar eclipse.[1] Meyer-Schwickerath first published the concept of using light to treat ocular tissues in 1949.[1] He would focus sunlight from the rooftop of his laboratory to treat ocular melanoma. Given the variability in access to sunlight, other sources were sought, and he moved on to use the high-intensity Beck arc.[2] This instrument had the disadvantages of gas and carbon liberation and the short life of the filaments. By the mid-1950s, Zeiss made the first commercially available xenon arc photocoagulator; however, this device was difficult to use clinically and produced large, severe burns.[1]

The concept of the laser (light amplification by stimulated emission of radiation) was developed by Einstein in 1917, but Arthur Townes and Charles Schawlow built the first device using optical light at the same time Russian physicists Alexander Prokhorov and Nicolai Basov described how a molecular beam of alkali halide in a resonating cavity might result in a microwave oscillator.[3,4] These scientists eventually won a Nobel Prize in physics for their work.[3] The first functioning ruby laser was produced by Theodore Maiman at the Hughes Laboratories in 1960.[1,5] Laser radiation had features that allow its clinical application in the treatment of ophthalmic diseases. In laser systems, photons demonstrate coherence and narrow wavelength and are collimated with improved control and predictability compared with the preceding arc photocoagulators.[1] The ruby laser had its limitations, and in 1964 the argon laser using the blue and green spectrum range (488–514 nm, respectively) was developed, also at Hughes Laboratories.[1]

The invention of the argon laser marked a new milestone in the advancement of retinal photocoagulation. The argon laser had the advantage of being absorbed by hemoglobin and melanin over the deep red wavelength of the ruby laser (694 nm).[1,6] To this day, argon laser is the foundation for treating numerous retinal disorders, including diabetic macular edema (DME) and proliferative diabetic retinopathy (PDR).

PRINCIPLES OF LASER TREATMENT

Lasers comprise the following basic elements: an active medium, a cavity, and a source of excitation (see Fig. 9.1). For light amplification to occur, stimulated emission of photons needs to occur more than absorption; hence, there should be more photons in the excited state than in the lower energy state (population inversion).[1,3] The excitation source stimulates the active medium inside the cavity to create the laser beam, and the cavity circulates the emitted light between the two mirrors. The light trapped inside the cavity stimulates the emission of new photons from the active medium, thus forming new photons. Once an excitation source is stimulated, a laser beam is created in one wavelength (monochromaticity), without divergence (collimation), and can be focused to a very small size (spatial coherence).[1]

LASER-TISSUE INTERACTIONS

There are three types of laser-tissue interactions: photochemical, photothermal, and photomechanical. Conventional laser for diabetic retinopathy utilizes photothermal effects, which include necrosis, coagulation,

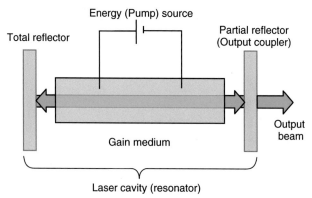

FIG. 9.1 Elements of laser. Basic laser configuration leading to a highly collimated beam of energy. https://timothytrespas.wordpress.com/2014/05/27/lasers-laser-technology-termsphysics-ans-information-to-help-targeted-individuals-understand-lasermaser-technology/.

vaporization, carbonization, and melting, depending of the duration and power selected.[3] Laser photocoagulation causes destruction of oxygen-utilizing cells by cell death and scarring, by an increase in tissue temperature by tens of degrees Celsius above body temperature.[3] This laser energy is absorbed primarily by melanin in the retinal pigment epithelium (RPE) and choroid.[3] The absorption of energy by tissue chromophores is dependent on the wavelength of the laser (see Laser Parameters section).[3] The pertinent chromophores in ocular tissues include water, proteins, melanin/pigments, and blood.[3] For example, at 532 nm green wavelength, approximately 5% of incident laser light on the retina is absorbed by neural retina; about half is absorbed in the RPE, and the rest in the choroid.[7] The heat generated by laser energy absorption in RPE and choroid diffuses into the retina and causes coagulation of the photoreceptors; it may also diffuse into the inner retina.[3] The use of shorter pulses and smaller spot sizes (as with the micropulse laser) helps limit heat diffusion to the photoreceptor layer, thus minimizing damage to the inner retina.[3] The extent of tissue damage has been evaluated via the Arrhenius model, which is a formula for the temperature dependence of reaction rates.[7] To prevent complications from laser procedures, it is important to understand that the width of the retinal photothermal lesion increases linearly with laser power and logarithmically with pulse duration.[3,7] Conversely the denaturation of proteins varies exponentially with temperature and linearly with pulse duration.[3]

To this day, the exact mechanism of tissue repair leading to treatment effect is poorly understood.[3,8] RPE defects can be filled by RPE cell spreading if the defect is small or by cell hyperplasia/proliferation if the defect is large.[9] The RPE cells can react to the tissue disruption induced by laser in differential ways, which allows ophthalmologists to take advantage of the different tissue reactions to treat both neovascularization of the retina and DME in diabetic retinopathy.

The effect of panretinal photocoagulation (PRP) laser is thought to be due to a combination of mechanisms. These mechanisms include facilitation of oxygen and nutrient transport from the choroid to the retina, facilitation of waste out of the retina, reduction of metabolic demand, and reduced sequestration of proangiogenic or permeability cytokines that accumulate in the photoreceptors in hypoxic conditions, thus reducing VEGF load.[3]

Focal laser's effect is presumed to be due to the stabilization of leaky microaneurysms by the stimulation of RPE to restore the retinal-blood barrier and secretion of cytokines that downregulate angiogenesis and vascular permeability.[3,9] When the diameters of retinal vessels were assessed before and after focal macular laser, the diameter of retinal arterioles, venules, and their macular branches showed a decrease in diameter status post laser. The macular arteriolar branches constricted 20.2%, and the venular branches constricted 13.8%. This was attributed to autoregulatory vasoconstriction from the improved retinal oxygenation caused after focal laser treatment–induced reduction of DME.[10]

DELIVERY SYSTEMS

Early laser systems were large bulky machines attached to direct monocular ophthalmoscopes.[11] Current systems can be attached via fiber-optic cables to the slit lamp, indirect ophthalmoscope, or vitrectomy console.[11] Slit lamp delivery systems produce a highly magnified fundus image with the benefit of ocular stability to accurately place photocoagulation near the fovea or

TABLE 9.1
Common Contact Lenses

Lens	Image Magnification	Laser Beam Magnification
Ocular Mainster Standard	0.95	1.05
Ocular Fundus Laser	0.93	1.08
Ocular Karichoff Laser	0.93	1.08
Ocular 3 Mirror Univ.	0.93	1.08
Ocular Mainster Wide	0.67	1.50
Ocular Mainster Ultra	0.53	1.90
Ocular Mainster 165	0.51	1.96
Rodenstock Panfundoscope	0.67	1.50
Volk G-3 Gonio	1.06	0.94
Volk Area Centralis	1.06	0.94
Volk TransEquator	0.69	1.44
Volk SuperQuad 160	0.5	2.00
Volk QuadraAspheric	0.51	1.97
Volk HRWF	0.5	2.00
Goldmann 3 Mirror	1.00	1.00

Adapted from http://www.aao.org/munnerlyn-laser-surgery-center/optical-properties-of-eye.

to the intended tissue target. Wide-field contact lenses offer a view of the peripheral retina, which is beneficial when performing PRP laser. A variety of contact lenses can be used (Table 9.1) providing differential magnification. It is important to be aware of the potential disparity between the spot size set on the laser and actual spot size when using a contact lens before placing the first laser spot. Some lenses, such as the Mainster focal grid and Volk Area Centralis (1.05× and 1.0×, respectively), do not magnify the spot size significantly, but other common lenses such as the Mainster PRP, Quadraspheric, SuperQuad, and Ultrafield (1.96×, 1.92×, 2.0×, and 1.89×, respectively) need compensation of the laser spot size to prevent large tissue burns.[11] Using the laser indirect ophthalmoscope (LIO) delivery system, a noncontact condensing lens, such as 28 D or 20 D lens, is used to focus the laser onto the peripheral retina and can be combined with scleral depression as needed. This method of delivery system does not offer the precise accuracy to administer laser to the macular region.

LASER PARAMETERS

The optimal laser power is typically titrated and depends on the ability of the target tissue to absorb the energy. The laser energy is converted to heat energy,

which is absorbed by melanin in the RPE and choroid, as well as vessels. Starting with a low power, the energy is increased until the effect of the laser is clinically evident as a gray-white lesion in the retina. The aim of photocoagulation is to optimize the therapeutic effect of the thermally induced laser spot while minimizing damage to the adjacent tissue. Effective retinal photocoagulation requires clear media for light to reach and be absorbed by pigment in the retinal tissue.[12] Melanin absorbs green, yellow, red, and infrared wavelengths; xanthophyll absorbs mostly blue wavelengths; hemoglobin absorbs blue, green, and yellow with minimal red wavelength.[12] The ability of a laser to create a visible laser burn is dependent on the tissue's ability to absorb the energy, which is dependent on the fundus pigmentation. In general, PRP, which is used to cover a larger surface area, employs larger spot sizes (200–500 μm). Focal laser, which is directed to small treatment areas or small vascular abnormalities, is optimized using smaller spot sizes (50–100 μm).[12–14]

LASER FOR DIABETIC RETINOPATHY

There are several laser types depending on the wavelength and the composition of the active medium, which can be gas (such as argon and krypton), solid

TABLE 9.2
Laser Types

Laser Type	Wavelength (nm)
Argon	488 (blue) and/or 514.5 (green)
Dye laser	Tunable 570–630 nm depending on dye
Diode	780–850 (infrared spectrum)
Double Frequency Nd:YAG	532
Krypton	568.2 (yellow) and/or 647.1 (red)

state (such as diode and neodymium-doped yttrium aluminum garnet/Nd:YAG), or liquid as in a tunable dye laser (Table 9.2).[15] Currently the most popular lasers used for retinal photocoagulation are the argon-green (532 nm), frequency-doubled Nd:YAG (532 nm) and yellow semiconductor lasers (577 nm).[8] Melanin absorbs energy at most wavelengths; therefore the selection of wavelength is less important when melanin is the primary tissue target.[8] To minimize the amount of energy that is lost through cataracts or vitreous opacities, longer wavelengths such as yellow may be used.[8] For treating lesions near the xanthophyll-rich macula, it is best to avoid wavelengths under 500 nm to prevent excessive damage to the nerve fiber layer.[8]

In preparation for treatment, informed consent should be obtained and the treatment eye should be marked. PRP treatment is most often performed in an office setting. To increase patient cooperation, it is important the patient is aware that the procedure may cause some discomfort. A topical anesthetic eye drop, such as tetracaine or proparacaine, should be applied. Rarely subconjunctival, peribulbar, or retrobulbar lidocaine injection may be required. Monitored or general anesthesia is rarely used for patients unable to cooperate. Proper patient and physician positioning is vital for comfort and improves compliance. The spot size should be adjusted depending on the contact lens used. For example, if using a Volk SuperQuad lens (magnification 0.5× and a laser spot of 2.0×), the slit lamp spot size should be set to 250 μm to obtain a 500 μm spot size on the retina.

PANRETINAL PHOTOCOAGULATION

Panretinal laser photocoagulation (PRP) has been considered the gold standard to treat proliferative vascular as well as ischemic changes in diabetes (Fig. 9.2 A color, B early FA, C late FA). PRP is associated with worsening of preexisting DME.[16] This secondary effect may be minimized with more peripheral placement of

PRP. In the setting of eyes with high-risk or florid PDR and DME, PRP combined with focal laser or PRP after focal laser and/or anti-VEGF therapy has been recommended.[17,18] The exact mechanism by which PRP aids in the treatment of PDR is hypothesized to be due to the secondary effects of peripheral retinal destruction, leading to a reduction of both oxygen demand and VEGF expression and an increased transport of oxygen and metabolic nutrients into the retina and choroid.[3]

As recommended by the Early Treatment Diabetic Retinopathy Study (ETDRS) and the Diabetic Retinopathy Study, the end point for the therapeutic effect is visualization of a gray-white spot on the retina, which is a result of thermal damage.[11,14,19] The recommended spot size for a PRP burn is 400–500 μm, with a spacing of one spot diameter apart, 100–150 ms duration, and laser setting adjustment based on the contact lens utilized.[14] A typical treatment would consist of 1200–1500 burns, but up to 2000 spots per eye is common and even more if the LIO is used given the smaller spot size with LIO. Treatment end point should be based on the minimal application to achieve a specific result, such as regression of neovascularization in PDR or reduction of macular edema in DME. PRP may be applied over a single or multiple sessions. Observational data from the DRCR.net Protocol F suggested PRP for PDR can be safely administered in a single sitting (compared with up to four sittings) in patients with relatively good visual acuity and no or mild preexisting center-involved macular edema only.[20] More PRP can be applied later, often termed "fill-in."

FOCAL/GRID LASER PHOTOCOAGULATION

In the early development of focal laser, Rubenstein and Myska recognized that DME was not only a consequence of local and distant leakage sites but in a broader sense also a consequence of retinal hypoxia.[21,22] Their studies showed favorable results when xenon arc laser was applied to ischemic zones (indirect treatment) as well as to areas of leakage and centers of circinate rings (direct treatment).[21] When the argon laser was developed, it changed the way DME was treated. With a 50-μm laser spot size, individual microaneurysms and foci as close as 300 μm from the fovea could be treated directly.[19] The rationale for grid laser is not fully understood, but its effect may be caused by retinal thinning, which would bring the retinal vessels closer to the choroid. This can cause vascular constriction by autoregulation, thus decreasing retinal edema.[23]

The ETDRS research group established the early guidelines for focal, grid, and scatter (PRP) laser. The initial ETDRS study started in December 1979 and was designed to evaluate argon laser photocoagulation and aspirin treatment in the management of eyes with nonproliferative diabetic retinopathy or early PDR.[24] This initial study also defined clinically significant macular edema (CSME) to designate severity.[24] In 1987 the ETDRS determined that focal laser was appropriate to treat all lesions 500–3000 μm from the center of the macula, which include microaneurysms that fill or leak on fluorescein angiography, intraretinal microvascular abnormalities, and short capillary segments, if they are felt to contribute to the macular edema or exudates.[22] The recommended spot size was 50–100 μm with a duration of 0.1 s and an end point of whitening or darkening of the microaneurysm.[19] The ETDRS reserved the grid laser for areas of diffuse leakage or capillary dropout consisting of light-intensity burns of 50–200 μm spot size spaced 1 burn width apart.[19,22] Areas of exclusion include within 500 μm of the fovea or within 500 μm of the disc margin.[19,22] Fig. 9.3A and B demonstrate resolution of a well defined area of CSME and exudates after focal laser to microaneurysms. The conclusion of the ETDRS report number four was that a combination of focal or grid laser led to a net effect of reducing visual acuity decline by approximately 50%–70% in eyes with foveal involving or threatening DME/exudate.[22]

The technique for applying focal/grid laser has evolved since the ETDRS recommendations. The early Diabetic Retinopathy Clinical Research Network (DRCR.net) protocols evaluated variables in laser for DME and developed the current standards as outlined by the "modified ETDRS focal/grid photocoagulation" technique in Table 9.3.[13,25] When compared with the mild macular grid (MMG) laser technique in DRCR.net Protocol A (Appendix 1), the MMG technique was less effective at reducing optical coherence tomography (OCT) measured retinal thickening than the modified

ETDRS laser technique at 12 months post laser. However, the visual acuity outcomes with both approaches were not substantially different.[26] DRCR.net established some other important concepts that shaped the way DME is treated. In 2010 the DRCR.net determined that intravitreal ranibizumab with prompt or deferred laser was more effective through year 1 compared with prompt laser alone for the treatment of DME (Protocol I).[27] DRCR.net investigators also published 2-year expanded outcomes from this study, which supported their original findings.[28] The Ranibizumab Monotherapy or Combined With Laser Versus Laser Monotherapy for Diabetic Macular Edema (RESTORE) study was a large randomized trial to assess the efficacy and safety of ranibizumab monotherapy compared with laser monotherapy.[29] The RESTORE trial was a head-to-head comparison to assess the superiority of three intervention outcomes: ranibizumab + sham laser, ranibizumab + focal laser, or focal laser + sham injection. The final outcome determined ranibizumab alone or combined with focal laser was superior to laser alone in improving the mean average change in best corrected visual acuity at 1 year.

PATTERN SCANNING

Computer-guided scanning systems are currently in use to apply multiple treatment pulses. Pattern scanning laser was first described by Blumenkranz and associates in 2006.[30] The pattern scanning laser photocoagulator (PASCAL) allows rapid delivery of short-pulse semiautomated burns in a predetermined pattern array. Unlike PRP, the PASCAL pulse duration is reduced to be 10–30 ms. A shorter pulse duration in a pattern array was chosen to increase speed of delivery, minimize damage to the inner retina and choroid by controlling depth, and reduce pain for the patient (Fig 9.2C).[3,7] It was estimated that by using a 6 × 6 or 7 × 7 array, the total treatment time theoretically could be reduced by 50-fold. In reality, a decrease of 7- to 10-fold treatment time could be achieved, reducing a single PRP session to 3–5 min.[30] Comparison of the PASCAL system with a 532-nm solid-state green laser showed that there was a significant reduction in application time, subjective pain, laser spot size at 3 months, and better preservation of visual fields with the PASCAL for PRP treatment.[31] Although the PASCAL laser has its benefits, it falls short when it is compared with the conventional PRP technique when the same number of spots is used. Chappelow et al. compared eyes receiving a similar number of PRP spots with either the PASCAL or argon green laser

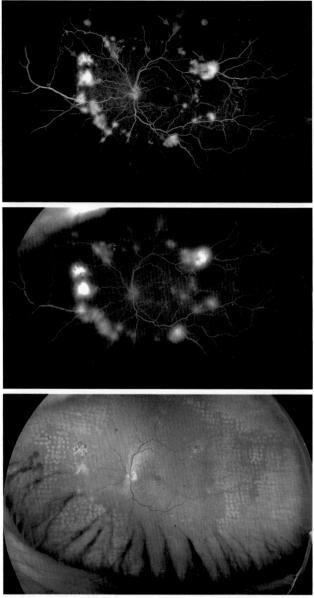

FIG. 9.2 A 38-year-old male with poorly controlled insulin-dependent diabetes mellitus presented with proliferative diabetic retinopathy without diabetic macular edema. Fluorescein angiography ((A) early 45 s; (B) late) confirms the presence of numerous hyperfluorescent foci of retinal neovascularization (*arrows*), large areas of peripheral capillary nonperfusion, and an irregular foveal avascular zone. He preferred laser treatment in view of his prior noncompliance with follow-up. (C) Color photograph taken 2 weeks after pattern scanning laser (PASCAL) panretinal photocoagulation (PRP) was applied to peripheral nonperfused retina with a 3 × 3 grid. Additional laser was required at subsequent visits to induce regression of neovascularization.

TABLE 9.3
Modified-ETDRS Focal Photocoagulation Technique

Burn Characteristic	Focal Photocoagulation (Modified-ETDRS Technique)
Direct treatment	Directly treat all leaking microaneurysms in areas of retinal thickening between 500 and 3000 μm from the center of the macula (although they may be treated between 300 and 500 μm of macula if center-involved edema persists after initial focal photocoagulation, but generally not if the visual acuity is better than 20/40)
Change in microaneurysm color with direct treatment	Not required, but at least a mild gray-white burn should be evident beneath all microaneurysms
Burn size for direct treatment	50 μm
Burn duration for direct treatment	0.1 s
Grid treatment	Applied to all areas with edema not associated with microaneurysms. If fluorescein angiography is obtained, the grid is applied to areas of edema with angiographic nonperfusion when judged indicated by the investigator
Area considered for grid treatment	500–3000 μm superiorly, nasally, and inferiorly from the center of macula; 500–3500 μm temporally from the macular center. No burns placed within 500 μm of disc
Burn size for grid treatment	50 μm
Burn duration for grid treatment	0.05–0.1 s
Burn intensity for grid treatment	Barely visible (light gray)
Burn separation for grid treatment	Two visible burn widths apart
Wavelength (grid and direct treatment)	Green to yellow wavelengths

The laser treatment "session" should generally be completed in a single sitting. This modified ETDRS treatment approach is commonly used in clinical practice in 2016.
Note: The investigator may choose any laser wavelength for photocoagulation within the green to yellow spectrum. The wavelength used is recorded, and any retreatment should use the same wavelength; Lenses used for the laser treatment cannot increase or reduce the burn size by more than 10%.
ETDRS, Early Treatment Diabetic Retinopathy Study.
Adapted from publicfiles.jaeb.org/drcrnet/Misc/ModifiedETDRSFocalPhotoTech10.23.06.pdf.

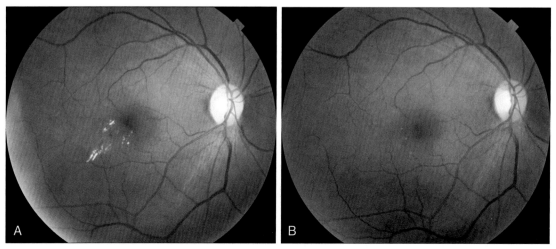

FIG. 9.3 **(A)** Color fundus photo of the right eye before focal laser. Note evidence of center-involving macular edema, exudates, and intraretinal hemorrhage. **(B)** Post focal laser treatment. Note improvement of macular edema and exudates.

and found PASCAL-treated eyes were more likely to have persistent or recurrent neovascularization within 6 months of the initial treatment. They also determined a 6 × 6 array delivered inconsistent burns for all spots on the grid.[32]

NAVIGATED LASER PHOTOCOAGULATION TECHNIQUE

Navigated laser photocoagulation is a newer technique guided by ancillary imaging and tracking software to compensate for patient movement. This allows for automated, safe, and accurate placement of focal as well as PRP laser. This technology is particularly valuable when applying focal laser, as the exact location of the offending microaneurysms can be targeted. Studies have shown that navigated laser photocoagulation can deliver 96% of the shots within 100 µm of the target on a per-protocol basis.[33] Another benefit of this system is that contact lenses do not need to be used, which increases patient comfort and decreases the time of application.

SUBTHRESHOLD MICROPULSE LASER

The concept of the micropulse laser treatment was developed by Birngruber and colleagues in 1986.[1] To limit the amount of damage to the retina and photoreceptors, this technique delivers laser in microsecond doses. The mechanism by which the photoreceptors and inner retina are spared is by focusing the energy to cause selective cellular damage to melanosomes in the RPE.[1,34] As micropulse laser uses a low-duty cycle and long off time between pulses, it causes no clinically visible evidence of laser lesions in contrast to the visible lesions from conventional laser photocoagulation.[35] Studies demonstrate a lack of retinal changes with high-resolution imaging after subthreshold micropulse.[36] Experimental rabbit models have shown histologically that micropulse lesions from 532- to 810-nm lasers showed tissue damage limited to the RPE, with sparing of the choriocapillaris and neurosensory retina.[37] When the micropulse laser is compared with the modified ETDRS Protocol l, subthreshold micropulse laser has been found to be more effective in treating DME.[38] Owing to the absence of full-thickness retinal tissue destruction, the utility of this technology is currently being assessed over a wide variety of ophthalmic conditions. The current subthreshold micropulse laser is commercially available in 810 nm infrared and 577 nm yellow.

LASER VERSUS INTRAVITREAL ANTI-VEGF INJECTION
Treatment for Center-Involving DME

Focal or grid laser photocoagulation has been shown to stabilize rather than improve visual acuity. In 1985 the ETDRS demonstrated that eyes assigned to immediate focal photocoagulation were about half as likely to lose 15 or more letters on the ETDRS eye chart compared with eyes assigned to deferral of photocoagulation.[22] The RESTORE study demonstrated gains of 0.8 letters with laser monotherapy,[29,39] and another study by Elman et al. reported gains of only 3 letters in the sham plus prompt laser group.[27] Multiple prospective randomized clinical control trials, such as RESTORE,[29] READ-2,[40] and DRCR.net protocol I,[28] have shown greater visual improvement with ranibizumab alone or in combination with laser over laser monotherapy for DME. The 2-year outcomes of the READ-2 and Protocol I were analyzed, and a similar trend toward improved visual acuity in the ranibizumab-treated patients versus laser monotherapy patients was seen.[28,41] The RESTORE study did not show the benefit of laser in combination with ranibizumab, but the 2-year outcomes of the READ-2 and DRCR.net Protocol I suggest the long-term effects of laser may reduce the number of intravitreal injections.[28,29,40] The Bevacizumab or Laser Therapy in the Management of Diabetic Macular Edema (BOLT) and DME and VEGF Trap-Eye: Investigation of Clinical Impact (DA VINCI) studies demonstrated a lack of vision improvement after conventional laser compared with intravitreal bevacizumab and aflibercept, respectively. These studies have established anti-VEGF agents as the preferred therapy over laser monotherapy for center-involving diabetic macular edema (CI-DME). Subsequent to the US Food and Drug Administration approval to treat DME with either 0.3 mg ranibizumab or 0.5 mg aflibercept, there is a current trend to treat CI-DME initially with intravitreal anti-VEGF injections ± focal/grid laser and to reserve focal/grid lasers for treating non-CI-DME or patients who do not have an adequate response to anti-VEGF injections.[42]

PRP VERSUS ANTI-VEGF THERAPY FOR PROLIFERATIVE DIABETIC RETINOPATHY: NONINFERIORITY STUDY

The DRCR.net published the results of Protocol S, which may change the way we manage diabetic retinopathy and DME . Protocol S compared PRP laser with 0.5 mg ranibizumab intravitreal injection for the treatment of PDR.[43] The primary objective was to evaluate the safety and efficacy of ranibizumab 0.5 mg to PRP with a primary end point of mean change in visual acuity. There were 394 eyes from 305 patients from 55 sites with active PDR randomized to treatment with either six injections of 0.5 mg ranibizumab monthly (n = 191) or PRP in one to three sessions over no more than an 8-week period (n = 203).[43] Patients in the PRP group could receive more PRP for increased neovascularization or ranibizumab injections for DME as needed. Inclusion criteria included age of 18 years or older, visual acuity greater or equal to 20/320, and no prior PRP.[43] Eyes with baseline CI-DME were included.[43] In the ranibizumab group, eyes were injected at baseline and every 4 weeks for 12 weeks. Retreatment was based on the investigator's assessment of neovascularization, and injections were required at week 16 and 20 unless the neovascularization resolved, otherwise the injection could be held.[44] At week 24, an injection was required unless there was resolution of neovascularization or the patient was determined to be stable over two consecutive injections.[44] Injections were resumed if neovascularization worsened, and PRP could be used for treatment failure.[44] At the 2-year end point, the ranibizumab group had a mean gain of +2.8 letters versus +0.2 letters in the PRP group.[43] The study concluded that ranibizumab was noninferior to PRP given a noninferiority limit of five letters.[43] In the patients with baseline DME, the ranibizumab group demonstrated a gain of eight letters compared with two letters in the PRP group (both arms received ranibizumab for DME).[43]

In addition, there were important secondary outcomes from Protocol S. Visual field loss was tested, and a mean of −23 dB loss versus −422 dB loss in the ranibizumab and PRP group was demonstrated, respectively.[43,44] Rates of vitrectomy were less in the ranibizumab group (4%) than in the PRP group (15%).[43] The ranibizumab group had a greater reduction in central thickness on OCT, and fewer eyes went on to develop CME in the ranibizumab group (9%) versus the PRP group (28%).

COMPLICATIONS OF LASER

Informed consent as to the potential complications and side effects of laser should be obtained (Table 9.4). PRP with conventional laser photocoagulation can be associated with potential adverse effects, including pain, loss of peripheral vision, and difficulty with night vision. Inadvertent laser to the fovea may result in the loss of central vision and can be minimized with proper technique and patient cooperation, although this is extremely rare. If excess PRP is applied, the inflammatory effect to the surrounding tissue may cause an

TABLE 9.4
Complications of Panretinal Photocoagulation
• Hemorrhages
• Anterior segment complications such as corneal or lenticular opacification
• Transient visual loss
• Misdirected laser/photocoagulation to the fovea or other structures
• Macular edema
• Subretinal fibrosis
• Choroidal effusion
• Color vision alterations
• Visual field defects and night vision problems
• Bruch membrane destruction leading to choroidal neovascularization (CNV)
• Expansion of laser scars

effusion, but utilizing multiple treatment sessions can reduce the risk of this complication. If inflammation develops, treatment with corticosteroids and cycloplegics is indicated. Choroidal neovascularization (CNV) is another visually threatening process that results from damage to the Bruch membrane. This complication is usually seen with focal laser whereby the energy is concentrated in a small spot size; therefore the intensity and duration should be titrated to the desired effect.[12]

SPECIAL CONSIDERATIONS

With the advent of intravitreal anti-VEGF injections, the need for laser treatments, especially in the foveal region, has been greatly reduced. However, there may be cases of incomplete response or contraindications to intravitreal injections with either anti-VEGF or steroids that make laser therapy an attractive alternative.

THE NONCOMPLIANT PATIENT

If a patient treated solely with anti-VEGF therapy for PDR fails to return for follow-up, there is risk of worsening PDR. There is no long-term study showing the stability of PDR in the patients treated solely with anti-VEGF injections, whereas there are data to show long-term stability of PRP in eyes with PDR.

PDR IN THE SETTING OF VITREOUS HEMORRHAGE

Initiating PRP can be difficult in the setting of vitreous hemorrhage. During the acute period, laser photocoagulation may be precluded by dispersed hemorrhage. After a trial of observation, if there is no continued hemorrhage, the view of the retina may clear enough to initiate PRP. Even in this setting, the inferior retina may not be available for laser treatment if it remains obscured by settled hemorrhage or debris. The DCRC.net Protocol N evaluated the benefit of ranibizumab in the setting of vitreous hemorrhage from PDR. Over the 16-week study, there was no clinically significant difference in the probability of requiring vitrectomies in the ranibizumab group (12%) versus the saline group (17%).[45] Although only the short-term effects were analyzed, the secondary outcomes of this initial study suggested there may be an increase in visual acuity, an increased likelihood of completing PRP treatment, and a reduced risk of recurrent hemorrhages in the ranibizumab group.[45] A 1-year follow-up study was performed on 82% of the original participants from the Protocol N study. There was still no significant difference in the cumulative probability of vitrectomy between the ranibizumab (35%) and saline (41%) groups.[45] At 52 weeks, both groups had similar visual acuities and reported recurrent hemorrhages. There was still an increased probability of needing to complete PRP in the ranibizumab group (55%) versus the saline group (42%) at 52 weeks.[45]

PDR IN THE SETTING OF DME

In the setting of DME, it is important to consider anti-VEGF injections before initiating PRP, as PRP has been known to potentially worsen DME. McDonald et al. demonstrated this correlation in the 1980s. PRP was performed on 175 eyes with PDR.[46] About 43% of the 175 eyes demonstrated increased macular edema 6–10 weeks post treatment with PRP as determined by the amount of leakage on fluorescein angiography.[46] Forty-seven of these patients had persistent macular edema after PRP, but only 16 patients experienced vision loss.[46] Prospective randomized studies such as READ-2, RESOLVE, RESTORE and Protocol I (reviewed in Chapter 7), all demonstrated the clinical benefit of ranibizumab when treating DME. In a patient with concomitant PDR and DME, it would be wise to consider using intravitreal injections of anti-VEGF, as it has been shown to not be inferior to PRP in the setting of PDR and beneficial when treating DME.

PREGNANCY

Intravitreal anti-VEGF medications are considered a category C drug in pregnancy, as there has been no investigation in a pregnant population. To date, there

have been approximately 11 case reports including approximately 20 female patients receiving intraocular injections published.[47] Three of these patients had a miscarriage early in the first trimester. Given that the rate of spontaneous abortion is estimated to be 11%–16% of recognized pregnancies,[47] there are not enough data to prove a correlation between intravitreal anti-VEGF administration and risk to the fetus. It is very important that there is a documented conversation about the potential risk of such a medication with women of childbearing age and in the setting of pregnancy. Intravitreal anti-VEGF medications should be considered only when the benefits outweigh the potential risk to the fetus. In this situation, other alternatives such as laser or intraocular steroids for non-CI-DME should be considered first.

SUMMARY

Intravitreal anti-VEGF injections have greater potential to improve vision in DME, thus surpassing focal/grid laser as first-line therapy. The role of PRP laser in PDR also appears to be changing. However, laser still remains appealing as an option to reduce treatment burden as well as the potential complications from intravitreal injections. Novel innovations in laser photocoagulation are being developed, especially to treat DME lesions previously considered too close to fixation.

REFERENCES

1. Palanker DV, Blumenkranz MS, Marmor MF. Fifty years of ophthalmic laser therapy. *Arch Ophthalmol.* 2011;129(12):1613–1619.
2. Meyer-Schwickerath G. History and development of photocoagulation. *Am J Ophthalmol.* 1967;63(6):1812–1814.
3. Blumenkranz MS. The evolution of laser therapy in ophthalmology: a perspective on the interactions between photons, patients, physicians, and physicists: the LXX Edward Jackson Memorial Lecture. *Am J Ophthalmol.* 2014;158(1):12–25. e11.
4. Basov N, Prokhorov A. Application of molecular beams for the radiospectroscopic study of rotational molecular spectra. *Zh Eksp Teor FizPis'ma Red.* 1954;27:431–438.
5. Yun SH, Adelman RA. Recent developments in laser treatment of diabetic retinopathy. *Middle East Afr J Ophthalmol.* 2015;22(2):157–163.
6. L'Esperance FA. Clinical comparison of xenon-arc and laser photocoagulation of retinal lesions. *Arch Ophthalmol.* 1966;75(1):61–67.
7. Sramek C, Paulus Y, Nomoto H, Huie P, Brown J, Palanker D. Dynamics of retinal photocoagulation and rupture. *J Biomed Opt.* 2009;14(3):034007.

8. Palanker D, Blumenkranz MS. Retinal laser therapy: bio-physical basis and applications. In: 5th ed. Ryan SJ, ed. *Retina.* Elsevier; 2013:748–758. vol. 1.

9. Glaser BM, Campochiaro PA, Davis JL, Jerdan JA. Retinal pigment epithelial cells release inhibitors of neovascularization. *Ophthalmology.* 1987;94(7):780–784.

10. Gottfredsdóttir MS, Stefánsson E, Jónasson F, Gíslason I. Retinal vasoconstriction after laser treatment for diabetic macular edema. *Am J Ophthalmol.* 1993;115(1):64–67.

11. Kozak I, Luttrull JK. Modern retinal laser therapy. *Saudi J Ophthalmol.* 2015;29(2):137–146.

12. Ip M, Puliafito C. Laser photocoagulation. In: Duker Y, ed. *Ophthalmology.* 3rd ed. 2008;522–523.

13. Modified-ETDRS Focal Photocoagulation Technique [publicfiles.jaeb.org/drcrnet/Misc/ModifiedETDRSFocalPhotoTech10.23.06.pdf].

14. Techniques for scatter and local photocoagulation treatment of diabetic retinopathy: early treatment diabetic retinopathy study report no. 3. The early treatment diabetic retinopathy study research group. *Int Ophthalmol Clin.* 1987;27(4):254–264.

15. Evans JR, Michelessi M, Virgili G. Laser photocoagulation for proliferative diabetic retinopathy. *Cochrane Database Syst Rev.* 2014;(11):CD011234.

16. Blankenship GW. A clinical comparison of central and peripheral argon laser panretinal photocoagulation for proliferative diabetic retinopathy. *Ophthalmology.* 1988;95(2):170–177.

17. Gaucher D, Fortunato P, LeCleire-Collet A, et al. Spontaneous resolution of macular edema after panretinal photocoagulation in florid proliferative diabetic retinopathy. *Retina.* 2009;29(9):1282–1288.

18. Early photocoagulation for diabetic retinopathy. ETDRS report number 9. Early treatment diabetic retinopathy study research group. *Ophthalmology.* 1991;98(suppl 5):766–785.

19. Treatment techniques and clinical guidelines for photocoagulation of diabetic macular edema. Early treatment diabetic retinopathy study report number 2. Early treatment diabetic retinopathy study research group. *Ophthalmology.* 1987;94(7):761–774.

20. Brucker AJ, Qin H, Antoszyk AN, et al. Observational study of the development of diabetic macular edema following panretinal (scatter) photocoagulation given in 1 or 4 sittings. *Arch Ophthalmol.* 2009;127(2):132–140.

21. Rubinstein K, Myska V. Pathogenesis and treatment of diabetic maculopathy. *Br J Ophthalmol.* 1974;58(2):76–84.

22. Photocoagulation for diabetic macular edema: Early treatment diabetic retinopathy study report no. 4. The early treatment diabetic retinopathy study research group. *Int Ophthalmol Clin.* 1987;27(4):265–272.

23. Wilson DJ, Finkelstein D, Quigley HA, Green WR. Macular grid photocoagulation. An experimental study on the primate retina. *Arch Ophthalmol.* 1988;106(1):100–105.

24. Photocoagulation for diabetic macular edema. Early treatment diabetic retinopathy study report number 1. Early treatment diabetic retinopathy study research group. *Arch Ophthalmol.* 1985;103(12):1796–1806.

25. Baker CW, Jiang Y, Stone T. Recent advancements in diabetic retinopathy treatment from the diabetic retinopathy clinical research network. *Curr Opin Ophthalmol.* 2016;27(3):210–216.

26. Fong DS, Strauber SF, Aiello LP, et al. Comparison of the modified Early Treatment Diabetic Retinopathy Study and mild macular grid laser photocoagulation strategies for diabetic macular edema. *Arch Ophthalmol.* 2007;125(4):469–480.

27. Elman MJ, Aiello LP, Beck RW, et al. Randomized trial evaluating ranibizumab plus prompt or deferred laser or triamcinolone plus prompt laser for diabetic macular edema. *Ophthalmology.* 2010;117(6):1064–1077.e1035.

28. Elman MJ, Bressler NM, Qin H, et al. Expanded 2-year follow-up of ranibizumab plus prompt or deferred laser or triamcinolone plus prompt laser for diabetic macular edema. *Ophthalmology.* 2011;118(4):609–614.

29. Mitchell P, Bandello F, Schmidt-Erfurth U, et al. The RESTORE study: ranibizumab monotherapy or combined with laser versus laser monotherapy for diabetic macular edema. *Ophthalmology.* 2011;118(4):615–625.

30. Blumenkranz MS, Yellachich D, Andersen DE, et al. Semiautomated patterned scanning laser for retinal photocoagulation. *Retina.* 2006;26(3):370–376.

31. Nagpal M, Marlecha S, Nagpal K. Comparison of laser photocoagulation for diabetic retinopathy using 532-nm standard laser versus multispot pattern scan laser. *Retina.* 2010;30(3):452–458.

32. Chappelow AV, Tan K, Waheed NK, Kaiser PK. Panretinal photocoagulation for proliferative diabetic retinopathy: pattern scan laser versus argon laser. *Am J Ophthalmol.* 2012;153(1). 137–142.e132.

33. Kernt M, Cheuteu RE, Cserhati S, et al. Pain and accuracy of focal laser treatment for diabetic macular edema using a retinal navigated laser (Navilas). *Clin Ophthalmol.* 2012;6:289–296.

34. Schuele G, Rumohr M, Huettmann G, Brinkmann R. RPE damage thresholds and mechanisms for laser exposure in the microsecond-to-millisecond time regimen. *Invest Ophthalmol Vis Sci.* 2005;46(2):714–719.

35. Vujosevic S, Martini F, Longhin E, Convento E, Cavarzeran F, Midena E. Subthreshold micropulse yellow laser versus subthreshold micropulse infrared laser in center-involving diabetic macular edema: morphologic and functional safety. *Retina.* 2015;35(8):1594–1603.

36. Luttrull JK, Sramek C, Palanker D, Spink CJ, Musch DC. Long-term safety, high-resolution imaging, and tissue temperature modeling of subvisible diode micropulse photocoagulation for retinovascular macular edema. *Retina.* 2012;32(2):375–386.

37. Yu AK, Merrill KD, Truong SN, Forward KM, Morse LS, Telander DG. The comparative histologic effects of subthreshold 532- and 810-nm diode micropulse laser on the retina. *Invest Ophthalmol Vis Sci.* 2013;54(3):2216–2224.

38. Lavinsky D, Cardillo JA, Melo LA, Dare A, Farah ME, Belfort R. Randomized clinical trial evaluating mETDRS versus normal or high-density micropulse photocoagulation for diabetic macular edema. *Invest Ophthalmol Vis Sci.* 2011;52(7):4314–4323.

39. Bandello F, Cunha-Vaz J, Chong NV, et al. New approaches for the treatment of diabetic macular oedema: recommendations by an expert panel. *Eye (Lond).* 2012;26(4):485–493.

40. Nguyen QD, Shah SM, Heier JS, et al. Primary end point (six months) results of the ranibizumab for edema of the mAcula in diabetes (READ-2) study. *Ophthalmology.* 2009;116(11):2175–2181.e2171.

41. Nguyen QD, Shah SM, Khwaja AA, et al. Two-year outcomes of the ranibizumab for edema of the mAcula in diabetes (READ-2) study. *Ophthalmology.* 2010;117(11): 2146–2151.

42. Jalkiewicz J. Lasers in DME. *Retin Physicians.* 2016;13: 19–21.

43. Beaulieu WT, Bressler NM, Melia M, et al. Panretinal photocoagulation versus ranibizumab for proliferative diabetic retinopathy: patient-centered outcomes from a randomized clinical trial. *Am J Ophthalmol.* 2016;170:206–213.

44. Gross JG, Glassman AR, Jampol LM, et al. Panretinal photocoagulation vs intravitreous ranibizumab for proliferative diabetic retinopathy: a randomized clinical trial. *JAMA.* 2015;314(20):2137–2146.

45. Network* DRCR. Randomized clinical trial evaluating intravitreal ranibizumab or saline for vitreous hemorrhage from proliferative diabetic retinopathy. *JAMA Ophthalmol.* 2013;131(3):283–293.

46. McDonald HR, Schatz H. Macular edema following panretinal photocoagulation. *Retina.* 1985;5(1):5–10.

47. Polizzi S, Mahajan VB. Intravitreal anti-VEGF injections in pregnancy: case series and review of literature. *J Ocul Pharmacol Ther.* 2015;31(10):605–610.

CHAPTER 10

Surgical Treatment of Diabetic Retinopathy

MARÍA H. BERROCAL, MD • ALEXANDRA ACABÁ

Diabetes is a significant health problem worldwide, with approximately 30 million patients with diabetes in the United States. Epidemiologic data suggest that over 50% of patients with diabetes can develop proliferative diabetic retinopathy (PDR) over time.[1,2] Without adequate treatment, a large percentage will experience severe visual loss (SVL). At present, PDR accounts for approximately 20,000 new cases of blindness in the United States.[3] Prevention programs, as well as adequate screening programs in underserved high-risk communities, can help reduce the devastating effects of this disease. Earlier treatment with new modalities can help reduce the ocular complications of diabetic retinopathy and the associated vision loss.

Surgical treatment of the sight-threatening complications of diabetic retinopathy has evolved substantially since the results of the Diabetic Retinopathy Study (DRS), Early Treatment of Diabetic Retinopathy Study (ETDRS), and the Diabetic Retinopathy Vitrectomy Study (DRVS) in the 1970s and 1980s.[4–9] Panretinal photocoagulation (PRP) has proved effective in reducing the risk of SVL in PDR.[4] However, retinal neovascularization may not regress or may even increase in some PRP-treated eyes, eventually requiring surgical intervention. The 5-year cumulative rate of vitrectomy in ETDRS patients was 5.3%, even with frequent retinal examinations and timely PRP treatment as per the study protocol.[9] Newer, more advanced surgical technologies have allowed for earlier intervention with reduced complications and improved visual acuity outcomes. Important advances include small-gauge vitrectomy platforms, chandelier intraocular illumination, wide-angle viewing systems, 3-D surgical viewing systems, illuminated lasers, small-gauge instrumentation, and anti-VEGF drugs. Despite all of these advances, the ocular complications of diabetes still remain the main cause of blindness among younger patients worldwide.

The largest National Institutes of Health–sponsored study that established the beneficial effect of pars plana vitrectomy (PPV) in the management of diabetic vitreous hemorrhage was the DRVS in the 1980s. At that time, vitrectomy machines were rudimentary, wide-angle viewing systems were unavailable, instrumentation was limited, and intraoperative endophotocoagulation was unavailable. Results of the DRVS cautioned for more conservative management of vitreous hemorrhage with prolonged observation, because complications of vitrectomy were considerable at that time. Optimized instrumentation and visualization systems during the past 2 decades have significantly reduced surgical complications and allowed for earlier, more aggressive management of diabetic retinal pathologies, with improved visual and anatomic outcomes. They has also vastly expanded the indications for vitrectomy surgery to include not only vitreous hemorrhage but also traction retinal detachment (TRD), combined traction and rhegmatogenous retinal detachment (CTRRD), diabetic macular edema (DME), macular hole associated to diabetic retinopathy, vitreomacular traction (VMT), neovascular glaucoma (NVG), and concomitant cataract and vitreous pathologies. Current objectives of vitrectomy in diabetic eyes include removal of vitreous opacities, separation and excision of the posterior thickened hyaloid, removal of fibrovascular proliferation and retinal traction, retinal reattachment, and treatment of retinal ischemia. As the pathology in PDR is related to internal vitreous traction and retinal neovascularization, the role of scleral bucking surgery is minimal. Diabetic retinopathy is a bilateral condition, so treatment decisions regarding the optimal timing of surgery should consider the disease status in each eye.

NEW TREATMENTS FOR PDR

The mainstay of treatment for PDR during the past 40 years has been PRP as per the DRS results.[4] Other treatment modalities have been explored in an attempt to reduce the complications of photocoagulation. Inhibitors of vascular endothelial growth factor (VEGF inhibitors, also known as anti-VEGF agents) have shown great efficacy in the treatment of DME and in the reduction of progression of diabetic eyes to proliferative disease.[10,11] Protocol S from the Diabetic Retinopathy Clinical Research Network (DRCR.net) compared prompt PRP with intravitreal ranibizumab with deferred PRP for PDR. This multisite trial randomized 394 eyes to baseline PRP or to monthly and prn ranibizumab injections. PRP was allowed as a rescue treatment for the ranibizumab treatment group. The 2-year study results showed that visual acuity outcomes were similar between the PRP and ranibizumab arms. However, more eyes in the PRP treatment arm required vitrectomy as well as treatment for DME in a statistically significant manner ($P<.001$). Despite how promising anti-VEGF treatment of diabetic retinopathy may seem, its main drawback is its transient effect and the treatment burden of frequent (often monthly) injections compared with the permanent effect of PRP.[12] Nevertheless, this is a treatment modality that may be the most promising in the future, particularly as adjunct treatment, and can expand our current armamentarium of treatment modalities for diabetic retinopathy.

The DRVS showed a benefit for early vitrectomy, particularly in younger patients with type 1 diabetes with vitreous hemorrhage, with almost twice as many patients (25%) achieving 20/40 visual acuity compared with conventional treatment (11%).[6] Earlier vitrectomy, particularly in young patients with PDR without vitreous hemorrhage, has been advocated as a means to prevent progression of retinopathy by removing the posterior hyaloid.[13] According to the DRVS, the most appropriate candidates for early vitrectomy were those with severe fibrovascular proliferation, extensive prior photocoagulation, and/or media opacities that prevented photocoagulation.[6] It is rare for neovascularization of the optic nerve and posterior pole to occur following surgical excision of posterior cortical vitreous.[14] Improvements in surgical technologies as well as visualization systems have reduced the potential complications of vitrectomy and simplified procedures. Thus earlier vitrectomy in high-risk PDR eyes may provide the best outcomes in the future to prevent progression to TRD in eyes with severe disease.

PREOPERATIVE CONSIDERATIONS

A thorough preoperative evaluation of diabetic eyes is essential to adequately plan the surgical procedure and avoid intraoperative complications. The patient's medical status is also important. It is ideal to optimize control of blood glucose as well as blood pressure. Poorly controlled hypertension during the surgery can cause considerable intraoperative and postoperative

bleeding, which can impair visibility and have adverse effects. Antiplatelet agents should be suspended if possible, particularly in very vascular and difficult tractional detachments where excessive bleeding can be catastrophic. In cases in which anticoagulation withdrawal is too risky systemically, preoperative injection of an anti-VEGF agent may be warranted, as this can be extremely useful to reduce intraoperative bleeding. Patients with poorly controlled diabetes who have renal disease are more likely to develop inflammation and fibrin in the postoperative period, as their blood-eye barrier is more compromised.

Slit lamp and gonioscopic evaluation of the iris and angle for neovascularization is very important, as these eyes may also benefit from presurgical antiangiogenic (anti-VEGF) agents. Funduscopic examination with scleral depression to detect peripheral pathology should be performed. In cases in which vitreous opacities preclude an adequate view of the retina, B-scan ultrasonography is essential to detect areas of detachment. Imaging technologies such as ultrawide-field photography and optical coherence tomography (OCT) can provide anatomic information, even in eyes with significant vitreous or lenticular opacities. Preoperative OCT is important to assess the macular surface and detect localized retinal detachment (Fig. 10.1) and lamellar holes and edema to plan the surgery adequately.[15] The status of the lens and angle are important, as well as the degree of ischemia and neovascularization present. Two newer imaging modalities

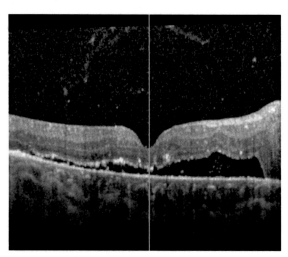

FIG. 10.1 Optical coherence tomography showing localized retinal detachment of the fovea in a 30-year-old associated with traction retinal detachment and sudden decrease in vision.

that can be useful to assess diabetic eyes preoperatively are OCT angiography (OCT-A) and ultrawide-field fluorescein angiography (Fig. 10.2).[16] Eyes with ischemia and capillary dropout in the foveal region as detected by OCT-A may show faster progression to PDR. Ultrawide-field angiography may reveal more extensive peripheral retinal ischemia than suspected with indirect viewing. If significant ischemia is present, more aggressive photocoagulation should be performed before or during surgery.

If many areas of florid neovascularization are present, presurgical treatment with anti-VEGF injection can help reduce intraoperative bleeding. The injection should be done within 5–7 days of the surgical intervention, as progression of hyaloidal traction has been described on occasion in eyes with an attached hyaloid.[17] Nevertheless, anti-VEGF injection is most useful in reducing intraoperative bleeding in eyes with significant neovascularization and areas of traction and is essential in eyes with anterior segment neovascularization and NVG.[18–22]

If a significant cataract that hinders adequate intraoperative visualization is present, concomitant removal with posterior chamber intraocular lens (IOL) implantation by phacoemulsification is ideal. It is risky to perform cataract surgery before vitrectomy in very ischemic eyes, as postoperative progression to iris and angle neovascularization can occur. There are dissenting views as to when the IOL should be placed when doing concomitant phacoemulsification and IOL surgery with vitrectomy. It can be placed initially, and then the PPV can be performed, or the phacoemulsification

can be done and the IOL placed at the end of the procedure. The advantage of the latter technique is increased visibility of the periphery in an aphakic state during the dissection parts of the vitrectomy. Pars plana lensectomy, popular in the past, has fallen into disuse because of the less-than-ideal placement of an IOL in the sulcus or anterior chamber, compared with the preferred placement of the IOL in the capsular bag in ischemic eyes. In eyes with preexisting macular edema undergoing cataract extraction, intravitreal corticosteroid or bevacizumab at the time of surgery results in a reduction of the foveal thickness and improved visual outcomes.[23] These modalities can be particularly useful in eyes undergoing combined cataract surgery and vitrectomy.

VITREOUS HEMORRHAGE AND PRERETINAL HEMORRHAGES

The first indication for PPV in patients with diabetes was nonclearing vitreous hemorrhage.[24] Waiting for clearing of dense hemorrhages made sense in the 1980s when complications of vitrectomy were many. At present, it can be dangerous to wait in PDR eyes with dense hemorrhages, as underlying pathologies can progress undetected and tractional and combined tractional and rhegmatogenous retinal detachments can ensue, particularly in younger patients with an attached hyaloid.[6,7] Diabetic eyes can develop retinal tears unrelated to the diabetic retinopathy, and a rhegmatogenous detachment can progress masked by the blood. At present, early vitrectomy is advocated for most large dense vitreous hemorrhages, eyes that have not had prior PRP or that have minimal PRP. Observation is reserved for milder cases that seem likely to clear spontaneously and for patients not amenable to surgery. Earlier vitrectomy may also be considered in eyes with subhyaloid premacular hemorrhage, as blood in this location can obscure foveal pathology and take a prolonged time to resorb. Hyaloid disruption with the Nd:Yag laser has been described to allow internal drainage of subhyaloid hemorrhage in select PDR eyes; however, this technique does not address the underlying pathologic vitreous traction and neovascularization.

In addition to the preoperative evaluation for cataract and anterior segment neovascularization, B-scan ultrasonography should be performed if the fundus is not visible to detect tractional or rhegmatogenous retinal detachment. If there is suspicion of a rhegmatogenous component, prompt vitrectomy should be performed. Pretreatment with VEGF inhibitors in the setting of vitreous hemorrhage should be utilized in

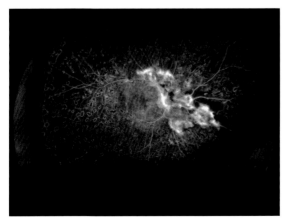

FIG. 10.2 Ultrawide-field fluorescein angiography in an eye with proliferative diabetic retinopathy and traction retinal detachment. Fibrovascular tissue continued to grow despite over 2000 spots of panretinal photocoagulation.

eyes with anterior segment neovascularization, NVG, and a posterior vitreous detachment by B-scan.

The surgical technique should include wide-angle viewing systems, either contact or noncontact, to allow for visualization of the periphery. Microincision vitrectomy surgery (MIVS) with valved trocar systems of 25 or 27 gauge are ideal for these cases, and improved outcomes have been demonstrated compared with 20 gauge.[25-28] The valved trocars are important because they help maintain constant intraocular pressures (IOPs) during the procedure, reduce turbulence, and help control intraoperative bleeding. Vitrectomy machines with IOP control are useful to maintain intraoperative pressure, reduce intraoperative bleeding, and prevent extremely high pressures that can damage the optic nerve. Removal of blood and vitreous behind the lens or IOL is important to allow for faster clearing in cases of postoperative rebleeding. Clearing the peripheral vitreous with the aid of wide-angle viewing and scleral depression is important to have proper visibility and check for peripheral tears, which, if untreated, an progress to postoperative retinal detachment. After all the vitreous is removed, the hyaloid should be separated from the retina if it is still attached. This prevents it from acting as a scaffold for neovascularization and also removes potential traction forces in the foveal area and the thickened hyaloid associated to macular edema. Although intraoperative OCT is limited in availability, it can be useful to assess pathology in the foveal area, particularly in cases in which the macula was not visible preoperatively.[15,41] Bleeding is common when fibrovascular tissue is cut and can be controlled by raising the intraoperative pressure, with diathermy or continuous laser to the bleeding vessel or by direct pressure on the bleeding vessel with the vitrectomy probe.

After all the blood is cleared and aspirated from the retinal surface, PRP should be applied from anterior to the arcades peripherally to the ora serrata. At the end of the procedure, the peripheral retina and sclerotomies should be inspected to detect vitreous incarceration and/or breaks. If breaks are present, these areas should be treated with laser followed by air-fluid exchange with long-acting gas tamponade. Most eyes are left filled with fluid, but in cases in which macular elevation, VMT, or epiretinal membrane (ERM) was present, an air-fluid exchange can be useful. In eyes with significant vascular tissue proliferation that are at a high risk of bleeding in the postoperative period, VEGF inhibitors can be injected at the end of the surgery. Preventing hypotony is important in diabetic eyes to prevent rebleeding in the perioperative period. Thus proper wound construction is paramount and leaking sclerotomies should be sutured.

TRACTION RETINAL DETACHMENT

TRD is very common, particularly in younger patients with diabetes. This is the most frequent indication, accounting for 40% of diabetic vitrectomies.[29] The posterior hyaloid is attached in younger patients, and neovascularization from the retina utilizes this as a scaffold to proliferate on the surface.[24] Progressive fibrovascular proliferation on the posterior hyaloid and contraction produces traction on the neurosensory retina, separating it from the retinal pigment epithelium (RPE). Further contraction causes areas of TRD. This type of detachment can be asymptomatic if it is distant from the fovea but can result in SVL if it progresses to involve the central fovea. If the retina is very ischemic and tractional forces are significant, retinal breaks can develop under traction and a CTRRD can occur. These eyes with CTRRD present with rapidly progressive visual loss and need prompt intervention.

Preoperative evaluation of TRDs is of utmost importance in the decision to perform and plan surgery. Ophthalmoscopy findings include a concave retina associated with fibrovascular proliferation. Biomicroscopy, ultrasonography, and OCT can aid in determining the degree of foveal involvement. OCT can show associated macular interface pathologies, such as ERM, edema, VMT, and atrophic macular holes.[30]

Localized areas of retinal traction that are nasal or distant to the fovea can be watched for progression. Office-based laser photocoagulation can be used to stabilize small extrafoveal TRDs, and the incidence of progression to involve the fovea in these eyes is 14% per year.[31] The use of anti-VEGFs as the sole treatment of eyes with TRD is a relative contraindication because increased contraction of the fibrovascular tissue can ensue and the TRD may progress in some cases and convert to a CTRRD.[32] Use of anti-VEGFs in this setting should be reserved as an adjunct to surgery for the preoperative reduction of vascularity or combined with PRP laser.

The objectives of vitrectomy are relieving retinal traction by releasing and removing the posterior hyaloid as well as fibrovascular tissue and treating areas of retinal ischemia to prevent VEGF production and subsequent neovascularization of the retina or iris. Indications for vitrectomy in eyes with TRDs include detachment involving or threatening the fovea and eyes with associated vitreous hemorrhage (Fig. 10.3). Small-gauge vitrectomy platforms are ideal for these cases, and the benefit of the smallest gauge (currently 27 gauge) instruments is their ability to more readily fit between tissue planes such that tissue can be

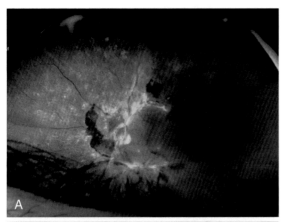

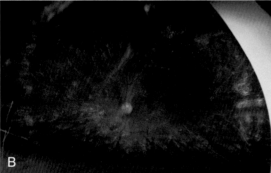

FIG. 10.3 **(A)** Preoperative fundus photo of a 30-year-old female with traction retinal detachment and vitreous hemorrhage; visual acuity was 20/200. **(B)** Six months after 27-gauge vitrectomy, visual acuity was 20/40. Residual preretinal fibrosis is present nasal to the optic nerve.

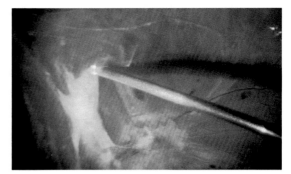

FIG. 10.4 Blunt dissection with a 25-gauge vitrector probe during a pars plana vitrectomy for a combined traction and rhegmatogenous diabetic retinal detachment.

removed in a safer fashion.[33] Three-port small-gauge vitrectomy with trocar placement is performed, and the periphery is initially cleared of vitreous. Often the hyaloid is partially detached in the periphery, and this area of vitreous should be cleared circumferentially. This usually can be done quickly with maximum aspiration and high cutting speed. This peripheral vitreous removal is important to prevent traction on the periphery from attached vitreous while membranes are removed as well as to visualize planes between the retina and the hyaloid/membrane complex. After all the vitreous is removed around the foci of fibrovascular tissue, an entry plane between the retina and the membrane is accessed. Newer techniques to achieve removal of fibrovascular tissue utilize the small-gauge vitrectomy probe for blunt dissection, for segmentation, and in lifting/cutting techniques (Fig. 10.4).[34,35] The degree and extent of adhesion of the fibrovascular

tissue determine the surgical complexity. Other factors that can make these cases challenging include degree of vascularity and ischemia of the retina. Eyes with extensive neovascularization benefit from preoperative injection of an anti-VEGF agent, and intravitreal bevacizumab (Avastin) has been effective in reducing intraoperative bleeding and simplifying the surgical technique (Fig. 10.5). Nevertheless, it should be administered from 1 to 6 days before surgery to avoid increased fibrovascular contraction.[32] Occasionally, tissues are so adherent that a plane cannot be safely found. This is common in areas where extensive fibrovascular tissue covers the posterior pole in a tabletop fashion. In these cases, lifting the fibrovascular attachments over the optic nerve with forceps and creating an opening in that area can allow for dissection to be performed from the inside out. Also viscoelastic dissection (viscodissection) with hyaluronic acid can be utilized starting near the optic nerve to delineate a plan (Fig. 10.6). This can be done with special retractable cannulas or with a bent-tip cannula. Despite the simplified techniques that are possible with MIVS, it is still essential to have on hand all the ancillary instrumentation that could be required, including chandeliers, scissors, forceps, and diathermy.

In the 20-gauge vitrectomy era, TRDs (and CTRRDs) were treated with segmentation, delamination, and en block dissection. These techniques require the use of multiple instruments, including intraocular scissors, chandeliers, illuminated instruments, or a tissue manipulator to control intraoperative bleeding. Segmentation utilizes scissors to cut fibrovascular tissue and relieve circumferential traction. Delamination is performed with curved scissors and involves dissecting the abnormal tissue from the surface of the retina

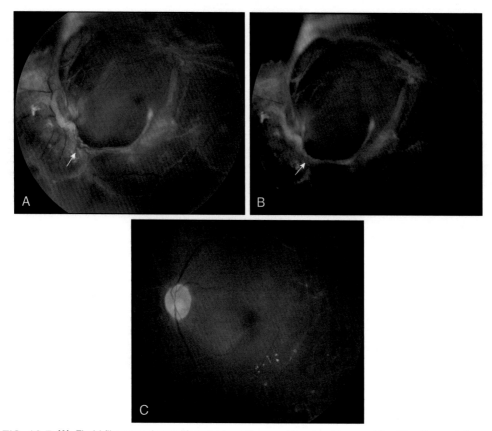

FIG. 10.5 **(A)**. Florid fibrovascular proliferation in a 38-year-old male with a combined traction and rheg-matogenous retinal detachment; visual acuity was hand motion. **(B)**. Five days after bevacizumab injection, there was regression of the vascular component of the preretinal fibrovascular tissue (arrow). The patient underwent 25-gauge pars plana vitrectomy 5 days after bevacizumab injection. **(C)**. Eight months after 25-gauge vitrectomy with C_3F_8 gas, visual acuity measured 20/80.

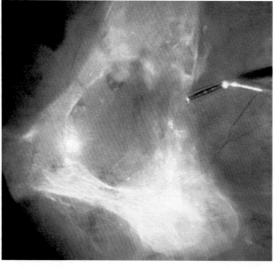

FIG. 10.6 Viscodissection with bent cannula for a traction retinal detachment with a large plaque of fibrous tissue. Preop-erative bevacizumab had been injected 5 days before vitrectomy.

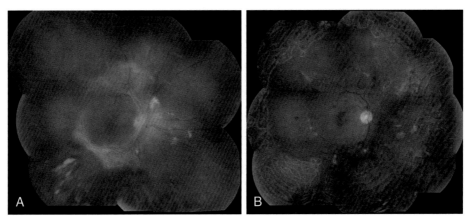

FIG. 10.7 **(A)** Preoperative fundus photo of a 40-year-old female with traction retinal detachment; visual acuity was 20/200. **(B)** Four months status post 25-gauge vitrectomy with air tamponade, vision improved to 20/70.

and cutting the epicenters of membranes. En block dissection utilizes the attached posterior hyaloid as a second hand to maintain traction on the hyaloid/membrane complex as this is dissected with scissors. With MIVS, segmentation and delamination can be performed with the small cutters instead of scissors and bleeding can be reduced either with preoperative anti-VEGFs or IOP control with valved cannulas. Illuminated instruments were common in 20-gauge surgeries, but with MIVS, chandeliers are preferred when bimanual surgery is needed. When 27- or 25-gauge instrumentation is not readily available, performing vitrectomy with a 23-gauge setup and utilizing a smaller 27- or 25-gauge vitrectomy cutter through the 23-gauge cannulas is a potential option to take advantage of the smaller cutter precision.

Very careful dissection of membranes should be performed because the occurrence of iatrogenic breaks reduces the visual outcomes in these cases. Also when iatrogenic breaks develop, it is then necessary to completely removal all of the surface fibrovascular tissue, making the management similar to a CTRRD. After all of the traction around the posterior pole is relieved, and intraoperative bleeding is controlled and treated, laser photocoagulation is applied peripherally to the ora serrata in attached retina (Fig. 10.7). Laser should be avoided in areas where the retina is not in contact with the RPE, as this can contribute to retinal breaks. Air-fluid exchange at the end of the procedure with prone positioning for a few days can be beneficial in eyes with preoperative traction in the foveal region. Peripheral fibrovascular tissue with localized traction areas away from the posterior pole does not need to be removed as long as there is no

rhegmatogenous component or iatrogenic breaks. Eyes with TRD often have associated thickened hyaloid, ERM, VMT, and/or macular edema. If available, intraoperative OCT can assess the status of the fovea and adequacy of membrane removal, and heads-up 3-D surgical viewing modalities may help visualize tissue planes by enhancing depth perception in these pathologies.[36]

Complications of vitrectomy for TRD include bleeding, poor visibility from corneal and lens opacities, and creation of iatrogenic breaks. Bleeding in the postoperative period is most common, occurring in 22% of eyes, but the most serious is the creation of iatrogenic retinal breaks.[37] It is critical to detect these intraoperatively and treat them adequately. Once a break occurs, it is imperative to free all areas of traction, remove all of the fibrovascular tissue, and treat the breaks with diathermy so that they can be visualized under air. Removal of all subretinal fluid by aspiration through the breaks is performed during an air-fluid exchange, and laser photocoagulation is applied around the created breaks. Either a long-acting gas or silicone oil can be utilized for intraocular tamponade at the end of the surgery. Long-acting gases such as perfluoropropane (C_3F_8) are preferred in postsurgical TRD eyes because of the higher buoyant forces (Figs. 10.8 and 10.9). Silicone oil has the drawback in that it maintains blood clots isolated on the surface of the retina contributing to periretinal proliferation, and a second surgical procedure is necessary for its removal. Nevertheless it is useful for patients who cannot position or who are monocular. If silicone oil is utilized, ideally it should be removed within 6 months to avoid long-term oil complications.[38]

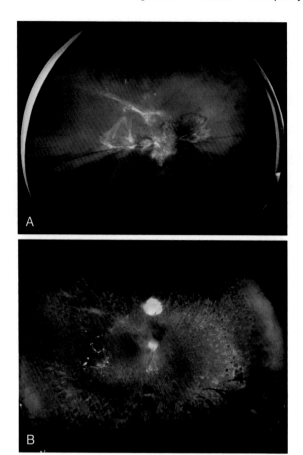

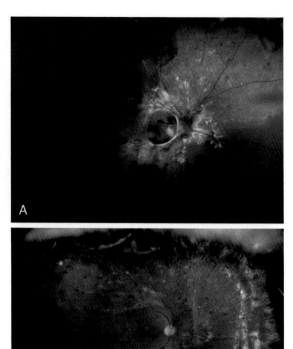

FIG. 10.8 **(A)** A 32-year-old with sudden loss of vision to hand motion because of vitreous hemorrhage and traction retinal detachment with a rhegmatogenous component. **(B)** One year post 27-gauge vitrectomy with C_3F_8 gas, the retina was reattached with residual hard exudates in the temporal fovea; vision was 20/40.

FIG. 10.9 **(A)** Preoperative fundus photo of a 36-year-old female with type 1 diabetes who presented with sudden decreased vision to 20/200 and florid fibrovascular tissue encircling vascular arcades. **(B)** Five months status post 27-gauge vitrectomy with C_3F_8 gas, vision is 20/50.

COMBINED TRACTIONAL WITH RHEGMATOGENOUS RETINAL DETACHMENT

CTRRDs are more common in young patients with diabetes with severe proliferative disease, significant ischemia, and attached hyaloid. Tractional forces exerted by partially detaching posterior hyaloid on fibrovascular tissue can threaten the retinal surface integrity. Contraction of the hyaloid exacerbates preexisting TRD and, as increasing forces are generated, can create breaks in ischemic retina. When a retinal break is formed in an area of traction, liquefied vitreous can access the subretinal space and separate the overlying retina from the RPE, resulting in a CTRRD. When this progression of

TRD to CTRRD occurs, the configuration of the retinal surface changes from concave to convex. If the macula is involved by CTRRD, acute loss of vision ensues.

Indirect ophthalmoscopy in CTRRD reveals whitening of the detached retina with bullous or mobile retina in some or all areas and a convex configuration (Fig. 10.5A and 10.8). Ultrawide-angle photography can be helpful, particularly in eyes with media opacities to visualize all the pathology and localize retinal breaks. Retinal breaks are usually localized posterior to the equator and adjacent to areas of fibrovascular proliferation in ischemic retina or in areas of photocoagulation. These breaks may be multiple and difficult to detect, and in contrast to horseshoe tears, there is usually no associated vitreous traction. OCT should be performed in all eyes with TRD or CTRRD to determine fovea status and if fibrous tissue is over the posterior pole.

Irrespective of whether the fovea is detached or not, eyes with CTRRDs should undergo prompt vitrectomy to prevent permanent visual loss.[39,40] These CTRRDs can present with associated anterior segment neovascularization and/or hypervascular retinal proliferation. In these cases, pretreatment with VEGF inhibitors can be useful to inhibit intraoperative bleeding in the retina or angle. The lens is ideally preserved, but in cases with significant cataract or peripheral pathology, combined phacoemulsification and vitrectomy can be performed for better visibility. In combined procedures, maintaining pupillary dilation throughout the vitrectomy is important to optimize visibility in these technically difficult cases.

CTRRDs are the most challenging diabetic surgeries, as they require complex maneuvers to remove tightly adherent fibrovascular tissue from detached, mobile, ischemic retina. Because these cases all have a rhegmatogenous component, it is essential to remove all abnormal fibrovascular tissue entirely, as residual areas of traction will prevent closure of retinal breaks and reattachment of the retina. Wide-angle viewing systems as well as MIVS platforms are particularly useful in these difficult cases. Smaller vitreous cutters can fit between tight tissue planes to help dissect abnormal fibrovascular tissue. These cases benefit the most from the small openings of 27-gauge vitrectors to carefully shave tissue from the retinal surface with reduced risk of iatrogenic breaks. High-speed vitrector cutting rates of up to 10,000 cuts per minute exert minimal traction over the detached retina and allow for shaving and peeling techniques from the retinal surface. Chandelier illuminators can be useful to enhance visualization and are necessary when bimanual tissue dissection is required, as it allows for the concomitant use of forceps with scissors or vitrectors. The chandelier can be placed at the 12-o'clock position or in small eyes inferonasally and can be changed and placed in the different cannulas to access different areas. Some eyes present with extensive plaques of fibrovascular tissue, which are very adherent to the underlying retina. These eyes benefit from viscodissection techniques with hyaluronic acid injected under the fibrovascular tissue to separate the membranes from the mobile retina, creating a potential space to allow for safe fibrovascular tissue removal. Bimanual dissection techniques are often necessary in eyes with very adherent, extensive proliferation, particularly if it extends toward the equator and periphery. Dissection of fibrovascular proliferation in the periphery is particularly challenging because access to the area is limited, visibility is more difficult, and the angles required for manipulation are cumbersome. The

peripheral retina is also thinner and more susceptible to iatrogenic tearing. The anatomic and visual acuity prognosis in these eyes is guarded. Nevertheless, preoperative factors associated with improved prognosis include shorter duration of detachment, particularly of foveal involvement, visual acuity of 5/200 or better, absence of rubeosis or NVG, and an attached macula.[35] Encircling buckles are rarely needed in diabetic vitrectomies. The only indication would be an eye with CTRRD and significant retinal shortening caused by peripheral pathology that cannot be relieved by dissection only or eyes with retinal redetachment with proliferative vitreoretinopathy. If an encircling buckle is utilized, it should be measured to avoid excessive tightness that can result in anterior segment ischemia in these predisposed eyes with retinovascular compromise. Retinectomies should be avoided as much as possible because shortening of the retina can occur from surface proliferation or blood clots on the surface.

PATHOLOGIES OF THE MACULAR INTERFACE

Eyes with diabetic retinopathy have a thickened hyaloid and are prone to pathologies of the vitreomacular interface. These include a thickened hyaloid associated with macular edema and/or traction, VMT with or without foveolar detachment, lamellar or full-thickness macular hole secondary to macular edema, and ERM. Many of these pathologies are associated with macular edema mechanically induced by the hyaloid, and there may also be a component of DME secondary to diabetic retinopathy. If significant edema is present, it should be treated before surgery with anti-VEGF or intravitreal corticosteroid injection. Eyes with large cysts from long-standing macular edema are more prone to progress to macular holes, and reducing the underlying edema before surgery reduces the risk of their formation during hyaloid and membrane removal. Preoperative OCT is imperative to assess surface relationships and establish a surgical plan, as localized detachments can be common (Fig. 10.1).

Intraoperative OCT is useful in patients with diabetes because often there are multiple layers of tissue over the posterior pole and it can be challenging to determine if all of the abnormal tissue has been removed.[41] Chromovitrectomy is the use of vital dyes to assist in the identification and removal of membranes and fine tissue during vitrectomy. The use of triamcinolone stain aids in visualization and removal of the posterior hyaloid, a step that should be considered in all diabetic eyes. Pigmented dyes are valuable when removal of the internal limiting membrane (ILM) is desired and for reverse staining to remove the ERM. The most commonly utilized dyes include indocyanine green or brilliant blue for ILM staining and triamcinolone acetonide or trypan blue for ERM and vitreous staining.[42]

Eyes with these macular pathologies often present with a modest and gradual reduction of visual acuity. In cases in which there is a sudden and dramatic reduction in visual acuity, a localized tractional foveolar detachment should be suspected and an OCT performed (Fig. 10.1). These eyes should undergo prompt vitrectomy. Microincisional techniques with 25 or 27 gauge are ideal for macular interface pathologies, as the small vitrectors allow for direct peeling of tissue from the retina. The surgical technique includes removal of the vitreous, detachment of the posterior hyaloid, and removal of preretinal membranes. Different techniques can be used for ERM removal, including direct forceps peeling with or without staining, probe peeling with 27-gauge vitrectomy probe in aspiration, or removal with a retractable loop. Intraoperative OCT is advantageous in these pathologies because often vitreoschisis can be present and multiple layers of tissue over the posterior pole can be seen. It is also useful to determine if a full-thickness macular hole is present after the hyaloid or membrane removal has occurred. If lamellar or full-thickness macular holes are present, the ILM should be removed and a gas tamponade utilized. The advantage of removal of ILM in diabetic eyes with edema or ERM but without macular holes remains controversial. Cases in which significant edema is present may benefit from corticosteroid injection at the end of the procedure, either with triamcinolone or a sustained release implant.

NEOVASCULAR GLAUCOMA

NVG is a devastating sequelae of poorly controlled diabetes and inadequately treated PDR. It is associated with poor glycemic control, systemic hypertension, and ischemic cardiovascular disease, and all patients should have evaluation for systemic ischemia. The degree of ocular ischemia can be assessed with iris and ultrawide-field fluorescein angiography if the media is clear. Gonioscopy reveals angle rubeosis with synechiae in many of these eyes that may require glaucoma surgery. When systemic vascular compromise is present, delayed fluorescein dye transit times can be seen on the affected side. Urgent management of this condition is imperative. NVG can often be treated with aggressive injection of anti-VEGF agents combined with PRP and glaucoma surgery.[43] If the fundus cannot be visualized

because of media opacities or hemorrhage, then PPV is required to clear the opacities and apply extensive photocoagulation. Eyes with NVG are pretreated with anti-VEGF injections and possibly corticosteroids to reduce inflammation and intraoperative bleeding, particularly in the anterior chamber from the iris or angle. Treatment of the IOP is important to prevent permanent optic nerve damage. A few days after anti-VEGF injection, vitrectomy can be performed with removal of all the vitreous and blood and application of extensive PRP. The periphery should be checked for retinal detachment, as these may be present in eyes with NVG. Vitrectomy can be combined with glaucoma surgery, or the later can be performed subsequently. Intravitreal steroids and/or anti-VEGFs can be injected at the end of surgery.

CATARACT SURGERY

Diabetic retinopathy may progress after uncomplicated cataract surgery with regards to diabetic retinopathy severity score as well as advancement to center-involving (CI) DME. The presence of non-central involving DME immediately before cataract surgery or a history of DME treatment increases the risk of developing CI-DME at 16 weeks after cataract extraction.[46] Injection of an anti-VEGF agent such as ranibizumab or bevacizumab before or at the completion of cataract surgery has been shown to reduce postsurgical exacerbation of CI DME.[23,47]

COMPLICATIONS OF DIABETIC VITRECTOMY

The most common complications of vitrectomy in diabetic eyes are early rebleeding in the postoperative period and residual nonclearing vitreous hemorrhage. Delayed hemorrhage can occur in 10% of eyes.[37] These complications can occur in all diabetic pathologies but are more frequent in eyes that have severe ocular neovascularization and extensive fibrovascular membranes, patients with uncontrolled hypertension, who are taking antiplatelet agents, or who present with hypotony on the first day postoperatively. With the advent of MIVS in which sclerotomies are not routinely sutured, it is important to have a low threshold for suturing if the sclerotomies are not closed at the end of the surgery. A partial fluid-air exchange can be performed to help assess patency of sclerotomies by the egress of air. If residual vitreous hemorrhage is not dense, it can resolve with observation. Cases that do not clear spontaneously, monocular patients who are limited by poor vision, or eyes that have large rebleeds can be managed with repeat vitrectomy in the operating room or rarely with an office-based air-fluid exchange.

Another postoperative complication that can occur in any eye is rhegmatogenous retinal detachment from an undetected iatrogenic break, a poorly treated break during the surgery, or reopening of a break in CTRRD. The incidence of this complication has been reported as 4.7%.[44] To avoid this complication, it is important to check the periphery meticulously at the end of the vitrectomy with scleral depression and to evaluate sclerotomies for vitreous incarceration. Peripheral breaks require photocoagulation, and vitreous traction to sclerotomies should be relieved. Cases of CTRRD that redetach are usually the result of missed or opened break secondary to residual traction or reproliferation of membranes. If no traction is perceived, office-based intravitreal gas and photocoagulation can be attempted, but if traction is present, reoperation with long-acting tamponade (either gas or silicone oil) is required.

Postoperative anterior segment neovascularization and NVG are challenging complications that require careful evaluation to determine the cause. They are more common in eyes with marked ischemia, reduced perfusion caused by vascular obstructions, or peripheral retinal detachment. Aggressive management with anti-VEGF injections, photocoagulation to ischemic areas, and repair of peripheral detachment if present is often necessary, as well as silicone oil tamponade in recalcitrant cases. Other frequent complications that can be seen in diabetic vitrectomies include corneal epithelial defects from trauma and neurotrophic factors and progression of cataract. Corneal trauma has been reduced with faster surgical times and noncontact viewing systems. The incidence of cataract extraction after diabetic vitrectomy has been reported at 15%, which is much lower than in eyes after macular hole surgery.[45]

Prevention of the most common postoperative complication, bleeding, can be achieved by meticulous treatment of bleeding vessels, optimal systemic hypertension control intraoperatively, and adequate sclerotomy closure to prevent postoperative hypotony. Prevention of postoperative redetachment and anterior segment neovascularization requires careful examination of the periphery for iatrogenic breaks and vitreous incarceration, thorough laser photocoagulation of the ischemic retina with emphasis on the periphery, and preoperative and perioperative anti-VEGF injections to reduce intra- and postoperative bleeding.

INTRAOPERATIVE CONSIDERATIONS AND COMPLICATIONS

Poor visibility during surgery was a significant problem in the past because of very lengthy procedures and limited visual technology. The advent of wide-angle viewing systems, improved microscopes, and shorter surgical times has reduced this complication. Microincision surgery (MIVS) has not only expedited and simplified diabetic vitrectomies, but also reduced the frequency of iatrogenic breaks. This reduction is related to the use of microcannulas that protect the vitreous base when instruments enter and exit the eye and to utilization of the vitrectomy probe as a multipurpose instrument with cutting rates up to 10,000 c/min that allow vitreous removal with minimal traction. The smaller sclerotomies of 25 and 27 gauge reduce inflammation as well as the incidence of fibrovascular ingrowth and neovascularization in the sclerotomy sites.[33,38] Reduced turbulence from valved cannulas and optimized IOP control are useful to reduce traction on the retina and vitreous and prevent bleeding. These technologic improvements have reduced surgical times and complications in these challenging diabetic eyes.

Intraoperative bleeding in diabetic eyes was a very common event in the past and the cause of many failed surgeries in diabetic eyes with severe pathologies. The advent of anti-VEGFs and their use before complicated diabetic vitrectomy with vascularized tissue have markedly reduced intraoperative bleeding and improved outcomes. Other innovations that have helped streamline the vitrectomy procedures as well as reduce bleeding include intraoperative pressure control systems in the vitrectomy machines and smaller sclerotomies with valved cannulas to maintain a stable intraocular environment.

CONCLUSION

Despite many advances in the diagnosis and treatment of diabetes, the ocular complications of this disease continue to be a devastating cause of blindness worldwide. Newer modalities of screening and treatment, including telemedicine, intravitreal anti-VEGF agents and steroids, MIVS, and earlier surgical interventions, will help expand the armamentarium of options that can be offered to diabetic patients. Late complications from diabetic retinopathy can result in severe pathologies that are very challenging to repair. Early vitrectomy to remove the posterior hyaloid is ideal to prevent the progression to TRD and CTRRD, particularly in young patients with diabetes.[8] MIVS platforms, preoperative use of anti-angiogenics, and advances in instrumentation and cutting rates have optimized the management of difficult diabetic pathologies. These advances have reduced complications and optimized outcomes, as well as allowed for more expedient interventions in these very challenging and potentially devastating diabetic retinopathy complications.

REFERENCES

1. Kempen JH, O'Colmain BJ, Leske MC, et al. The prevalence of diabetic retinopathy among adults in the United States. *Arch Ophthalmol.* 2004;122:552–563.
2. Klein R, Klein BE, Moss SE. A population-based study of diabetic retinopathy in insulin-using patients diagnosed before 30 years of age. *Diabetes Care.* 1985;8(suppl 1): 71–76.
3. Writing Committee for the Diabetic Retinopathy Clinical Research Network, Gross JG, Glassman AR, et al. Panretinal photocoagulation vs intravitreous ranibizumab for proliferative diabetic retinopathy: a randomized clinical trial. *JAMA.* 2015;314:2137–2146.
4. Photocoagulation treatment of proliferative diabetic retinopathy. Clinical application of Diabetic Retinopathy Study (DRS) findings, DRS report number 8. The Diabetic Retinopathy Study Research Group. *Ophthalmology.* 1981;88:583–600.
5. Early vitrectomy for severe proliferative diabetic retinopathy in eyes with useful vision. Clinical application of results of a randomized trial–Diabetic Retinopathy Vitrectomy Study Report 4. The Diabetic Retinopathy Vitrectomy Study Research Group. *Ophthalmology.* 1988;95(10):1321–1334.
6. Early vitrectomy for severe vitreous hemorrhage in diabetic retinopathy. Two-year results of a randomized trial. Diabetic Retinopathy Vitrectomy Study Report 2. The Diabetic Retinopathy Vitrectomy Study Research Group. *Arch Ophthalmol.* 1985;103(11):1644–1652.
7. Early vitrectomy for severe vitreous hemorrhage in diabetic retinopathy. Four-year results of a randomized trial: Diabetic Retinopathy Vitrectomy Study Report 5. *Arch Ophthalmol.* 1990;108(7):958–964.
8. Early vitrectomy for severe proliferative diabetic retinopathy in eyes with useful vision. Results of a randomized trial–Diabetic Retinopathy Vitrectomy Study Report 3. The Diabetic Retinopathy Vitrectomy Study Research Group. *Ophthalmology.* 1988;95(10):1307–1320.
9. Flynn HW, Chew EW, Simmons BD, Barton FB, Remaley NA, Ferris FL. Early Treatment Diabetic Retinopathy Study Research Group: pars plana vitrectomy in the Early Treatment Diabetic Retinopathy Study. ETDRS report number 17. *Ophthalmology.* 1992;99:1351–1357.
10. Ip MS, Domalpally A, Hopkins JJ, Wong P, Ehrlich JS. Long-term effects of ranibizumab on diabetic retinopathy severity and progression. *Arch Ophthalmol.* 2012; 130:1145–1152.
11. Ip MS, Domalpally A, Sun JK, Ehrlich J. Long-term effects of therapy with ranibizumab on diabetic retinopathy severity and baseline risk factors for worsening retinopathy. *Ophthalmology.* 2015;122:367–374.
12. Kiss S, Liu Y, Brown J, et al. Clinical utilization of anti-vascular endothelial growth-factor agents and patient monitoring in retinal vein occlusion and diabetic macular edema. *Clin Ophthalmol.* 2014;8:1611–1621.
13. Stefánsson E. Physiology of vitreous surgery. *Graefes Arch Clin Exp Ophthalmol.* 2009;247:147–163.
14. Davis MD. Vitreous contraction in PDR. *Arch Ophthalmol.* 1965;74(6):741–751.
15. Massin P, Duguid G, Erginay A, Haouchine B, Gaudric A. Optical coherence tomography for evaluating diabetic macular edema before and after vitrectomy. *Am J Ophthalmol.* 2003;135(2):169–177.
16. Nagiel A, Lalane RA, Sadda SR, Schwartz SD. Ultra-widefield fundus imaging: a review of clinical applications and future trends. *Retina.* 2016;36(4):660–678.
17. Yeh PT, Yang CM, Lin YC, Chen MS, Yang CH. Bevacizumab pretreatment in vitrectomy with silicone oil for severe diabetic retinopathy. *Retina.* 2009;29:768–774.
18. Oshima Y, Shima C, Wakabayashi T, et al. Microincision vitrectomy surgery and intravitreal bevacizumab as a surgical adjunct to treat diabetic traction retinal detachment. *Ophthalmology.* 2009;116:927–938.
19. Chen E, Park CH. Use of intravitreal bevacizumab as a preoperative adjunct for tractional retinal detachment repair in severe proliferative diabetic retinopathy. *Retina.* 2006;26:699–700.
20. Rizzo S, Genovesi-Ebert F, Di Bartolo E, Vento A, Miniaci S, Williams G. Injection of intravitreal bevacizumab (avastin) as a preoperative adjunct before vitrectomy surgery in the treatment of severe proliferative retinopathy (PDR). *Graefes Arch Clin Exp Ophthalmol.* 2008;246: 837–842.
21. da R Lucena D, Ribeiro JA, Costa RA, et al. Intraoperative bleeding during vitrectomy for diabetic tractional retinal detachment with versus without preoperative intravitreal bevacizumab (IBeTra study). *Br J Ophthalmol.* 2009;93:688–691.
22. Pokroy R, Desai UR, Du E, Li Y, Edwards P. Bevacizumab prior to vitrectomy for diabetic traction retinal detachment. *Eye.* 2011;25:989–997.
23. Lim LL, Morrison JL, Constantinou M, et al. Diabetic macular edema at the time of cataract surgery trial: a prospective, randomized clinical trial of intravitreous bevacizumab versus triamcinolone in patients with diabetic macular oedema at the time of cataract surgery – preliminary 6 month results. *Clin Exp Ophthalmol.* 2016;44(4):233–242.
24. Smiddy WE, Flynn Jr HW. Vitrectomy in the management of diabetic retinopathy. *Surv Ophthalmol.* 1999;43: 491–507.
25. Lakhanpal RR, Humayan MS, De Juan Jr E, et al. Outcomes of 140 consecutive cases of 25-gauge transconjunctival surgery for posterior segment disease. *Ophthalmology.* 2005;112:817–824.

26. Kellner L, Wimpissinger B, Stolba U, Brannath W, Binder S. 25-gauge vs 20-gauge system for pars plana vitrectomy: a prospective randomized clinical trial. *Br J Ophthalmol.* 2007;91:945–948.

27. Recchia FM, Scott IU, Brown GC, Brown MM, Ho AC, Ip MS. Small-gauge pars plana vitrectomy: a report by the American Academy of Ophthalmology. *Ophthalmology.* 2010;117:1851–1857.

28. Oshima Y, Wakabayashi T, Sato T, Ohji M, Tano YA. 27-gauge instrument system for transconjunctival suture-less microincision vitrectomy surgery. *Ophthalmology.* 2010;117:93–102.

29. Arevalo JF, Sanchez JG, Saldarriaga L, et al. Retinal detachment after bevacizumab. *Ophthalmology.* 2011;118(11): 2304 e3–2304 e7.

30. Robaszkiewicz J, Chmielewska K, Figurska M, Wierzbowska J, Stankiewicz A. Triple therapy: phaco-vitrectomy with ILM peeling, retinal endophotocoagulation, and intraoperative use of bevacizumab for diffuse diabetic macular edema. *Med Sci Monit.* 2012;18(4):CR241–CR251.

31. Charles S, Flinn CE. The natural history of diabetic extramacular traction retinal detachment. *Arch Ophthalmol.* 1981;99:66–68.

32. Arevalo JF, Maia M, Flynn Jr HW, et al. Tractional retinal detachment following intravitreal bevacizumab (avastin) in patients with severe proliferative diabetic retinopathy. *Br J Ophthalmol.* 2008;92(2):213–216.

33. Khan MA, Shahlaee A, Toussaint B, et al. Outcomes of 27 gauge microincision vitrectomy surgery for posterior segment disease. *Am J Ophthalmol.* 2016;161:36–43.

34. Yeoh J, Williams C, Allen P, et al. Avastin as an adjunct to vitrectomy in the management of severe proliferative diabetic retinopathy: a prospective case series. *Clin Exp Ophthalmol.* 2008;36:449–454.

35. Thompson JT, de Bustros S, Michels RG, Rice TA. Results and prognostic factors in vitrectomy for diabetic traction-rhegmatogenous retinal detachment. *Arch Ophthalmol.* 1987;105:503–507.

36. Eckardt C, Paulo EB. Heads-up surgery for vitreoretinal procedures: an experimental and clinical study. *Retina.* 2016;36(1):137–147.

37. Yorston D, Wickham L, Benson S, et al. Predictive clinical features and outcomes of vitrectomy for proliferative diabetic retinopathy. *Br J Ophthalmol.* 2008;92:365–368.

38. Oshima Y, Shima C, Wakabayashi T, et al. Microincision vitrectomy surgery and intravitreal bevacizumab as a surgical adjunct to treat diabetic traction retinal detachment. *Ophthalmology.* 2009;116:927–938.

39. Yang CM, Su PY, Yeh PT, Chen MS. Combined rhegmatogenous and traction retinal detachment in proliferative diabetic retinopathy: clinical manifestations and surgical outcome. *Can J Ophthalmol.* 2008;43:192–198.

40. Rice TA, Michels RG, Rice EF. Vitrectomy for diabetic rhegmatogenous retinal detachment. *Am J Ophthalmol.* 1983;95(1):34–44.

41. Falkner-Radler CI, Glittenberg C, Gabriel M, Binder S. Intrasurgical microscope-integrated spectral domain optical coherence tomography-assisted membrane peeling. *Retina.* 2015;35(10):2100–2106.

42. Hisatomi T, Enaida H, Matsumoto H, et al. Staining ability and biocompatibility of brilliant blue G: preclinical study of brilliant blue G as an adjunct for capsular staining. *Arch Ophthalmol.* 2006;124(4):514–519.

43. Olmos LC, Sayed MS, Moraczewski AL, et al. Long-term outcomes of neovascular glaucoma treated with and without intravitreal bevacizumab. *Eye (London).* 2016;30(3):463–472.

44. Schrey S, Krepler K, Wedrich A. Incidence of rhegmatogenous retinal detachment after vitrectomy in eyes of diabetic patients. *Retina.* 2006;26:149–152.

45. Smiddy WE, Feuer W. Incidence of cataract extraction after diabetic vitrectomy. *Retina.* 2004;24:574–581.

46. Baker CW, Almukhtar T, Bressler NM, et al. Macular edema after cataract surgery in eyes without pre- operative central-involved diabetic macular edema. *JAMA Ophthalmol.* 2013;131(7):870–879.

47. Chae JB, Joe SG, Yang SJ, et al. Effect of combined cataract surgery and ranibizumab injection in postoperative macular edema in nonproliferative diabetic retinopathy. *Retina.* 2014;34(1):149–156.

Treatment of Diabetic Retinopathy in Pregnancy

AVNI P. FINN, MD, MBA • LEJLA VAJZOVIC, MD

INTRODUCTION

The evaluation and treatment of diabetic retinopathy in pregnancy deserves special consideration. A growing number of women are at risk for complications of diabetes in pregnancy because of a rise in the prevalence of diabetes mellitus, the younger age of onset of type 2 diabetes, and an increase in maternal age.[1] Diabetes currently affects about 17% of pregnancies worldwide, and progression of retinopathy is frequently observed in pregnant women with diabetes.[2] Those with type 1 diabetes are at highest risk of developing proliferative diabetic retinopathy (PDR) when compared with nonpregnant women.[3] As such, the prevalence of diabetic retinopathy in pregnant women with type 1 diabetes is estimated to be as high as 34%–72% compared with around 15% in those with type 2 diabetes.[4–7]

RISK FACTORS FOR THE PROGRESSION OF DIABETES DURING PREGNANCY

Pregnancy itself is an independent risk factor for the progression of diabetic retinopathy because of metabolic and hormonal changes within the body. Glycemic control becomes more difficult in early pregnancy owing to the rapidly changing, high metabolic demands of pregnancy. This is coupled with changes in systemic vasculature, including increased cardiac output and decreased peripheral vascular resistance, resulting in retinal hyperperfusion. This hyperdynamic flow state in pregnancy along with poor endothelial function and autoregulation of retinal blood flow in patients with diabetes increases endothelial cell damage at the capillary level and may lead to worsening of retinopathy.[8,9] Furthermore, hormonal changes in pregnancy, including increased levels of human placental lactogen, estrogen, and progesterone, induce vascular changes through increased levels of insulin-like growth factor 1, placental growth factor, and endothelin-1 that may potentiate retinopathy.[10–12]

Other risk factors associated with the progression of diabetic retinopathy during pregnancy include the severity of retinopathy at conception, duration of diabetes, adequacy of treatment before pregnancy, and the presence of other vascular disorders. In women with moderate to severe nonproliferative diabetic retinopathy (NPDR), 30% experienced progression in one study compared with 3% of those without significant retinopathy.[3] Similarly, in the Diabetes in Early Pregnancy Study, 29% of patients with moderate NPDR progressed to have proliferative changes in pregnancy, whereas only 6.3% of those with minimal NPDR progressed to proliferative changes.[6] A longer duration of diabetes at the time of conception correlated significantly with the development of more severe retinopathy during pregnancy.[3,6,13] Retinopathy progressed to proliferative disease in 39% with diabetes mellitus for greater than 15 years versus 18% of those with less than 15 years.[6] Consequently, patients with type 1 diabetes are at an increased risk of retinopathy progression compared with those with type 2 diabetes given the earlier age of disease onset and typically longer duration of disease at the time of pregnancy.

There is an additional correlation between the degree of disease control around pregnancy and the progression of retinopathy during pregnancy. In a study of 155 pregnant women with insulin-dependent diabetes, those with better diabetic control before pregnancy had less progression of diabetic retinopathy during pregnancy. However, an improved glucose control during pregnancy may lead to worsening retinopathy. Intensive glucose control early in pregnancy has been associated with an increased progression of retinopathy.[4,14] Despite this finding, the long-term benefits of optimizing glucose control, particularly for the health of the mother and fetus, outweigh this increased risk of retinopathy progression. To reduce potential complications to the fetus (such as preterm delivery and intrauterine growth retardation) and worsening of retinopathy, achieving good glycemic control before conception is strongly recommended.[15] Lastly, preeclampsia and hypertension during pregnancy augment worsening of retinopathy. About 50%–55% of diabetic women with preeclampsia compared with 8%–25% without preeclampsia had progression of retinopathy; thus vigilant control of blood pressure is advised.[16,17]

SCREENING GUIDELINES FOR DIABETIC WOMEN

Diabetic women should be counseled on the risk of progression of retinopathy during pregnancy and the benefits of achieving good glucose control before pregnancy. The initial examination during pregnancy should occur shortly after conception or early in the first trimester. The timing of subsequent examinations is dictated by the level of diabetic retinopathy. Earlier treatment may be indicated in those who may not be able to follow up frequently because of other comorbidities or social issues during pregnancy. Women who develop gestational diabetes do not require an eye examination during pregnancy and are not at increased risk of developing retinopathy.[6] Table 11.1 offers a guide for ophthalmologic screening recommendations in pregnant women with diabetes.

DIAGNOSTIC AND TREATMENT CONSIDERATIONS DURING PREGNANCY

All mydriatic and cycloplegic eye drops are categorized as pregnancy category C medications. Category C means that not enough research has been done to determine a drug is safe for humans during pregnancy. Neither animal nor human studies have been performed with drops such as cyclopentolate, tropicamide, or phenylephrine. When necessary, their use is thought to be safe; however, patients should be made aware of unknown potential risks and punctual occlusion is recommended after administration to limit systemic absorption.

Adjunctive imaging, such as fundus photography, optical coherence tomography (OCT), and fluorescein angiography (FA), is often used to aid in the staging and treatment of patients with diabetes with retinopathy. In pregnant women, the fluorescein dye crosses the placenta and enters fetal circulation, posing an unknown potential risk to the fetus.[18] Thus FA should be used with extreme caution and only if absolutely required during pregnancy. The physician should also alert nursing women that fluorescein dye is present in breast milk for 72 h. Although teratogenic effects have not been reported, the US Food and Drug Administration has classified fluorescein

	Screening for Patients With Type 1 or 2 Diabetes During Pregnancy	Need for Treatment
No retinopathy or mild NPDR	Every 3–6 months	No
Moderate NPDR	Every 3 months	No
Severe NPDR or worse	Every 1–2 months	Sometimes • PRP
High-risk PDR, vitreous hemorrhage	Every 1–2 months	Usually • PRP laser • vitrectomy in select cases
DME	Every 1–2 months	Usually • focal laser • intravitreal or posterior subtenon triamcinolone acetonide
Postpartum	6 months postpartum, sooner if retinopathy was present during pregnancy as above	As above

TABLE 11.1
Recommendations for Ophthalmologic Evaluation in Pregnant Women With Diabetes

DME, diabetic macular edema; *NPDR*, nonproliferative diabetic retinopathy; *PDR*, proliferative diabetic retinopathy; *PRP*, panretinal photocoagulation.
Retinal evaluation is recommended preconception to maximize control of systemic factors and treat preexisting retinopathy. Then retinal examination should be done shortly after conception or early in the first trimester, and subsequent examinations should be directed based on the level of diabetic retinopathy and risk factors.

dye as a pregnancy category C drug, implying that insufficient studies have been performed on this drug. Fluorescein use in pregnant women has been reported in two series of 22 and 105 pregnant women. In both studies, there were no adverse effects to the fetus; however, it is worth noting that only a limited number of FAs were performed during the first trimester when teratogenic potential is likely the greatest.[19,20] It is typically unnecessary to obtain FA in current practice in diabetic pregnant women, and its use is contraindicated during the first trimester.

An excellent clinical examination along with OCT and fundus photography is likely sufficient for the diagnostic and diabetic treatment decision made during pregnancy. Interestingly, indocyanine green dye does not cross the placenta and has been used in pregnant women for other indications.[21] OCT angiography is a noninvasive modality to image the retinal and choroidal vasculature that may add additional information without the risk of systemic dye injection as an alternative to FA in pregnancy.

TREATMENT OF PROLIFERATIVE DIABETIC RETINOPATHY

The indications for the treatment of PDR during pregnancy follow similar guidelines to the treatment in nonpregnant patients, with two important caveats: patients with PDR that is treated before pregnancy may experience reduced progression of retinopathy during pregnancy, and there is some, albeit conflicting, evidence that diabetic retinopathy occurring in pregnancy may regress in the final trimester or postpartum period. Optimization of the treatment of PDR before pregnancy has been shown to reduce progression during pregnancy. Sunness and colleagues showed those with panretinal photocoagulation (PRP) before pregnancy had a 26% rate of progression during pregnancy compared with 58% in those without PRP.[18] However, about half of patients may need additional PRP during pregnancy despite prior treatment.[22] For this reason, preconception retinal evaluation that reveals severe NPDR or low-risk PDR may warrant earlier treatment with PRP to prevent progression during pregnancy. The natural history of PDR during pregnancy remains somewhat controversial, as some studies have shown regression occurring during the third trimester or postpartum period; however, others have required aggressive postpartum treatment because of lack of regression.[23,24]

Laser PRP remains the standard of care for PDR in pregnancy, as retinal laser is safe and effective without risks to the fetus. Eyes should be classified by the level of diabetic retinopathy as in nonpregnant patients. PRP is recommended for all cases of high-risk PDR in pregnancy just as in nonpregnant patients.[25] For those patients with severe NPDR and non-high-risk PDR, other risk factors, including duration of disease, prior glycemic control, baseline severity of disease, coexisting morbidities such as hypertension or preeclampsia, and patient ability to follow up, should be taken into account to direct how aggressive to be with laser treatment or deferring treatment in favor of close follow-up.

In rare cases, vitreoretinal surgery may be necessary during pregnancy, such as in the case of bilateral vitreous hemorrhage, for visual rehabilitation. It is imperative to involve the obstetrician in the care of the patient, and local anesthesia is preferable. Lidocaine is safe to use as a peribulbar or retrobulbar block; however, bupivacaine and mepivacaine should be avoided in pregnancy. Silicone oil is also considered safe for use in pregnancy when needed and may be advantageous in the pregnant patient because of positioning difficulties.[26,27]

TREATMENT OF DIABETIC MACULAR EDEMA

Patients who develop diabetic macular edema (DME) in pregnancy may have a different disease course and prognosis compared with those who are not pregnant. DME can occur during any trimester of pregnancy, at a reported incidence between 5% and 27%.[7,28,29] Physiologic changes, such as increased blood volume and fluid retention, in the pregnant state may contribute to macular edema in pregnant diabetic patients.[18,30] Thus, resolution of DME without treatment may occur in the postpartum period and result in improved visual acuity compared with nonpregnant patients. In one study of 29% of eyes that developed macular edema during pregnancy, 88% had postpartum improvement in visual acuity and resolution of DME without treatment.[31] Others may have such a florid presentation of DME during pregnancy that treatment is necessary as in Fig. 11.1. Sight-threatening or progressive DME should be treated with focal laser during pregnancy and may necessitate adjunctive agents during and after pregnancy. In cases of non-sight-threatening, nonprogressive DME, it may be reasonable to observe closely for potential improvement or until after pregnancy when anti–vascular endothelial growth factor (VEGF) medications may be safely used.

The use of anti-VEGF medications during pregnancy and their safety remain questionable. Anti-VEGF medications approved for the treatment of DME (ranibizumab and aflibercept) are designated pregnancy class C agents as they have not been formally evaluated in pregnancy. Intravitreal administration does limit systemic exposure; however, the mechanism of action of the drugs poses potential teratogenic and embryotoxic effects in animal studies.[32,33] There is a potential increased risk of systemic exposure because of both the breakdown of the blood-retinal barrier in diabetic retinopathy and the increased cardiac output and circulation in pregnancy. A literature review of publications related to anti-VEGF agents for the treatment of other conditions during pregnancy revealed two reports of fetal loss after intravitreal bevacizumab and four patients receiving bevacizumab for choroiditis during pregnancy without any teratogenic effects on the infants.[34,35] Given the potential teratogenic effects to the fetus, particularly during the first trimester, progressive DME with visual decline may require treatment with focal laser during pregnancy, holding adjunctive anti-VEGF use until after delivery. Although there are no recommendations on the administration of anti-VEGF agents in nursing mothers, published reports show no free bevacizumab or ranibizumab has been detected in breast milk after intravitreal injection. However, there are safety concerns about the effects of these agents on VEGF-A levels in infants. Ranibizumab lowers VEGF-A levels in the breast milk to a lesser extent compared with bevacizumab after intravitreal injection, potentially arguing for the increased safety of administering ranibizumab in nursing mothers.[36,37]

For symptomatic DME cases that may be refractory to laser during pregnancy, intravitreal steroids may be an option. The injection of triamcinolone formulations into the vitreous for DME remains an off-label indication, although there is moderate experience utilizing it for DME during pregnancy. It is notable that Triesence (triamcinolone acetonide injectable suspension, Alcon, Fort Worth, TX, USA) is labeled pregnancy drug class D based on findings that maternal systemic corticosteroid use during the first trimester was associated with an increased rate of orofacial clefts and topical corticosteroids were associated with decreased birth weight.[38] Because serum levels of triamcinolone acetonide have been shown to be minimal from other studies, intravitreal triamcinolone is considered a relatively safe option for the treatment of refractory DME in pregnant patients, especially after the first trimester.[39,40] The dexamethasone implant (Ozurdex, Allergan, CA, USA) has also been used safely and effectively in pregnant women with DME.[41] In addition, posterior subtenon Kenalog (PSTK) injection has been widely used in uveitic conditions in pregnancy, but no reports have been published to date with regards to DME in pregnancy.[42–44] Fig. 11.1 outlines a pregnant woman presenting at 31 weeks gestational age with PDR and DME who was successfully treated with PRP and PSTK.

CONCLUSION

Women with diabetes should be counseled on the risk factors associated with the progression of diabetic retinopathy during pregnancy, including baseline level of retinopathy, glucose control at conception, duration of disease, and coexisting hypertension or illnesses. As postpartum regression of retinopathy is variable, high-risk PDR and progressive severe NPDR should be treated during pregnancy with PRP laser. DME during pregnancy is variable with less definitive treatment guidelines. As DME may improve in the postpartum period, milder cases may be watched unless it is progressive or vision threatening, at which time focal laser is preferred and local triamcinolone acetonide may be considered in refractory cases. Anti-VEGF medications should be avoided in the first trimester, and their use remains quite controversial at any time during pregnancy. Careful monitoring in the postpartum period for 6–12 months is indicated, as there is still some risk for retinopathy progression during this time.

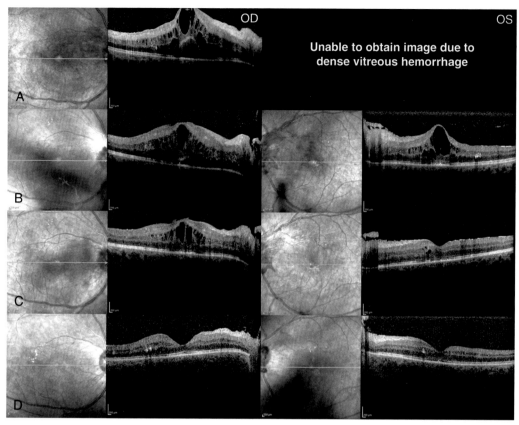

FIG. 11.1 A 34-year-old woman who was 31 weeks pregnant with poorly controlled type 2 diabetes presented acutely with vitreous hemorrhage in both eyes, more dense in the left eye (OS) than in the right (OD). She had no known history of diabetic retinopathy. Once the hemorrhage began to clear, examination revealed intraretinal hemorrhages, florid neovascularization of the disc, and diabetic macular edema (DME) in both eyes. Anti–vascular endothelial growth factor (VEGF) was not used because of pregnancy and she was treated with bilateral panretinal photocoagulation (PRP) along with posterior subtenon Kenalog (PSTK) injection to treat and reduce exacerbation of DME related to PRP. **(A)** At presentation, acuity was 20/200 OD and optical coherence tomography (OCT) showed severe diffuse DME with intraretinal and subretinal fluid. Visual acuity was counting fingers OS, and dense vitreous hemorrhage precluded OCT imaging. PRP and PSTK injection were performed OD. **(B)** One month later, there was some improvement in subretinal fluid OD. The vitreous hemorrhage began to clear OS, and OCT revealed DME OS. PRP and PSTK injection were performed OS. **(C)** After she delivered, intravitreal anti-VEGF injections were given in both eyes for persistent DME. **(D)** Visual acuity improved to 20/30 OD and 20/40 OS after three anti-VEGF injections in each eye postpartum.

REFERENCES

1. Lawrence JM, Contreras R, Chen W, Sacks DA. Trends in the prevalence of preexisting diabetes and gestational diabetes mellitus among a racially/ethnically diverse population of pregnant women, 1999-2005. *Diabetes Care.* 2008;31(5):899–904.
2. Aschner P, Colagiuri R, Mohan C. *Global Perspectives on Diabetes;* 2014.
3. Temple RC, Aldridge VA, Sampson MJ, Greenwood RH, Heyburn PJ, Glenn A. Impact of pregnancy on the progression of diabetic retinopathy in Type 1 diabetes. *Diabetes Med.* 2001;18(7):573–577.
4. Rasmussen KL, Laugesen CS, Ringholm L, Vestgaard M, Damm P, Mathiesen ER. Progression of diabetic retinopathy during pregnancy in women with type 2 diabetes. *Diabetologia.* 2010;53(6):1076–1083.
5. Axer-Siegel R, Hod M, Fink-Cohen S, et al. Diabetic retinopathy during pregnancy. *Ophthalmology.* 1996;103(11):1815–1819.
6. Chew EY, Mills JL, Metzger BE, et al. Metabolic control and progression of retinopathy. The diabetes in early pregnancy study. National Institute of Child Health and Human Development Diabetes in Early Pregnancy Study. *Diabetes Care.* 1995;18(5):631–637.

7. Vestgaard M, Ringholm L, Laugesen CS, Rasmussen KL, Damm P, Mathiesen ER. Pregnancy-induced sight-threatening diabetic retinopathy in women with Type 1 diabetes. *Diabetes Med.* 2010;27(4):431–435.

8. Chen HC, Newsom RS, Patel V, Cassar J, Mather H, Kohner EM. Retinal blood flow changes during pregnancy in women with diabetes. *Invest Ophthalmol Vis Sci.* 1994;35(8):3199–3208.

9. Tooke JE. Microvascular function in human diabetes. A physiological perspective. *Diabetes.* 1995;44(7):721–726.

10. Gibson JM, Westwood M, Lauszus FF, Klebe JG, Flyvbjerg A, White A. Phosphorylated insulin-like growth factor binding protein 1 is increased in pregnant diabetic subjects. *Diabetes.* 1999;48(2):321–326.

11. Khaliq A, Foreman D, Ahmed A, et al. Increased expression of placenta growth factor in proliferative diabetic retinopathy. *Lab Invest.* 1998;78(1):109–116.

12. Best RM, Hayes R, Chakravarthy U, Archer DB, Hadden DR. Plasma levels of endothelin-1 in diabetic retinopathy in pregnancy. *Eye.* 1999;13(2):179–182.

13. Lauszus F, Klebe JG, Bek T. Diabetic retinopathy in pregnancy during tight metabolic control. *Acta Obstet Gynecol Scand.* 2000;79(5):367–370.

14. Diabetes Control and Complications Trial Research Group. Effect of pregnancy on microvascular complications in the diabetes control and complications trial. The Diabetes Control and Complications Trial Research Group. *Diabetes Care.* 2000;23(8):1084–1091.

15. Early worsening of diabetic retinopathy in the diabetes control and complications trial. *Arch Ophthalmol (Chicago, Ill 1960).* 1998;116(7):874–886.

16. Lövestam-Adrian M, Agardh C-D, Åberg A, Agardh E. Pre-eclampsia is a potent risk factor for deterioration of retinopathy during pregnancy in type 1 diabetic patients. *Diabetes Med.* 1997;14(12):1059–1065.

17. Rosenn B, Miodovnik M, Kranias G, et al. Progression of diabetic retinopathy in pregnancy: association with hypertension in pregnancy. *Am J Obstet Gynecol.* 1992;166(4):1214–1218.

18. Sunness JS. The pregnant woman's eye. *Surv Ophthalmol.* 1988;32(4):219–238.

19. Soubrane G, Canivet J, Coscas G. Influence of pregnancy on the evolution of background retinopathy. Preliminary results of a prospective fluorescein angiography study. *Int Ophthalmol.* 1985;8(4):249–255.

20. Greenberg F, Lewis RA. Safety of fluorescein angiography during pregnancy. *Am J Ophthalmol.* 1990;110(3):323–325.

21. Rubinchik-Stern M, Shmuel M, Bar J, Eyal S, Kovo M. Maternal–fetal transfer of indocyanine green across the perfused human placenta. *Reprod Toxicol.* 2016;62:100–105.

22. Reece EA, Lockwood CJ, Tuck S, et al. Retinal and pregnancy outcomes in the presence of diabetic proliferative retinopathy. *J Reprod Med.* 1994;39(10):799–804.

23. Moloney JB, Drury MI. The effect of pregnancy on the natural course of diabetic retinopathy. *Am J Ophthalmol.* 1982;93(6):745–756.

24. Chan WC, Lim LT, Quinn MJ, Knox FA, McCance D, Best RM. Management and outcome of sight-threatening diabetic retinopathy in pregnancy. *Eye.* 2004;18(8):826–832.

25. Diabetic Retinopathy PPP – Updated 2016-of American Academy Ophthalmology. https://www.aao.org/preferred-practice-pattern/diabetic-retinopathy-ppp-updated-2016.

26. Charters L. *How to Manage Retinal Disease in Pregnant Patients;* 2017.

27. Ashish M, Alok S, Elesh J, Shubhi T. Considerations in management of rhegmatogenous retinal detachment in one eyed pregnant females: a report of two cases. *Ann Med Health Sci Res.* 2015;5(6):480–482.

28. Arun CS, Taylor R. Influence of pregnancy on long-term progression of retinopathy in patients with type 1 diabetes. *Diabetologia.* 2008;51(6):1041–1045.

29. Hampshire R, Wharton H, Leigh R, Wright A, Dodson P. Screening for diabetic retinopathy in pregnancy using photographic review clinics. *Diabet Med.* 2013;30(4):475–477.

30. Johnson MW. Etiology and treatment of macular edema. *Am J Ophthalmol.* 2009;147(1):11–21. e1.

31. Sinclair SH, Nesler C, Foxman B, Nichols CW, Gabbe S. Macular edema and pregnancy in insulin-dependent diabetes. *Am J Ophthalmol.* 1984;97(2):154–167.

32. *Genentech I. Lucentis Prescribing Information;* 2016. https://www.gene.com/download/pdf/lucentis_prescribing.pdf.

33. Regeneron I. *Eylea Prescribing Information;* 2016. https://www.regeneron.com/sites/default/files/EYLEA_FPI.pdf.

34. Petrou P, Georgalas I, Giavaras G, Anastasiou E, Ntana Z, Petrou C. Early loss of pregnancy after intravitreal bevacizumab injection. *Acta Ophthalmol.* 2010;88(4):e136.

35. Tarantola RM, Folk JC, Boldt HC, Mahajan VB. Intravitreal bevacizumab during pregnancy. *Retina.* 2010;30(9):1405–1411.

36. McFarland TJ, Rhoads AD, Hartzell M, Emerson GG, Bhavsar AR, Stout JT. Bevacizumab levels in breast milk after long-term intravitreal injections. *Retina.* 2015;35(8):1670–1673.

37. Ehlken C, Martin G, Stahl A, et al. Reduction of vascular endothelial growth factor a in human breast milk after intravitreal injection of bevacizumab but not ranibizumab. *Arch Ophthalmol.* 2012;130(9):1226.

38. Oren D, Nulman I, Makhija M, Ito S, Koren G. Using corticosteroids during pregnancy. Are topical, inhaled, or systemic agents associated with risk? *Can Fam Physician.* 2004;50:1083–1085.

39. Fazelat A, Lashkari K. Off-label use of intravitreal triamcinolone acetonide for diabetic macular edema in a pregnant patient. *Clin Ophthalmol.* 2011;5:439–441.

40. Degenring RF, Jonas JB. Serum levels of triamcinolone acetonide after intravitreal injection. *Am J Ophthalmol.* 2004;137(6):1142–1143.

41. Concillado M, Lund-Andersen H, Mathiesen ER, Larsen M. Dexamethasone intravitreal implant for diabetic macular edema during pregnancy. *Am J Ophthalmol.* 2016;165:7–15.

42. Thirupathy A, Tajunisah I. Rubella-related intermediate uveitis in pregnancy—a rare presentation. *Ocul Immunol Inflamm.* 2011;19(3):156–157.

43. Nakamura T, Keino H, Okada AA. Sub-Tenon triamcinolone acetonide injection in a pregnant patient with vogt–koyanagi–harada disease. *Retin Cases Brief Rep.* December 2016:1.

44. Wadhwani M, Gogia V, Kakkar A, Satyapal R, Venkatesh P, Sharma Y. A case of frost branch angitis in pregnancy: an unusual presentation. *Nepal J Ophthalmol.* 2014;6(2): 234–236.

CHAPTER 12

Novel Treatments for Diabetic Retinopathy

DAVID EICHENBAUM, MD

Progress and innovation in the treatment of diabetic macular edema (DME) and diabetic retinopathy (DR) has accelerated at an increasing rate over the past decade. There has been increased research and pharmacologic development for the treatment of DME, along with other medical retinal conditions, such as age-related macular degeneration (AMD) and branch retinal vein occlusion. Current theories into the pathogenesis of DR and DME include vascular, inflammatory, and neurodegenerative hypotheses. Further delineation of the mechanism may enable precise pharmacologic targeting or even prophylaxis. Investigational therapies for DR are initially evaluated with laboratory and animal models of ischemia and neovascularization. However, very few of these early promising therapies progress to large-scale human trials or commercialization. Some of the past and current novel agents and their mechanism of action are discussed.

BACKGROUND OF MODERN DR AND DME TREATMENT

It is important to understand what has led to the current evolution in DR treatment. Before 2000, laser was the mainstay of therapy for decades for DME and DR. However, the visual results after laser were less than satisfying and recurrences of DME and/or progressive loss of vision frequently complicated the clinical scenario. With thermal laser photocoagulation as monotherapy, many patients did not gain significant vision. Intravitreal injection of corticosteroid was the first, local pharmacologic therapy for DR, in particular targeted to treat DME. Some of the first reports that demonstrated efficacy of intravitreal corticosteroid to reduce DME were published by Jonas[1] and Martidis.[2] Subsequent large prospective clinical data supported the utility of intravitreal triamcinolone (IVT) as an alternative or adjunct to laser therapy for center-involving DME.[3,4] Despite the reasonable efficacy of intravitreal corticosteroid, widely known adverse events included a moderate incidence of elevated intraocular pressure as well as cataract

advancement. Intraocular corticosteroid development has continued with progress in research and adoption of sustained-release corticosteroid delivery devices. Intravitreal dexamethasone (Ozurdex, Allergan)[5] as well as intravitreal fluocinolone (Iluvien, Alimera)[6] sustained-release implants are now commercially available for DME treatment. Modern sustained-release drug delivery implants do not escape the corticosteroid side-effect profile that was reported with IVT in the early 2000s, and their potential adverse effect limits their application. The search for DR therapies with minimal side-effect profiles and greater efficacy, along with the established success of molecular therapy, has stimulated explosive research growth in the DME and DR disease state.

The concept of achieving the broad-ranging anti-permeability effects of steroids without the potential for steroid-mediated ocular adverse events is desirable. A novel idea employing the knowledge gained from the clinical research that established the efficacy of corticosteroids was the development of angiostatic cortisene. The design innovation was the provision of the multiple target angiostatic activity of conventional corticosteroids but with a compound free of glucocorticoid activity.[7] The concept was to relieve the common adverse events associated with periocular and intraocular steroid administration. Anecortave acetate (Retaane, Alcon Laboratories) was a synthetic cortisone designed with the removal of the 11β-hydroxyl group and an addition of a 21-acetate group. Juxtascleral delivery of anecortave acetate was studied in DR[8] and rubeosis iridis[9] in two Phase 1 open-label studies, but both were terminated before planned completion because of an absence of drug effect.

An innovative approach to intraocular steroid delivery is the exploration of the effects of triamcinolone acetonide when the drug is deposited into the suprachoroidal space (SCS). Clearside Biomedical (Alpharetta, Georgia) is exploring a proprietary micro-injector designed for access to the SCS. Their preservative-free formulation of triamcinolone, Zuprata, initiated a Phase I/II trial in DME in 2016. Their concept is that suprachoroidal injection may limit exposure of the anterior segment to steroid and potentially reduce steroid-mediated adverse effects.[10]

An older medication that has been pursued to achieve broad-ranging antipermeability corticosteroid benefits without steroid-mediated adverse events is Danazol (Optina, Ampio Pharmaceuticals). Danazol was initially approved in 1971 as a treatment for endometriosis. Danzol has a complex pharmacology, and part of its mechanism of action includes effects on endothelial cells to reduce vascular leakage. In its traditional formulation, administration of Danazol is burdened with notable androgenic side effects, including masculinization and elevated lipid levels.[11] An ultralow dose formulation of Danazol (known as Optina) is being evaluated in an attempt to mitigate the unfavorable side-effect profile while maintaining its membrane-stabilizing properties. Optina has shown safety and efficacy in a 12-week, double-masked, randomized-controlled trial and is currently being considered as an investigative target in a Phase III study, likely as an adjunct or rescue treatment for DME refractory to anti–vascular endothelial growth factor (VEGF) injections.[12,13]

SOMATOSTATIN ANALOGUES

One of the first pharmacotherapies targeted toward DME unrelated to corticosteroids was the use of somatostatin analogues. Octreotide (Sandostatin, Novartis Pharmaceuticals) is a synthetic octapeptide that mimics somatostatin and was first synthesized in 1979. Octreotide inhibits growth hormone and insulin-like growth factor 1. There were several small, open-label trials of systemic administration of octreotide in its standard and long-acting forms (Sandostatin LAR, Novartis Pharmaceuticals) to treat various stages of DME and DR, and results of these preliminary trials were generally positive.[14,15] Octreotide was subjected to two parallel, Phase III, prospective, randomized, placebo-controlled trials. Type 1 and 2 diabetic subjects with severe nonproliferative (NPDR) and proliferative diabetic retinopathy (PDR) were randomized, with the active treatment subjects receiving either 20 or 30 mg long-acting octreotide by intramuscular injection. Neither study showed a beneficial effect on visual acuity or in the reduction of DME.[16] Octreotide has not been pursued as a treatment for DME since the completion of these Phase III studies because of its failure to meet its primary end points.

ANTI-VEGF TREATMENT

The subsequent inflection point in the development of therapy for DME and DR was the clinical success, commercialization, and widespread adoption of anti-VEGF biologic therapy. In the current era, the most common first-line therapy for center-involving DME with vision loss is serial intravitreal injections of anti-VEGF medication. Clinical efficacy has been demonstrated for each of the following anti-VEGF agents: ranibizumab (Lucentis, Genentech, San Francisco, CA, USA), bevacizumab (Avastin, Genentech), and aflibercept (Eylea, Regeneron, Tarrytown, NY, USA). Intravitreal steroids have moved to be second line of therapy since the mid-2000s because of the superior ocular adverse event profile and tolerability of sequential intravitreal anti-VEGF injections. The caveat with current commercially available anti-VEGF agents is that to achieve results on par with published trials, frequent, near-monthly injections for the first 1–2 years of treatment are commonly required. Over one-third of treated patients in the best-performing groups also continue to have intraretinal edema over 2 years of treatment on anti-VEGF monotherapy. Only about one-third of patients have a profound increase in vision.[17] Although commercially available anti-VEGF medications have been shown to induce regression of severe NPDR and PDR, the treatment burden required to achieve regression remains quite high in the first 2 years of treatment.[18,19] Regardless, current anti-VEGF medications have been a substantial advance in the treatment of DME and DR and currently have earned their place as the first-line therapeutic strategy for DME. Recent data also argue that anti-VEGF biologics can be considered for first-line treatment in PDR with appropriate, high-frequency dosing and ongoing close monitoring.[17,20] The apparent ceiling affect to current therapy, as well as the limited target profile of commercially available intravitreal large molecule medications, still leaves a large unmet need in the treatment of DR.

Two important concepts have emerged regarding DR treatment from the current data on commercially available anti-VEGF injections. The first is that the current medications have limitations to their efficacy. Through multiple reproducible prospective, randomized, controlled trials,[16–18] there is general consensus that frequent intravitreal injections are necessary to produce visual and anatomic benefits. One of the major factors leading to this high treatment burden is the limited half-life of these protein-based treatments in the ocular environment.[21,22] Potential solutions to this problem are wide-ranging, and options include increasing the potency or molar concentrations of the drug with each injection, sustained-release drug delivery devices, and more faculty—such as a greater range of therapeutic targets—built into each injection. As more targets are explored, there may be a synergistic effect revealed, and combining certain therapeutic targets may yield a better outcome than affecting an individual target in isolation. More novel, futurist options are in the early stages of development, such as genetic therapy that would allow the native ocular tissue to produce effective therapeutic proteins.

The second concept that has emerged from data is the relative safety and tolerability of local intravitreal injection of medication, even with the current high burden of treatment. In large-scale clinical trials involving thousands of intravitreal injections, there is a remarkably low incidence of serious ocular adverse events, such as retinal tear, retinal detachment, endophthalmitis, or iatrogenic cataract. There is also a high retention rate in pivotal trials, which is reflective of the rapid, widespread adoption of serial intravitreal injections. Although there may be other routes of therapeutic administration, the future of pharmacotherapy is likely to include intravitreal medication as a backbone of any armamentarium, and our current experience supports the reliability of this technique for drug delivery. Although this list is in a constant state of flux, Table 12.1 outlines some of the novel agents and delivery devices being evaluated to treat DR.

EXTENDED-RELEASE ANTI-VEGF TECHNOLOGY

A drug delivery device to allow longer-acting anti-VEGF effect may serve as a means to reduce the frequency of anti-VEGF injections. There are a number of modalities in development, including intravitreal implants, microspheres, and encapsulated cell technology. In patients with wet AMD, a Phase I clinical trial using a refillable, nonbiodegradable, long-term drug delivery implant (ForSight/Genentech) has been completed. In this design, the self-retaining implant is placed via a 3.2-mm surgical incision without sutures under the conjunctiva in the pars plana in the operating room. The implant can be refilled with concentrated ranibizumab in as-needed intervals in an office procedure similar to an intravitreal injection. Results using this implant showed an improvement in visual acuity of 10 letters in neovascular AMD, which was maintained throughout 1 year.[23] This implant is currently in Phase II study for wet AMD,

but it could easily be used for patients with DME if the implant proves safe and effective. Risks with a surgically implanted drug delivery device of any type are likely to be different than with serial anti-VEGF injections, and the results of ongoing larger prospective, randomized clinical trials will not only focus on comparable efficacy but will assess the safety of a surgically implantable device compared with the potential reduction of treatment burden. There are several other preclinical approaches under investigation for sustained-release injectable drug devices that may prolong the anti-VEGF effect, including early pipeline products from Ocular Therapeutix (Bedford, MA, USA) and pSivida (Watertown, MA, USA). Ocular Therapeutix is in a strategic partnership with Regeneron for further development of its hydrogel-based sustained-release drug delivery platform. Potentially, their hydrogel product could release small or large molecule therapeutics over a longer period of time than commercially available large molecule intravitreal injections.[24] pSivida's innovative product for extended-release therapy focuses on silicon nanostructuring in a product called Tethadur, which is being developed to potentially adapt to a wide variety of large molecule therapy.[25]

NOVEL ANTI-VEGF AGENTS

Another step forward is to investigate more potent and/or durable intravitreal anti-VEGF medications for the treatment of diabetic eye disease. Anti-VEGF designed ankyrin repeat protein (DAPRin) biologic therapy has the potential to deliver these desirable qualities via VEGF inhibition. DARPin molecules can be designed with specificity and affinity that can surpass antibody-based treatments and have improved potential because of their solubility, stability, and aggregation resistance.[26] A Phase II trial evaluating the efficacy and safety of the anti-VEGF DARPin abicipar (Allergan Laboratories, Parsippany-Troy Hills, NJ, USA) versus commercially available ranibizumab therapy for center-involving DME with decreased visual acuity has been completed. The study evaluated abicipar at a reduced injection frequency versus monthly ranibizumab per its registration trial protocol. Abicipar at various doses, including as infrequently as every 12 weeks, compared favorably with ranibizumab. However, there was more intraocular inflammation in the abicipar group.[27] Further refinement of the abicipar preparation followed by upcoming Phase III registration trials will inform on its potential efficacy for DME. Another potential

TABLE 12.1
Novel Pharmacologic Agents or Devices for Treatment of Diabetic Retinopathy

Agent	Company	Class of Drug	Mechanism of Action	Mode of Delivery
Abicipar	Allergan	DARPin-based novel anti-VEGF	Specific blockage of VEGF-A	Intravitreal injection
Brolucizumab (RTH-258)	Alcon	Novel anti-VEGF	Specific blockage of VEGF-A	Intravitreal injection
RO6867461	Hoffmann-LaRoche/ Genentech	Anti-angiopoietin2 and anti-VEGF combination	Specific antibody blockade of Ang2	Intravitreal injection
REGN910-3	Regeneron	Anti-angiopoietin2 and anti-VEGF combination	Specific blockade of Ang2	Intravitreal injection
Danazol	Ampio	Synthetic modified testosterone derivative	Increases endothelial cell barrier function	Oral
AKB-9778	Aerpio	Vascular endothelial tyrosine phosphatase beta inhibitor	Improvement of Tie-2 signaling	Subcutaneous injection
Luminate (ALG-1001)	Allegro Ophthalmics	Integrin peptide	Targets integrin receptors involved in cell signaling and regulation, downstream protein regulation, dual mechanism of antiangiogensis and vitreolysis	Intravitreal injection
Ocriplasmin	ThromboGenics	Protease cleaving fibronectin and laminin	Enzymatic vitreolysis	Intravitreal injection, FDA approved for symptomatic vitreomacular adhesion (VMA)
Squalamine (OHR-102)	Ohr Pharmaceuticals	Inhibits multiple growth factors, including anti-VEGF, anti-PDGF, anti-bFGF	Sequestration of intracellular calmodulin	Topical therapy
TG10081	TargeGen	Tyrosine kinase inhibitor	Inhibits VEGF	Topical therapy
Pazopanib	Votrient/ GlaxoSmithKline	Tyrosine kinase inhibitor	Inhibits VEGFR and PDGF	Topical therapy, FDA-approved oral agent for cancer
Ruboxistaurin	Eli Lilly	Protein kinase C β inhibition	Blocking signal transduction for VEGF binding	Oral, failed to meet primary outcome in 2005 trial
PF-g55	Quark	Small interfering RNA that inhibits the RTP801 gene	Target-specific pathways to block signal transduction	Intravitreal injection
Infliximab	Janssen	NSAID, TNF inhibitor	Decrease multiple interleukins, chemotactic proteins, VEGF	Intravenous administration
Rapamycin (Sirolimus)	MacuSight	Macrolide antibiotic and immunosuppressive agent	Inhibits activation of T cells and B cells by reducing production of IL-2, via action on mTOR	Sunconjunctival, oral
Minocycline		Tetracycline antibiotic	Inhibits microglial activation	Oral
DRUG DELIVERY				
Zuprata	Clearside Biomedical	Corticosteroid, preservative-free triamcinolone (Zuprata)	Antiinflammatory	Suprachoroidal injection
Ranibizumab	ForSight/ Genentech	Sustained release of anti-VEGF agent	Specific blockage of VEGF-A	Implantable port for intravitreal drug delivery
Intraocular hydrogel	Ocular Therapeutix	Sustained release of anti-VEGF and other drugs	Partnership with Regeneron	Intravitreal injection
Tethadur	pSivida	Silicon-based nanostructure for sustained drug release	Biodegradable and biocompatible, designed for biologic agents to be loaded into the matrix, and released at a controlled rate as Tethadur dissolves	Intravitreal placement

bFGF, basic fibroblast growth factor; *FDA*, US Food and Drug Administration; *IL*, interleukin; *mTOR*, mechanistic target of rapamycin; *NSAID*, nonsteroidal anti-inflammatory drug; *PDGF*, pigment-derived growth factor; *TNF*, tumor necrosis factor; *VEGF*, vascular endothelial growth factor; *VEGFR*, VEGF receptor.

advance in VEGF inhibition is RTH-258 (ESBA1008), which is a very low-molecular-weight antibody fragment with a high affinity for VEGF. It is currently in Phase III trial compared with aflibercept for neovascular AMD, with potential extension between injections as far as 12 weeks.[28] It is possible that RTH-258 will be employed for DME treatment as well if it shows efficacy in AMD.

BROAD-SPECTRUM GROWTH FACTOR SUPPRESSION

Another potential option is to consider broad-spectrum agents that inhibit action or production of multiple growth factors in addition to VEGF. The antiproliferative and immunosuppressive agent rapamycin (Sirolimus, MacuSight, Inc., Union City, CA, USA) is a macrolide antibiotic that can block upstream VEGF production. Its mechanism of action is via downregulation of multiple intracellular signaling pathways that ultimately lead to VEGF production, as well as inhibition of inflammatory genes that lead to interleukin (IL) production. A Phase I study of a single subconjunctival treatment has shown an improvement in vision and a decrease in macular thickness in a small trial.[29] A natural compound called decursin has been shown to phosphorylate the VEGF-Receptor2,[30] inhibiting neovascularization. Decursin is isolated from the root of *Angelica gigas* Nakai and has shown treatment effect on animal models of proliferation.[31] Neither of these treatments has seen further development, but they are examples of potential future therapeutics from nontraditional pipelines.

ANGIOPOIETIN PATHWAY MODULATION

Multi-modal inhibition is a potential mechanism for future intravitreal therapeutics, via inhibition of pathologic proteins other than VEGF combined with existing anti-VEGF agents. An example of a distinct target is the Tie-2 pathway. Angiopoietins are growth factors that bind to the tyrosine kinase Tie-2 receptor on the endothelium. The activity of this pathway is regulated by angiopoietin (Ang1) and angiopoietin 2 (Ang2), and, when functioning normally, this pathway serves to protect retinal vasculature, preserve endothelial cell structure, and reduce vascular leakage. When this pathway is pathologically activated in hyperglycemic states in diabetic animal models, Ang2 is upregulated and leads to perturbation of the pathway, increased vascular permeability, problems with

endothelial tight junctions, and potentiation of VEGF-mediated pathologic vascular changes.[32] Alternatively, animal models exposed to Ang1 show a reduction in pathologic vascular leakage.[33] The uniqueness of the approach to inhibiting both VEGF and Ang2 is that the downstream regulation of Ang2 progresses to mediate inflammatory cytokines. In a sense, an inhibitor of Ang2 could be considered a type of protein-specific nonsteroidal antiinflammatory (NSAID) drug. Both Genentech and Regeneron are investigating combinations of their anti-VEGF and anti-Ang2 intravitreal agents compared with their commercial anti-VEGF agent alone for DME.

In addition to pursuing the Tie-2 pathway as a target with intravitreal agents, a systemic agent targeting this pathway is under investigation. The TIME-2 study is Phase II trial evaluating AKB-9778 (Aerpio Therapeutics, OH, USA) which is a tyrosine phosphate β inhibitor that restores Tie-2 signaling without molecular inhibition of angiopoietin proteins. Administration of subcutaneous AKB-9778 in combination with intravitreal ranibizumab, showed a benefit when compared with ranibizumab monotherapy. The benefit of combination therapy in TIME-2 was realized with improved retinal thickness on optical coherence tomography and back-steps in DR level, with a trend toward better visual acuity. This study also showed a reduction in DR severity in the nonstudy eyes of individuals who received the systemic AKB-9778 agent, implying that there is proof of concept for mediating the Tie-2 pathway.[34] AKB-9778 is self-administered by subcutaneous injection, and Phase III testing has been planned. Although the potential benefits include improved systemic health status and reduced treatment burden, there is potential for systemic drug-related adverse events and noncompliance with self-administration in diabetic patients who have already exhibited poor control of their disease leading to their DR.

NOVEL LARGE MOLECULE THERAPY

Another avenue for inhibition of angiogenesis and vascular permeability with protein therapy is introducing a protein that inhibits angiogenesis directly instead of blocking proteins that promote established pathologic angiogenesis. One option is pigment-epithelium derived growth factor (PEGF), with research suggesting it is a key endogenous anti-angiogenic protein[35] that can alter neovascularization in animals.[36] Specific molecular development targeting PEGF is in its infancy as a different route for protein treatment for DR.

A similar unique option for future intravitreal protein therapeutics is to more directly approach the underlying vascular disease associated with DR instead of proteins that are increased after disease has set in. As retinal vascular disease is a result of microvascular endothelial decompensation, therapy to treat the endothelium has a specific, anatomic appeal. Integrin peptide therapy, as an integrin antagonist, has the potential to change cell functions and cell-to-cell interactions between cells and the extracellular matrix (ECM). In diabetic retinal disease, integrins can increase proteolytic pathways, leading to damaged endothelium and downstream vasogenic protein overproduction. Inhibiting the reaction between integrin peptides and their targets in the ECM may downregulate latter protein production. A Phase I study of integrin peptide therapy ALG-1001 (Allegro Ophthalmics, San Juan Capistrano, CA, USA) showed results lasting up to 3 months in some subjects. These preliminary results suggest that this distinct target may yield substantially more durable treatment than the current anti-VEGF therapy. An added potential benefit of ALG-1001 is that it can induce vitreolysis and vitreous detachment. Vitreous detachment may reduce the risk of progression to new PDR events by releasing the posterior hyaloid scaffold. This compound is completing several Phase II studies in a variety of settings, including a comparison with bevacizumab and focal laser treatment in DME.[37] Results of the noninferiority comparison with bevacizumab are positive, with ALG-1001 showing durability and top-line results similar to bevacizumab in this trial's design.[38] Enrollment in another Phase II trial evaluating the induction of posterior vitreous detachment (PVD) in ALG-1001 monotherapy has been completed.

ENZYMATIC VITREOLYSIS

Ocriplasmin is a recombinant protease enzyme that targets laminin and fibronectin and is being studied in NPDR. Its target is primarily the vitreoretinal interface in the posterior hyaloid, and it is approved by the US Food and Drug Administration for symptomatic vitreomacular adhesion. In 2016, ThromboGenics initiated the CIRCLE Phase II trial of ocriplasmin in the induction of PVD in patients with NPDR without DME. The study hypothesis is that separation of the vitreous from the inner retina surface may reduce the risk of DR progression by eliminating the scaffold for neovascularization and also

by improving retinal oxygenation. The study involves multiple doses of ocriplasmin, and the primary end point is the proportion of patients with a confirmed PVD on progression of DR. The current study plan is to randomize 230 patients to either ocriplasmin or sham control group.[39]

TOPICAL TREATMENTS

Self-administration with topical investigational proteins is also being explored as a potential treatment for DR and DME. Topical administration of eye drops for ocular disease is well established as glaucoma therapy. Squalamine (OHR-102, Ohr Pharmaceuticals) is a small molecule drug that has activity against multiple vasogenic growth factors, including VEGF, pigment-derived growth factor, and basic fibroblast growth factor. The broad efficacy of OHR-102 is attributed to its ability to actively enter cells and sequester intercellular calmodulin to impact many, but not all, intracellular VEGF pathways. There are only very preliminary data of topical squalamine in diabetic eye disease from investigator-initiated trials.[40] Other topical medications in early development for possible treatment of DME are tyrosine kinase inhibitors TG10081 (TargeGen, Inc., San Diego, CA, USA), which have been well-tolerated in human subjects,[41] and the tyrosine kinase inhibitor pazopanib (Votrient, GlaxoSmithKline, East Durham, NY, USA), which has shown efficacy in an animal model of DR.[42]

PROTEIN KINASE C β INHIBITION

An alternative route to angiogenic protein treatment is attacking signal transduction pathways that are initiated by VEGF protein binding. These pathways have physiologic effects downstream and have been implicated in the advancement of DR. Hyperglycemia activates the enzyme protein kinase C β (PKC β) by inducing de novo synthesis of diacylglycerol, resulting in diabetic microvascular complications in the eyes, nerves, and kidneys. A generation ago, both basic science and animal models showed that PKC β inhibition prevented VEGF-mediated proliferation in vitro,[43] and animal studies supported that PKC β inhibition treated vascular leakage.[44] Inhibition of PKC β with ruboxistaurin (RBX, Eli Lilly, Indianapolis, IN, USA) was investigated in a randomized controlled trial. Results in 2005 showed that RBX reduced the risk of vision loss but did not prevent the progression of DR and failed to meet that primary outcome. Aside from the failure to meet the primary end point, the data from the study were mixed. There was a benefit in the reduction in vision loss in patients with baseline DME, but there was not a reduction in the progression to new PDR events.[45] Based on the results of that trial, inhibition of PKC β has not been pursued further as a treatment option for DR.

SMALL INTERFERING RNA

Another novel path to intravitreal therapy affecting VEGF without specifically targeting VEGF is small interfering RNA (siRNA) targeting genetic pathways implicated in retinal vascular disease. This approach is similar to signal transduction interference inasmuch as it seeks to turn off the "faucet" instead of "sopping up the water." PF-655 (Quark Pharmaceuticals, Fremont, CA, USA) is an siRNA that inhibits the RTP801 gene, which has been shown to be expressed in neovascular AMD and DME. PF-655 showed efficacy in diabetic models of lower mammals. Early dose escalation studies showed safety and some improvement in vision in patients with DME. The DEGAS trial was designed to compared intravitreal PF-655 to laser photocoagulation for DME but was terminated early due to inability to achieve study objectives.[46]

NONSTEROIDAL ANTIINFLAMMATORY THERAPY

As development has moved forward with protein-based therapy for DR, work has continued to show the ongoing role of inflammation in the diabetic disease process. The inflammation of diabetes has been described as sustained, low-level chronic inflammation, as opposed to an acute inflammatory vasculitis. Increased leukostasis is an early hallmark of the inflammation associated with DR.[47] Elevated levels of neutrophils as well as increased number of macrophages have been demonstrated in the retinal and choroidal vessels as well as in extravascular retinal tissues in both human and animal studies.[48–50] In addition to high levels of VEGF, extreme elevations in monocyte chemotactic protein (MCP) and ILs have been demonstrated in the vitreous of eyes with both DR and DME. Elevations in both VEGF and these inflammatory markers are also proportional to angiographic leakage in DME, implying a positive correlation between DME severity and inflammation.[51]

Aqueous concentrations of inflammatory MCP and multiple ILs have been shown to be unaffected by a single injection of bevacizumab but, as predicted, were significantly reduced with intravitreal triamcinolone acetate, whereas VEGF was more strongly inhibited by the specific anti-VEGF activity of bevacizumab.[52] It is reasonable to continue to explore novel antiinflammatory treatments, as anti-VEGF monotherapy does not optimally benefit all patients with DME, with only about one-third of patients gaining >15 letters[53] and a similar one-third having persistent intravitreal fluid.[16]

Topical and systemic broad-spectrum NSAID therapies have shown limited efficacy in treating DME. Commercially available topical and systemic medications include cyclooxygenase and prostaglandin inhibitors. The oldest agent studied for DR is systemic aspirin. In 1991, the Early Treatment Diabetic Retinopathy Study (ETDRS) found no effect of high-dose aspirin (650 mg/day) in the prevention of vision loss in DME or severe NPDR.[54] Case series have shown that any apparent time to effect and the impact with topical NSAID treatment are less profound than with intravitreal steroid therapy.[55] The randomized controlled Phase II study (DRCR Protocol R, Appendix A) evaluating nepafenac 0.1% eye drops for 1 year showed no meaningful difference in visual outcome or central retinal thickness in patients with non-center-involving DME.[56] Oral and topical NSAID therapies have not been pursued as potent treatment options because of these limitations. Existing specific NSAIDs inhibiting the molecule tumor necrosis factor-α (TNF- α) have had some limited success as potential future treatments for DR. TNF-α is a known key mediator of leukostasis, monocyte regulation, and intracellular adhesion molecules. Infliximab (Remicade, Janssen Biotech, Horsham, PA, USA) is a monoclonal antibody approved for the treatment of various inflammatory diseases, such as rheumatoid arthritis and ankylosing spondylitis, and is known to block the inflammatory molecule TNF-α. TNF-α inhibition does not affect VEGF levels.[57] A small randomized controlled crossover trial of 11 patients with DME resistant to laser treatment showed significant functional and anatomic improvement with intravenous infliximab (5 mg/kg).[58] Owing to the high systemic adverse effect rate with systemic anti-TNF-α administration, it is unlikely that intravenous TNF-α therapy is a realistic approach for DME treatment. Potential applications of existing antiinflammatory technology with local dosing formulation remain a challenge for DR treatment.

A future direction in approaching DR from an antiinflammatory treatment includes specifically targeting some of the known proinflammatory proteins that have been measured in high concentrations in the vitreous of patients with DR.[30] Animal studies have started to evaluate some specific receptor antagonists, with data emerging on targeting the MCP receptor showing some effect. Translating the basic science data implicating multiple inflammatory factors in DR to safe and effective specific human treatment is only in its infancy.

CONCLUSION

Diabetic eye disease is multifaceted, with vasogenic, inflammatory, ischemic, and mechanical factors existing in combination in the diabetic eye. The future aim for DR therapy is to develop novel new agents with prolonged effect that lead to stable improvement in vision with minimal adverse effects. This may occur by increasing the durability of current therapies, combining agents and/or developing new agents that can be effective in halting the development or progression of DR. Novel therapeutic strategies under development may be evaluated to treat not only DR, but also a variety of ocular disorders.

REFERENCES

1. Jonas JB, Sofker A. Intraocular injection of crystalline cortisone as adjunctive treatment of diabetic macular edema. *Am J Ophthalmol.* 2001;132:425–427.
2. Martidis A, Duker JS, Greenberg PB, et al. Intravitreal triamcinolone for refractory diabetic macular edema. *Ophthalmology.* 2002;109:920–927.
3. Gillies MC, Sutter FK, Simpson JM, Larsson J, Ali H, Zhu M. Intravitreal triamcinolone for refractory diabetic macular edema: two-year results of a double-masked, placebo-controlled, randomized clinical trial. *Ophthalmology.* 2006;113:1533–1538.
4. Diabetic Retinopathy Clinical Research Network. A randomized trial comparing intravitreal triamcinolone acetonide and focal/grid photocoagulation for diabetic macular edema. *Ophthalmology.* 2008;115:1447–1449.
5. Boyer DS, et al. Three-year, randomized, sham-controlled trial of dexamethasone intravitreal implant in patients with diabetic macular edema. *Ophthalmology.* 2014;121 (10):1904–1914.
6. Campochiaro PA, Nguyen QD, Hafiz G, et al. *Ophthalmology.* 2013;120(3):583–587.
7. Clark AF. Mechanism of action of the angiostatic cortisone anecortave acetate. *Surv Ophthalmol.* 2007;52(suppl 1): S26–S34.
8. Yannuzzi LA. *Treatment of Diabetic Retinopathy with Open Label Anecortave Acetate Sterile Suspension (15 mg).* ClinicalTrials gov Identifier: NCT00211406; 2007.
9. Yannuzzi LA. *Treatment of Rubeosis Iridis with Open-Label Anecortave Acetate Sterile Suspension (15 mg).* ClinicalTrials gov Identifier: NCT00211471; 2007.
10. Suprachoroidal Injection of CLS-TA Alone or with Aflibercept in Subjects with Diabetic Macular Edema (HULK). https://clinicaltrials.gov/ct2/show/NCT02949024?term=cle arside&rank=5.
11. Howard WJ, John AR. *Te Linde's Operative Gynecology.* Wolters Kluwer Health; July 10, 2015:1327–1330.
12. Amirkiai T. *Ampio Pharmaceuticals Announce Additional Statistically Significant Study Results for Optina in the Treatment of Diabetic Macular Edema (DME)*Ampiopharma. com22; June 2015. http://ampiopharma.com/news/am pio-pharmaceuticals-announces-additional-statistically-significant-study-results-for-optina-in-the-treatment-of-diabetic-macular-edema-dme/.
13. thepharmaletter.com. *Ampio Pharma Updates on Path to FDA Approval for DME Drug Optina;* October 14, 2015. http:// www.thepharmaletter.com/article/ampio-pharma-updates-on-path-to-fda-approval-for-dme-drug-optina.
14. Kuijpers RWAM. Treatment of cystoid macular edema with octreotide. *N Engl J Med.* 338:624–626.
15. Grant MB, Mames RN, Fitzgerald C, et al. The efficacy of octreotide in the therapy of severe nonproliferative and early proliferative diabetic retinopathy. *Diabetes Care.* 23:504–509.
16. Grant MB, Caballero Jr S. The potential role of octreotide in the treatment of diabetic retinopathy. *Treat Endocrinol.* 2005;4(4):199–203.
17. Wells JA, Glassman AR, Ayala AR, et al. Aflibercept, bevacizumab, or ranibizumab for diabetic macular edema: two-year results from a comparative effectiveness randomized clinical trial. *Ophthalmology.* 2016;123(6): 1351–1359.
18. Diabetic Retinopathy Clinical Research Network. Panretinal photocoagulation vs intravitreous ranibizumab for proliferative diabetic retinopathy: a randomized trial. *JAMA.* 2015;314(20):2137–2146.
19. Eichenbaum D, Ruiz K, Hill L, Haskova Z. *Regression of Diabetic Retinopathy with Ranibizumab in Patients with Diabetic Macular Edema and Highest-Risk Non-proliferative Diabetic Retinopathy.* Poster presented at the America Academy of Ophthalmology Annual Meeting; October 15–16, 2016 (Chicago, IL).
20. Heier JS, Brown DM, Chong V, et al. Intravitreal aflibercept (VEGF trap-eye) in wet age-related macular degeneration. *Ophthalmology.* 2012;119:2537–2548.
21. Bakri S, Snyder M, Reid J, Pulido J, Ezzat M, Singh R. *Pharmacokinetics of Intravitreal Bevacizumab (Avastin).* American Society of Retinal Specialists meeting; September 2006. Cannes, France; Combined Retina Society and Jules Gonin Club meeting, October 2006, Capetown, South Africa; and American Academy of Ophthalmology meeting, November 2006, Las Vegas, Nevada.

22. Bakri S, Snyder M, Reid J, Pulido J, Ezzat M, Singh R. Pharmacokinetic of intravitreal ranibizumab (lucentis). *Ophthalmology*. 2007;114:2179–2182.
23. Rubio R. *Phase I Clinical Trial Using a Refillable, Non-biodegradable Long-Term Drug Delivery Implant of Ranibizumab*. Tokyo, Japan: World Congress of Ophthalmology; 2014.
24. Ocular Therapeutix Press Release. http://investors.ocutx.com/phoenix.zhtml?c=253650&p=irol-newsArticle&ID=2211419.
25. pSivida Corp Products/Tethadur. http://www.psivida.com/products-tethadur.
26. Plückthun A. Designed ankyrin repeat proteins (DARPins): binding proteins for research, diagnostics, and therapy. *Annu Rev Pharmacol Toxicol*. 2015;55:489–511.
27. Abicipar Pegol PALM Study Phase 2 Data in Diabetic Macular Edema (DME) Presented at 2016 AAO Annual Meeting. http://www.molecularpartners.com/abicipar-pegol-palm-study-phase-2-data-in-diabetic-macular-edema-dme-presented-at-2016-aao-annual-meeting.
28. Efficay and Safety of RTH-258 versus Aflibercept. Clinicaltrials.gov. https://clinicaltrials.gov/ct2/show/NCT02307682.
29. Blumenkranz M. Sirolimus Demonstrates Favorable Safety Profile and Improvements in Visual Acuity. In: *40 Annual Meeting of the Retina Society*; 2007. Boston, MA.
30. Yang Y, Yang K, Li Y, et al. Decursin inhibited proliferation and angiogenesis of endothelial cells to suppress diabetic retinopathy via VEGFR2. *Mol Cell Endocrinol*. 2013;378:46–52.
31. Shen J, Yang X, Xiao WH, Hackett SF, Sato Y, Campochiaro PA. Vasohibin is up-regulated by VEGF in the retina and suppresses VEGF receptor 2 and retinal neovascularization. *FASEB J*. 2006;20:723–725.
32. Rangasamy S, Srinivasan R, Maestas J, et al. A potential role of angiopoietin-2 in the regulation of the blood retinal barrier in diabetic retinopathy. *Invest Ophthalmol Vis Sci*. 2011;52:3784–3791.
33. Joussen AM, Poulaki V, Tsujikawa A, et al. Suppression of diabetic retinopathy with angiopoietin-1. *Am J Pathol*. 2002;160:1683–1693.
34. Campochiaro PA, Khanani A, Singer M, et al. Enhanced benefit in diabetic macular edema from AKB-9778 Tie2 activation combined with vascular endothelial factor suppression. *Ophthalmology*. August 2016;123(8):1722–1730.
35. Dawson DW, Volpert OV, Gillis P, et al. Pigment epithelium-derived factor: a potent inhibitor of angiogenesis. *Science*. 1999;285:245–248.
36. Gao G, Li Y, Fant J, Crosson CE, Becerra SP, Jx Ma. Difference in ischemic regulation of vascular endothelial growth factor and pigment epithelium – derived factor in brown Norway and sprague dawley rats contributing to different susceptibilities to retinal neovascularization. *Diabetes*. 2002;51:1218–1225.
37. Allegro Ophthalmics Begins Phase 2 Clinical Trial of Luminate® (Alg-1001) for the Treatment of Diabetic Macular Edema. Available at: http://www.allegroeye.com/press/.
38. Allegro Ophthalmics Announces Positive Topline Results from DEL MAR Phase 2b Trial Evaluating Luminate® in Patients with Diabetic Macular Edema. Allegro Ophthalmics. http://www.allegroeye.com/press-release/allegro-ophthalmics-announces-positive-topline-results-from-del-mar-phase-2b-trial-evaluating-luminate-in-patients-with-diabetic-macular-edema/.
39. *Thrombogenics Business Update – H1*. Thrombogenics; 2016.
40. Squalamine Lactate Eye Drops in Combination with Ranibizumab in Patients with Diabetic Macular Edema (DME). Clinicaltrials.gov.
41. A Phase 1 Safety Study of TG100801 Eye Drops in Healthy Volunteers. Clinicaltrials.gov; http://www.clinicaltrials.gov/ct2/show/NCT00414999.
42. Thakur A, Scheinman RI, Rao VR, Kompella UB. Pazopanib, a multitargeted tyrosine kinase inhibitor, reduces diabetic retinal vascular leukostasis and leakage. *Microvasc Res*. 2011;82:346–350.
43. Aiello LP, Bursell SE, Clermont A, et al. Vascular endothelial growth factor–induced retinal permeability is mediated by protein kinase C in vivo and suppressed by an orally effective beta-isoform-selective inhibitor. *Diabetes*. 1997;46:1473–1480.
44. Ishii H, Jirousek MR, Koya D, et al. Amelioration of vascular dysfunctions in diabetic rats by an oral PKC beta inhibitor. *Science*. 1996;272:728–731.
45. The PKC-DRS Study Group, PKC-DRS Study Group, Aiello LP, et al. The effect of ruboxistaurin on visual loss in patients with moderately severe to very severe nonproliferative diabetic retinopathy. *Diabetes*. 2005;54:2188–2197.
46. Nguyen QD, Schachar RA, Nduaka CI, et al. Dose-ranging evaluation of intravitreal siRNA PF-04523655 for diabetic macular edema (the DEGAS study). *Invest Ophthalmol Vis Sci*. 2012;53(12):7666–7674.
47. Miyamoto K, Khosrof S, Bursell SE, et al. Prevention of leukostasis and vascular leakage in streptozotocin-induced diabetic retinopathy via intercellular adhesion molecule-1 inhibition. *Proc Natl Acad Sci USA*. 1999;96:10836–10841.
48. McLeod DS, Lefer DJ, Merges C, Lutty GA. Enhanced expression of intracellular adhesion molecule-1 and P-selectin in the diabetic human retina and choroid. *Am J Pathol*. 1995;147:642–653.
49. Kim SY, Kim SY, Johnson MA, et al. Neutrophils are associated with capillary closure in spontaneously diabetic monkey retinas. *Diabetes*. 2005;54:1534–1542.
50. Rangasamy S, McGuire PG, Franco Nitta C, et al. Chemokine mediated monocyte trafficking into the retina: role of inflammation in alteration of the blood-retinal barrier diabetic retinopathy. *PLoS One*. 2014;9:e108508.
51. Funatsu H, et al. *Ophthalmology*. 2009;119:73–79.
52. Sohn HJ, et al. Changes in aqueous concentrations of various cytokines after intravitreal triamcinolone versus bevacizumab for diabetic macular edema. *Am J Ophthalmol*. 2011;152(4):686–694.
53. Brown DM, et al. *Ophthalmology*. 2013;120:2013–2022.

54. ETDRS Group. Effects of aspirin treatment on diabetic retinopathy. ETDRS report no. 8. Early Treatment Diabetic Retinopathy Study Research Group. *Ophthalmology.* 1991;98:757–765.

55. Callanan D, Williams P. Topical nepafenac in the treatment of diabetic macular edema. *Retina.* 2010;30:459–467.

56. Friedman SM, Almukhtar TH, Baker CW, et al. Topical nepafenac in eyes with noncentral diabetic macular edema. *Retina.* 2015;35:944–956.

57. Adamis AP, Berman AJ. Immunological mechanisms in the pathogenesis of diabetic retinopathy. *Semin Immunopathol.* 2008;30:65–84.

58. Sfikakis PP, Grigoropoulos V, Emfietzoglou I, et al. Infliximab for diabetic macular edema refractory to laser photocoagulation: a randomized, double-blind, placebo-controlled, cross-over, 32 week study. *Diabetes Care.* 2010;33:1523–1528.

CHAPTER 13

Clinical Scenarios: Introduction

CHARLES C. WYKOFF, MD • DAVID EICHENBAUM, MD • DARIN R. GOLDMAN, MD• CAROLINE R. BAUMAL, MD

Since 2006, there has been a dramatic increase in the number of treatment options for diabetic retinopathy. Where once there was only laser therapy, medical treatments have become first line for most eyes. However, there are limited universal guidelines to assist clinicians regarding initial therapeutic choices, when to change therapies, the role of combination therapy, and when treatment can be stopped or minimally maintained without risk for visual loss. The rigorous treatment regimens adhered to in study protocols are usually difficult or impossible to duplicate in real-world scenarios. Issues such as the patient's compliance and ability to return for frequent evaluations need to be taken into account. Overall there is no standard cookbook approach for each patient. Familiarization with the clinical studies as well as risks and benefits will assist to devise an individualized approach to treatment of diabetic retinopathy. The following is a collection of actual patient scenarios in which differential approaches may have been utilized and are discussed.

CASE 1: TREATMENT OF DIABETIC MACULAR EDEMA WITH ANTI–VASCULAR ENDOTHELIAL GROWTH FACTOR INJECTION AND A SUSTAINED-RELEASE STEROID IMPLANT

A 68-year-old female with type 2 diabetes mellitus, poorly controlled blood sugar (HbA1c 10%), chronic renal failure, and hypertension presented with gradual onset of bilateral reduced vision. Her acuity was 20/160 and 20/80 in the right and left eyes, respectively. Slit lamp examination revealed bilateral 2+ nuclear sclerotic cataracts. She had bilateral moderate nonproliferative diabetic retinopathy (NPDR) with foci of capillary nonperfusion (Fig. 13.1 right eye/Fig. 13.2 left eye: A, early-; B, mid-; and C, late-phase fluorescein angiogram, FA).

Optical coherence tomography (OCT) revealed center-involving diabetic macular edema (DME) with intraretinal cysts and subretinal fluid, more prominently in the right eye than in the left eye (Fig. 13.3 right eye, Fig. 13.4 left eye).

The treatment options for DME discussed with the patient included pharmacologic treatment or focal macular laser. Given the extensive nature of the center-involving edema, especially in the right eye, intravitreal injection of anti–vascular endothelial growth factor (VEGF) was preferred and bilateral bevacizumab injections were given. The right eye response was negligible at 4 weeks after the initial bevacizumab injection (Fig. 13.5), and the right eye treatment plan was switched to use aflibercept for intravitreal injection. In contrast, DME in the left eye showed some initial improvement after bevacizumab, so she was maintained on this medication in her left eye for financial reasons (Fig. 13.6).

After five monthly injections (one bevacizumab then four aflibercept), the right eye had persistent DME with minimal improvement on the OCT cube scan (Fig. 13.7). The DME completely resolved in her left eye after five bevacizumab injections (Fig. 13.8). Acuity measured 20/80-2 in the right eye and 20/50 in the left eye.

Fluorescein angiography (FA) was repeated. There appeared to be a reduced number of microaneurysms in the posterior pole bilaterally and less perifoveal leakage in the left eye (Figs. 13.9 and 13.10, A, early; B, mid; C, late).

At this point, the patient expressed concern that she would not be able to continue with monthly injections because of time and financial constraints. Her treatment plan was adjusted, and a sustained-release intravitreal dexamethasone implant (Ozurdex, Allergan) was injected in the right eye, whereas the interval between bevacizumab injections was extended for the left eye. She was evaluated 14 weeks after Ozurdex placement in the right eye, and the DME had completely resolved for the first time during her clinical course and vision improved to 20/50 (Fig. 13.11). The left eye remained stable without recurrent DME and extension of the bevacizumab injection interval (Fig. 13.12).

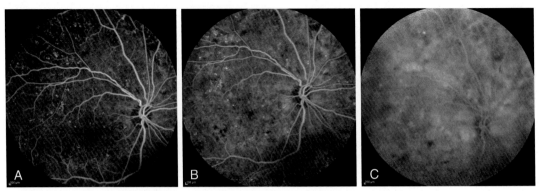

FIG. 13.1 FA right eye at presentation reveals NPDR and DME (A, early, B mid, C late phase).

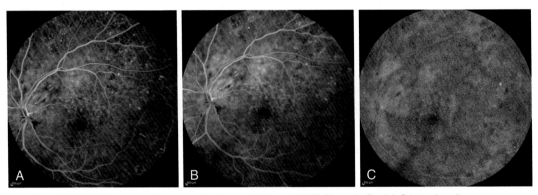

FIG. 13.2 FA left eye prior to treatment shows NPDR and DME (A, early, B mid, C late phase).

Discussion

The first-line treatment for most individuals with center-involving DME is intravitreal injection of an anti-VEGF agent as supported by multiple studies such as the DRCR.net Protocol I, Protocol H, Bevacizumab or Laser Therapy in the Management of Diabetic Macular Edema Study (BOLT), Ranibizumab Monotherapy or Combined With Laser Versus Laser Monotherapy in Asian Patients with Diabetic Macular Edema (REVEAL), and Intravitreal Administration of VEGF Trap-Eye (Aflibercept) in Patients with Diabetic Macular Edema (VIVID/VISTA). There are some exceptions when macular laser photocoagulation or intravitreal corticosteroid may be considered for initial therapy, for example, with pregnancy, inability to return for monthly injections, or noncentral DME. Anti-VEGF therapy requires education regarding the potentially prolonged treatment regimen as well as patient commitment to return for repeat injections, which may be bilateral as in this case. An advantage of anti-VEGF therapy is its beneficial effect on retinopathy as noted by the improvement in

the diabetic retinopathy severity score in the Ranibizumab Injection in Subjects with Clinically Significant Macular Edema with Center-Involvement Secondary to Diabetes Mellitus (RISE/RIDE) and VIVID/VISTA studies. This effect is apparent in this case, with a reduced number of microaneurysms in the fluorescein angiogram after anti-VEGF treatment (Figs. 13.9 and 13.10) compared with before treatment. Studies have reported successful DME treatment with all anti-VEGF agents. DRCR.net Protocol T provides some guidance as to the initial choice of anti-VEGF agent (Chapter 7, Appendix A). Economic considerations and availability based on geographic location also play a role.

Approximately one in five eyes with DME does not completely respond to anti-VEGF therapy. This is because the complex pathophysiology of DME involves not only VEGF but also other mediators and potentially unknown factors. Response of DME to anti-VEGF therapy has been classified as complete, partial/incomplete, or refractory/lack of response. There is no consensus definition on the number of injections before one is

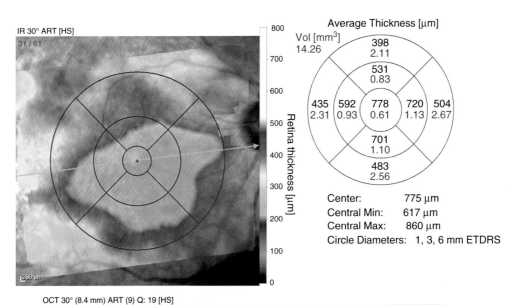

IR 30° ART [HS]
31 / 61

Retina thickness [µm]

Average Thickness [µm]

Vol [mm³]
14.26

398
2.11

531
0.83

435   592   778   720   504
2.31   0.93   0.61   1.13   2.67

701
1.10

483
2.56

Center: 775 µm
Central Min: 617 µm
Central Max: 860 µm
Circle Diameters: 1, 3, 6 mm ETDRS

OCT 30° (8.4 mm) ART (9) Q: 19 [HS]

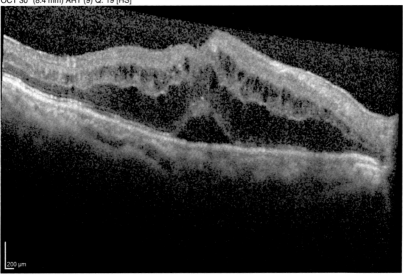

FIG. 13.3 OCT right eye pre-treatment shows center-involved DME with intraretinal cysts and subretinal fluid.

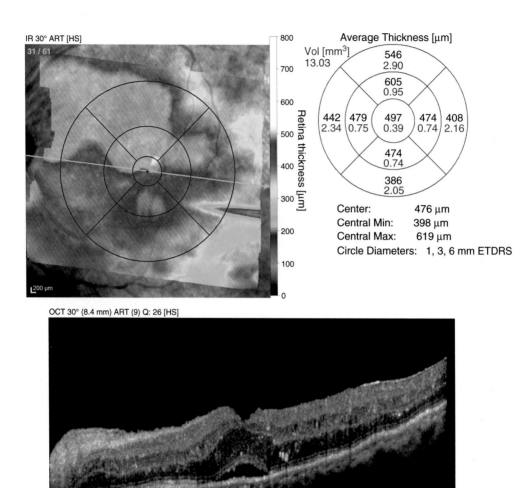

FIG. 13.4 OCT Left eye pre-treatment reveals DME with retinal thickening , subretinal fluid and intraretinal hyperreflective dots.

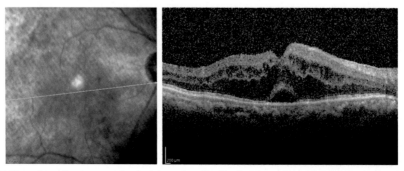

FIG. 13.5 There is no improvement noted 4 weeks after the first bevacizumab injection in the right eye.

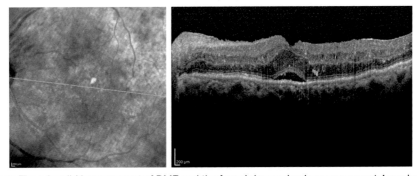

FIG. 13.6 There is mild improvement of DME and the foveal depression is now apparent 4 weeks after the initial bevacizumab injection in the left eye.

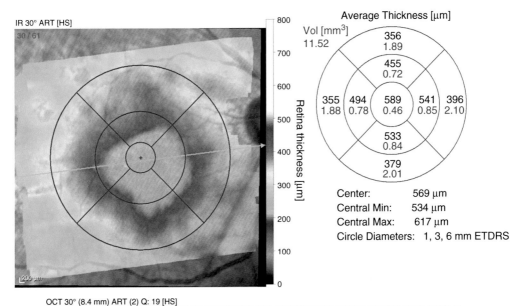

IR 30° ART [HS]

30 / 61

Retina thickness [µm]

Average Thickness [µm]

Vol [mm³]
11.52

	356 1.89	
355 1.88	455 0.72	
494 0.78	589 0.46	541 0.85	396 2.10
	533 0.84	
	379 2.01	

Center: 569 µm
Central Min: 534 µm
Central Max: 617 µm
Circle Diameters: 1, 3, 6 mm ETDRS

OCT 30° (8.4 mm) ART (2) Q: 19 [HS]

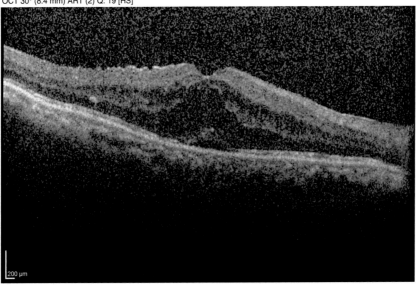

FIG. 13.7 DME persists right eye after 5 monthly anti-VEGF injections.

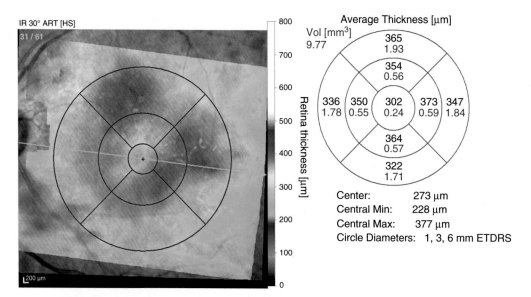

IR 30° ART [HS]

31 / 61

Retina thickness [μm]

200 μm

Vol [mm³]
9.77

Average Thickness [μm]

	365 / 1.93	
336 / 1.78	354 / 0.56	347 / 1.84
350 / 0.55	302 / 0.24	373 / 0.59
	364 / 0.57	
	322 / 1.71	

Center: 273 μm
Central Min: 228 μm
Central Max: 377 μm
Circle Diameters: 1, 3, 6 mm ETDRS

OCT 30° (8.4 mm) Q: 19 [HS]

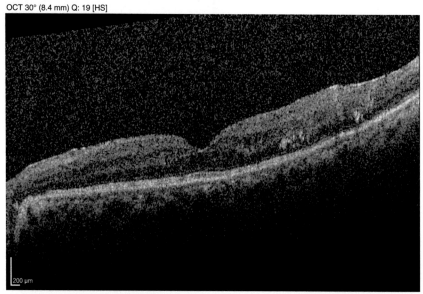

200 μm

FIG. 13.8 DME has resolved left eye after 5 monthly bevacizumab injections.

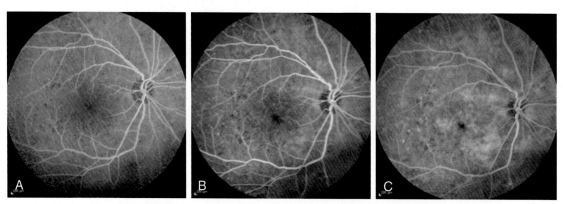

FIG. 13.9 FA shows reduced severity of diabetic retinopathy right eye and less leakage (A, early, B mid, C late phase).

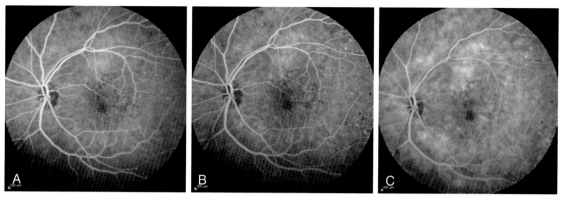

FIG. 13.10 FA shows reduced severity of diabetic retinopathy left eye (A, early, B mid, C late phase).

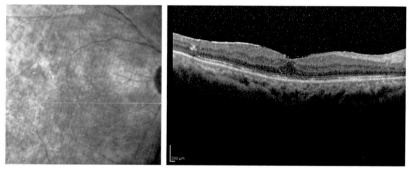

FIG. 13.11 For the first time in her clinical course, DME was completely resolved in her right eye seen on OCT 14 weeks after Ozurdex. Vision improved to 20/50.

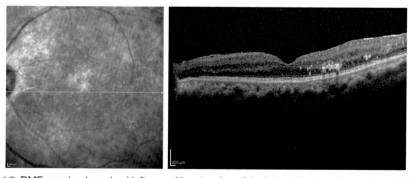

FIG. 13.12 DME remained resolved left eye with extension of the interval between bevacizumab injections.

considered to have DME refractory to anti-VEGF therapy. Most clinicians start with three monthly anti-VEGF injections and closely follow the OCT and visual acuity for response. If the clinician suspects the patient is not responding to an anti-VEGF agent, it may be useful to repeat the OCT within 7 days of an anti-VEGF injection when the medication level in the vitreous is high. If the OCT does not show improvement, the patient may not be responsive to that anti-VEGF agent. It is important to rule out vitreomacular traction and other causes of macular edema as contributing to the appearance of DME. Many clinicians consider changing therapy for DME that is refractory to an anti-VEGF after anywhere between three and seven injections, keeping in mind that it can take a prolonged course of an anti-VEGF for complete resolution of DME.

In this case, the clinician switched to aflibercept after a single bevacizumab injection because of lack of response on OCT and based on her poor acuity using protocol T criteria. The persistent DME in the right eye after five anti-VEGF injections and her limited ability for follow-up led to switching to another treatment modality with potential for longer duration of action with a slightly greater side-effect profile. Retrospective studies have shown positive results with a variety of switching or combination protocols for refractory DME. Ultimately the decision when to switch from a particular anti-VEGF agent to another therapy is made by the clinician with patient input and support from clinical studies. In addition to incomplete or lack of clinical response using OCT and acuity, other reasons to change the treatment plan include the inability to extend the anti-VEGF treatment interval without recurrence of fluid and patient and insurance issues.

CASE 2: ASYMMETRIC DIABETIC RETINOPATHY WITH PROLIFERATIVE DIABETIC RETINOPATHY AND NON-CENTER-INVOLVING DIABETIC MACULAR EDEMA

A 62-year-old man with a 15-year history of non-insulin-dependent diabetes mellitus was referred for evaluation of proliferative diabetic retinopathy (PDR). He denied symptoms. Vision was 20/20 bilaterally. The right eye had moderate NPDR (Fig. 13.13A) and non-center-involving DME, with extrafoveal thickening noted on the macular cube OCT scan (Fig. 13.13H). The left eye

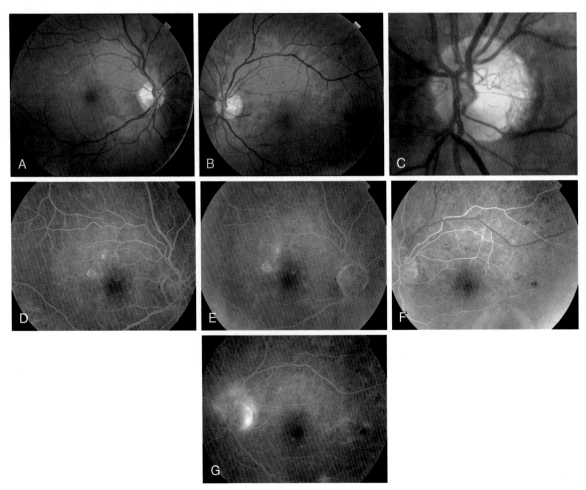

FIG. 13.13 **(A)** Moderate NPDR right eye, **(B)** PDR with NVD left eye, **(C)** Magnified NVD left eye, **(D)** Early FA right eye shows moderate NPDR, **(E)** Late FA right eye shows non-central DME, **(F)** Early FA left eye shows microaneurysms and blocked fluorescence from retinal hemorrhage, **(G)** Late FA confirms NVD with leakage

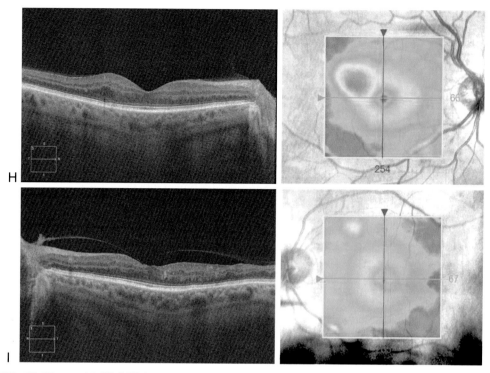

FIG. 13.13, cont'd **(H)** OCT right eye shows non-central DME, **(I)** OCT left eye shows mild vitreomacular traction

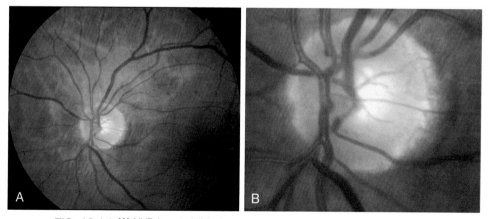

FIG. 13.14 **(A)** NVD is not visible 4 weeks after bevacizumab, **(B)** Magnified view

had neovascularization of the disc (NVD) over one-third of the optic nerve surface (Fig. 13.13B and C magnified image).

FA did not reveal any occult proliferative changes in the right eye (Fig. 13.13D early, Fig. 13.13E late FA) and confirmed that NVD indeed was present in the left eye (Fig. 13.13F early, Fig. 13.13G late).

OCT of the left eye did not show DME but showed focal vitreomacular traction and a small attachment of the posterior hyaloid to the neovascular tissue at the optic nerve margin (Fig. 13.13I).

Options for PDR with high-risk characteristics (HRC) included panretinal photocoagulation (PRP) or anti-VEGF therapy. Four weeks after one injection of bevacizumab in the left eye, the NVD was no longer apparent (Fig. 13.14A, close up Fig. 13.14B). The right eye was observed. The patient returned 8 weeks after the single bevacizumab injection, and a few neovascular fronds were now visible on the optic nerve of the left eye. The options of observation, anti-VEGF injection, or panretinal therapy were discussed. At this time, he preferred to commence peripheral panretinal laser photocoagulation and deferred another intravitreal injection. His main concern was to the the need for more frequent follow-up evaluations with anti-VEGF therapy.

Discussion

Although diabetic retinopathy can be asymmetric, consultation with the primary care physician for the evaluation of systemic factors such as carotid stenosis or ocular ischemic is indicated in this situation. Any factor, either systemic or local, that can produce poor ocular blood flow has the potential to exacerbate diabetic retinopathy. Regression of visible NVD occurred after one anti-VEGF injection. However, this effect may be impermanent and further treatment may be indicated either in the form of panretinal laser photocoagulation or additional anti-VEGF injection. Patient reliability and the ability to follow-up can play a major role in the treatment decision.

CASE 3: PROLIFERATIVE DIABETIC RETINOPATHY AND NON-CENTER-INVOLVING DME, TREATED WITH LASER FOLLOWED LATER BY ANTI-VEGF INJECTION

A 38-year-old white male with type I diabetes mellitus and well-controlled hypertension presented with increasing floaters for 3 months. He was diagnosed with diabetes at age 14 years, and his HbA1c had ranged from 7 to 12 over the last 10 years. He stated he has episodes where he is dedicated to optimizing his blood sugar but then fluctuating periods when he is discouraged and noncompliant with his medications. He stated that for the last few months, he had been compliant with medication and insulin use but had not been attentive to optimal dietary habits. His current HbA1c was 9.5%. He had never seen a retina specialist.

At initial examination, visual acuity was 20/25 in both eyes with mild myopic correction. He had minimal nuclear sclerosis and normal anterior segments. He had mild non-center-involving DME (Fig. 13.15A and B, OCT E and F) in both maculas, with more hard exudates in the left eye (Fig. 13.15B) than in the right eye. There were scattered microaneurysms, intraretinal hemorrhages, and subtle flat retinal neovascularization.

Wide-field FA revealed neovascularization of the retina evident as white hyperfluorescent foci adjacent to the arcades with peripheral small vessel pruning, staining, and peripheral capillary nonperfusion (Fig. 13.15C and D).

The options for management discussed with the patient included observation, pharmacologic treatment with anti-VEGF intravitreal injections, or application of limited PRP in both eyes. Given the patient's concern for potential noncompliance, he preferred treatment with PRP laser in both eyes. PRP was targeted anteriorly, remaining at and anterior to the equator without encroachment into the macula.

His floaters subsided and he was lost to follow-up until 2 years later when he noted recurrent bilateral floaters and returned for evaluation. Anterior segment and visual acuity were stable. Peripheral PRP laser spots were appreciated in both eyes (Fig. 13.16A and B). Repeat wide-field FA documented a substantial increase in the number of foci of retinal neovascularization in both eyes with new NVD in the left eye (Fig. 13.16 C, right eye; D, left eye). The mild non-center-involving DME in the right eye remained stable (Fig 13.16E). The DME and associated hard exudates in the left eye were increased, although they still did not involve the central fovea. Mild vitreomacular traction was present on the OCT line scan, with extrafoveal thickening on the cube scan of the left eye (Fig 13.16F).

The options for management were again discussed, including observation, pharmacologic treatment with intravitreal anti-VEGF injections, or application of additional PRP laser in both eyes. Given the possibility for side effects with additional more posteriorly placed PRP, the patient elected for initiation of anti-VEGF intravitreal injections.

Discussion

This case highlights options for a patient presenting with PDR and non-center-involving mild DME. It is probable that neovascularization of the retina induced fleeting microscopic vitreous hemorrhage in this 38-year-old man, thus fulfilling criteria for PDR with HRC. Treatment with PRP laser is supported by the Diabetic Retinopathy Study (DRS). Another option includes anti-VEGF injections as supported by Protocol S from the DRCR.net, which demonstrated the noninferiority of a series of anti-VEGF injections compared with PRP for PDR at 2 years. The status of the macula should be considered in eyes with PDR. PRP laser may exacerbate DME; however, studies have shown that this adverse secondary effect may be limited with peripheral or nasal placement of PRP.[1] Although intravitreal anti-VEGF

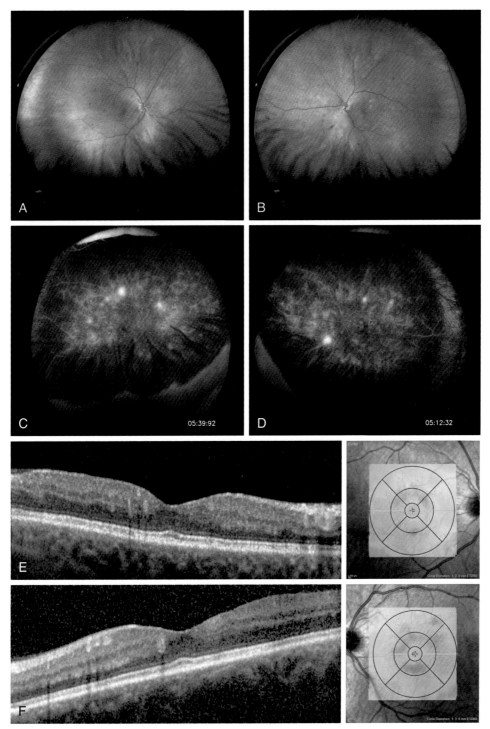

FIG. 13.15

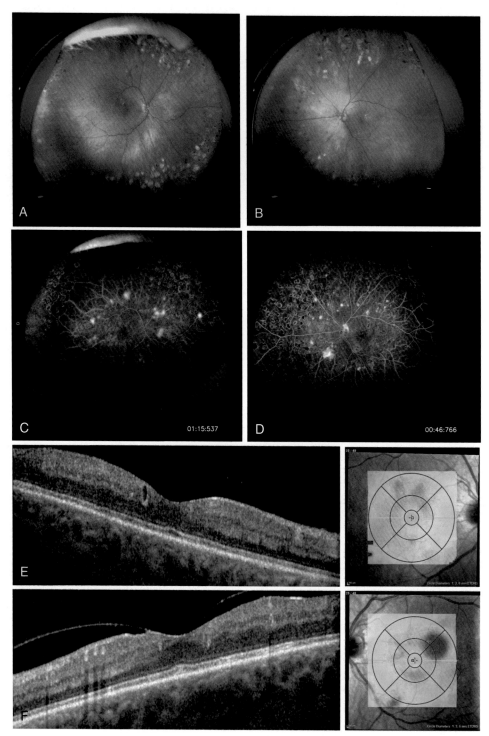

FIG. 13.16

injection alone may treat both the retinal neovascularization and DME simultaneously, patient compliance is critical, as both neovascularization and DME can recur without a series of injections. It is not known if or when the risk of reactivation of retinal neovascularization is eliminated after anti-VEGF injections. Another alternative in eyes with PDR and DME may be a combination treatment with PRP laser and anti-VEGF injection either at the same time or in close proximity, to induce more rapid stabilization in these eyes with severe disease. This patient initially chose PRP laser for its potential for long-term stability without the need for frequent follow-up. The laser was placed peripherally to reduce exacerbation of DME and also to limit secondary visual field constriction from laser. When he returned for follow-up 2 years later, he elected for anti-VEGF injection, which is reasonable based on some worsening of DME in the left eye and his concern about secondary PRP laser effects. It is notable that his left eye later showed mild vitreomacular traction, which needs to be considered when interpreting the anti-VEGF effect on the OCT.

CASE 4: RAPIDLY PROGRESSIVE PROLIFERATIVE DIABETIC RETINOPATHY TO TRACTIONAL RETINAL DETACHMENT IN PREGNANCY

A 30-year-old African American female who was 10 weeks pregnant presented with mild symptomatic vitreous hemorrhage in the right eye. She had a 15-year history of insulin-dependent diabetes mellitus with poor glucose control (hemoglobin AIc 10%) and chronic hypertension (blood pressure 220/150). Three months before presentation, she developed renal failure requiring dialysis. She had not previously had an examination of the retina or treatment.

Presenting vision was 20/25 and 20/30 in the right and left eyes, respectively. She had active NVD extending into the peripapillary region bilaterally and mild vitreous hemorrhage in the right eye Fig. 13.17A right eye, 13.17 B left eye, montage of seven standard color fields. There were cotton wool spots, venous beading, and sclerotic vessels in the macula in both eyes (Fig. 13.17C right eye and E left eye posterior pole image). There was no DME clinically, and this was confirmed with OCT (Fig. 13.17D right eye and F left eye one line macula OCT). Based on her presentation with PDR and HRC, PRP was performed. As she was in her first trimester of pregnancy, FA was not done, as it would not have altered management. Intravitreal anti-VEGF injection was not considered because of unknown potential risks in the first trimester.

She was treated with bilateral PRP peripheral to the arcades and initially stabilized. In the second trimester, PDR and NVD worsened in in both eyes with subhyaloid hemorrhage in the left eye (fig 13.18A right eye, 13.18B left eye).

Despite two additional sessions of fill-in PRP in the left eye, there was progressive fibrovascular prolif- eration and development of an extramacular tractional retinal detachment over the next 4 weeks (Figure 13.19A color) Vision decreased to 5/200 in the left eye. OCT showed the hyaloid attachment to the fovea and vitreous debris (Figure 13.19B OCT).

After discussion of the options, risks, and benefits with the obstetrician and patient, low-dose ranibizumab was given (0.15 mg), followed 6 days later with pars plana vitrectomy, laser, removal of fibrovascular tissue, and silicone oil tamponade (Fig. 13.20). Anesthesia was consulted, and surgery was performed with local anesthesia.

Her right eye had four sessions of PRP during her pregnancy, with subsequent development of DME with loss of the fovea depression on OCT (Fig. 13.21A and B).

She had a planned Caesarian section at 33 weeks and delivered a healthy infant. Post partum, her right eye was treated with ranibizumab 0.3 mg injections and OCT showed improved DME, residual eccentric cysts, and a small focal area where the retinal layers are indistinct (Fig. 13.22).

Silicone oil was removed 1 year later from the left eye (Fig. 13.23). The final acuity was 20/40 and 20/50 in the right and left eyes, respectively, before she was lost to follow-up.

Discussion

This case highlights multiple variables that need to be considered when treating diabetic retinopathy. Systemic medical conditions in this case include pregnancy, renal failure on dialysis, hypertension, and poor glycemic control. The risks and benefits of FA and anti- VEGF injection in pregnancy need to be considered as outlined in chapter 11. Low-dose ranibizumab was given 6 days before vitrectomy to reduce intraoperative bleeding during dissection of membranes. Ranibizumab was used, as it seems to have less effect on systemic VEGF levels, although this finding is from nonpregnant subjects. The bilateral nature of diabetic retinopathy is apparent, as the right eye developed mild center-involving DME after PRP, which is a known secondary effect. Development of DME may also be related to systemic changes in pregnancy. Treatment with anti-VEGF injections were commenced postpartum when

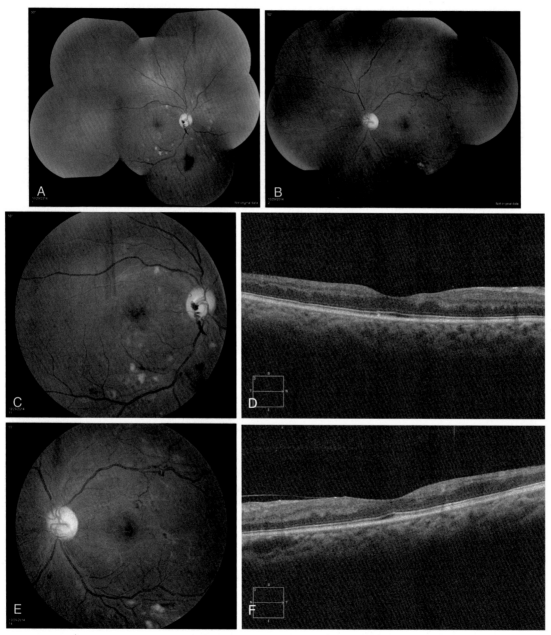

FIG. 13.17 **(A)** montage of 7 standard photos of the right eye with PDR, **(B)** Montage left eye, **(C)** Standard color photo right eye with NVD, cotton wool spots and sclerotic vesslels, **(D)** OCT right eye shows mild indistinct inner retinal layers, **(E)** Standard color photo left eye with venous beading, PDR and NVD, **(F)** OCT left eye shows mild inner retinal layer disorganization temporal to the fovea.

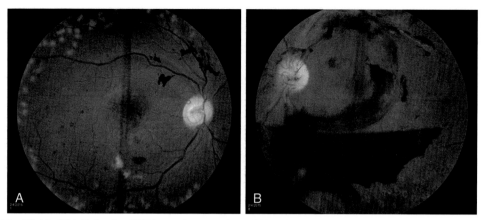

FIG. 13.18 **(A)** initially after PRP laser, there was less NVD in the right eye although some is apparent superior to the optic nerve, **(B)** There is boat shaped preretinal hemorrhage, NVD and early fibrovascular tissue.

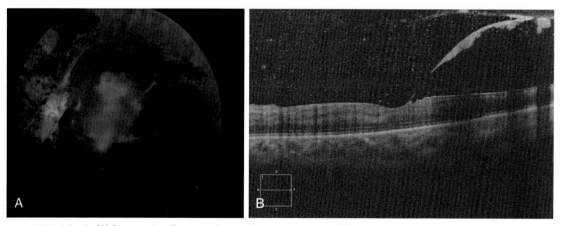

FIG. 13.19 **(A)** Progressive fibrovascular traction, extramacular TRD, preretinal hemorrhage and NVD right eye, **(B)** OCT shows vitreous hemorrhage and elevated hyaloid temporal to the macula.

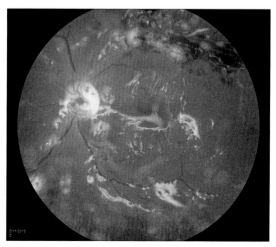

FIG. 13.20 After PPV with silicone oil, the retina is attached with resolution of the TRD.

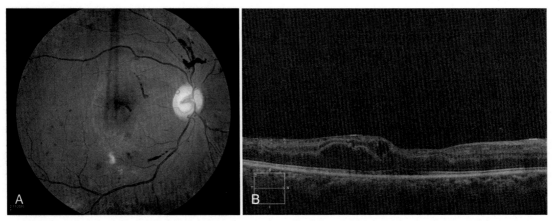

FIG. 13.21 **(A)** PDR was stable in the right eye after 4 sessions of PRP, **(B)** DME developed as seen on OCT.

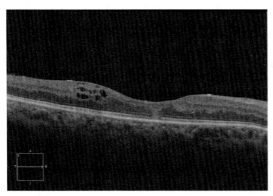

FIG. 13.22 DME improved postpartum after ranibizumab 0.3mg injections right eye.

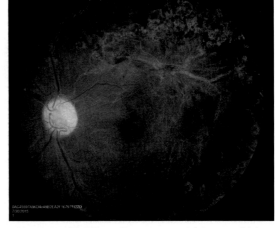

FIG. 13.23 **(A)** Af0ter silicone removal right eye with inactive PDR and resolution of TRD.

the DME did not resolve. Intravitreal anti-VEGF injections would also be favorable to induce regression of any residual PDR. Lastly, the patient presented late in the course of severe PDR without prior retinal evaluations and eventually did not return for follow-up, an all too common scenario in these patients with complicated medical issues.

REFERENCE

1. Blankenship GW. A clinical comparison of central and peripheral argon laser panretinal photocoagulation for proliferative diabetic retinopathy. *Ophthalmology.* 1988;95: 170–177.

Summary of Diabetic Retinopathy Clinical Research Network (DRCR.net) Protocols

CAROLINE R. BAUMAL, MD • XUEJING CHEN, MD

The Diabetic Retinopathy Clinical Research Network (DRCR.net) is a research organization comprising academic and private ophthalmology practices in North America. It is funded by the National Eye Institute/National Institutes of Health and also receives support from health agencies and industry. The DRCR.net has directed multiple trials evaluating relevant issues in the management of diabetic retinopathy. Each protocol is alphabetized and pertinent study details are outlined in this table. Various study types have been performed, including observational, pilot, and Phase I, II, and III studies. The evolution of DRCR study topics parallels our increasing knowledge and newly available therapeutic modalities for diabetic retinopathy since 2000. Many of the protocols and publication details are available to the public at the website www.drcr.net.

Protocol	Evaluation of	Study Group(s)	Outcome(s)	Results	Clinical Application
A	Phase II: Comparison of 2 laser techniques for DME	1. Modified ETDRS laser 2. MMG	• Change in CST on OCT at 1 year • Change in VA	1. MMG is less effective at reducing retinal thickening than modified ETDRS laser 2. VA similar with both techniques	Modified ETDRS laser remained standard for DME
B	Phase III: IVT versus focal/grid laser for DME	1. Laser 2. 1 mg IVT 3. 4 mg IVT	• VA at 2 years • CST • Complications	1. IVT 4 mg was most effective at 4 months, but laser became the most effective at 2 years 2. Treatment group differences could not be attributed solely to cataract formation 3. Laser had the least side effects	Focal/grid laser remained the standard for DME
C	Observational study: Diurnal variation of retinal thickening in DME	Eyes with CI-DME	• CST, which was measured 6 times between 8 a.m. and 4 p.m.	6% decrease in CST during the day	Although there was a slight decrease in CST during the day, most eyes with DME have little clinically significant change in CST between 8 a.m. and 4 p.m.
D	Observational study: Vitrectomy outcomes in eyes with DME and VMT	Eyes with CI-DME with VA 20/63–20/400 and VMT	• VA at 1 year after PPV ± ERM or ILM removal • CST • Complications	1. CST was reduced in most eyes 2. 28%–49% expected to have VA improvement versus 13%–31% expected VA worsening 3. Low complications rates	These estimates of surgical outcomes serve as a reference for future studies of PPV for DME in eyes with VMT
E	Phase II: ST TA ± focal laser for mild DME (VA 20/40 or better)	1. Anterior ST TA (20 mg) 2. Anterior ST TA (20 mg) + focal laser after 4 weeks 3. Posterior ST TA (40 mg) 4. Posterior ST TA (40 mg) + focal laser after 4 weeks 5. Focal laser	• Change in VA and CST at 34 weeks	No difference between treatment groups at 34 weeks	For mild DME, peribulbar TA unlikely to provide additional benefit Based on this, a Phase III trial to evaluate these treatments for mild DME was deferred

Protocol	Evaluation of	Study Group(s)	Outcome(s)	Results	Clinical Application
F	Observational study: Development of CME after one versus four sessions for PRP placement	1. Single-sitting PRP 2. Four-sitting PRP	• CST • VA	1. CST was slightly greater in the 1-sitting group than in the 4-sitting group at 3 days & 4 weeks 2. At 34 weeks, CST slightly greater in the 4-sitting group 3. VA paralleled CST changes	Minimal difference between PRP placement in 1 versus 4 sessions
G	Cross-sectional study: Retinal thickness in diabetic patients with minimal or no DR compared with normals	Eyes with no or minimal DR and no CI-DME	• CST	1. Male retinas are thicker than female retinas 2. CST similar between people with and without DM	Furthered understanding of retinal thickness in diabetes
H	Phase II: IVB ± focal laser for DME	1. Focal laser 2. IVB 1.25 mg at baseline and 6 weeks 3. IVB 2.5 mg at baseline and 6 weeks 4. IVB 1.25 mg at baseline and sham at 6 weeks 5. IVB 1.25 mg at baseline and 6 weeks with laser at 3 weeks	• CST and VA at 12 weeks	1. IVB 1.25 mg or 2.5 mg at baseline at 6 weeks had greater CST reduction than focal laser monotherapy 2. No difference between 1.25 and 2.5 mg IVB 3. Combining focal laser to IVB did not have short-term benefit	Results showed IVB can reduce DME in some eyes This short, small study was not designed to determine IVB efficacy
I	Phase III: Comparison of IVR + prompt or deferred laser versus IVT + prompt laser for DME	1. IVR 0.5 mg + prompt laser 2. IVR 0.5 mg + deferred laser 3. Sham injection + prompt laser (+/- very deferred IVR) 4. IVT 4 mg + prompt laser (± very deferred IVR)	• Change in BCVA at 1 year • Change in CST & retinal volume • Number of injections • Study was extended up to 5 years	1. VA and CST improvement with IVR ± laser are sustained over 5 years 2. Eyes receiving deferred IVR, while improved, did not do as well as eyes that received IVR as first-line treatment	IVR is more beneficial for DME than laser or IVT + laser. This study offered support of IVR as first-line therapy

Continued

Protocol	Evaluation of	Study Group(s)	Outcome(s)	Results	Clinical Application
J	Phase III: Short-term effects of IVR versus IVT on DME following focal/grid laser in eyes also receiving PRP	All eyes received focal/grid laser for DME and PRP for DR plus the following: 1. Sham injection at baseline & 4 weeks 2. IVR 0.5 mg at baseline & 4 weeks 3. IVT 4 mg at baseline + sham at 4 weeks	• Change in VA and CST at 14 weeks • Safety data at 56 weeks	1. VA & CST changes were better with IVR and IVT than sham at 14 weeks	Short-term exacerbation of DME from PRP in eyes also receiving focal can be reduced by IVR or IVT Whether continued long-term intravitreal treatment is beneficial cannot be determined from this study
K	Observational study: If eyes with DME that responded to focal/grid laser continue to improve if retreatment is deferred	Starting 16 weeks after laser and continuing every 8 weeks, eyes were assessed for retreatment and additional laser was deferred if the visual acuity letter score improved ≥5 letters or OCT CST decreased ≥10% compared with the visit 16 weeks prior	• VA & CST up to 48 weeks	16 weeks following focal/grid laser for DME, in eyes with a definite reduction, but not resolution, of central edema, 23%–63% will continue to improve without additional treatment	Results limited by small numbers An RCT would be needed to evaluate whether deferring treatment for improving eyes is of greater benefit than retreatment
L	Comparison of VA measurement using manual versus autorefraction	VA after autorefraction was compared with research protocol manual refraction	• VA	1. VA measurements tended to be worse with autorefraction 2. Results varied, depending on autorefractor used 3. Even with more favorable autorefractors, variability between auto & manual refraction was greater than test-retest for manual refraction	With current instruments, autorefraction is not an acceptable substitute for manual refraction for clinical trials
M	Phase III: Effect of diabetes education during ophthalmology visits on diabetes control	1. Patients receiving diabetes assessment & education 2. Patients undergoing usual care	• Change in HbA1c in 1 year • BMI, BP, diabetes self-management practices, & attitudes survey	1. Long-term optimization of glycemic control is not seen in the majority of patients 2. Personalized education during retinal examination visits did not improve HbA1c over 1 year	These data suggest that optimizing glycemic control remains a substantive challenge

Protocol	Evaluation of	Study Group(s)	Outcome(s)	Results	Clinical Application
N	Phase II/III: Evaluating IVR or saline for VH from PDR	Eyes with VH preventing PRP 1. IVR 0.5 mg 2. Intravitreal saline	• Cumulative probability of vitrectomy within 16 weeks • VA	1. Cumulative probability of vitrectomy was 12% in IVR and 17% in saline 2. Recurrent VH within 16 weeks occurred in 6% IVR and 17% saline	IVR does not appear to reduce vitrectomy rates compared with saline for VH from PDR
O	Cross-sectional study: Reproducibility of SD-OCT & TD-OCT in DME	Eyes underwent 2 Stratus scans and 2 Cirrus/Spectralis scans	• CST & macular volume	1. Reproducibility is best on the Spectralis 2. Conversions between SD and TD are possible	Furthered understanding between different generations of software-generated CST measurements
P	Observational study: Individuals with DME undergoing cataract surgery	Preoperative, intraoperative, and postoperative assessments up to 16 weeks	• Feasibility of an RCT • VA • CST	1. Study concluded early due to slow enrollment rate 2. As many as 50% had no meaningful improvement or worsened VA after cataract surgery	Low recruitment rates may limit a RCT Lack of standardization in DME management limited definitive conclusions
Q	Observational study: Assess for DME after cataract surgery in eyes with NC-DME operative	Patients with DR without definitive CI-DME treatment undergoing cataract surgery	• Development of CI-DME at 16 weeks	1. 10% of patients with NC-DME developed CI-DME 2. History of DME treatment was associated with development of CI-DME	Presence of NC-DME immediately before cataract surgery or history of DME treatment may increase risk of developing CI-CME 16 weeks after cataract extraction
R	Phase II: Topical nepafenac in eyes with NC-DME	1. Nepafenac 0.1% TID 2. Placebo TID	• Change in retinal volume at 12 months	1. No difference in VA 2. Clinically insignificant changes in retinal volume were seen at 12 months	Nepafenac does not have a meaningful effect on retinal thickness
S	Phase III: PRP versus IVR for PDR	1. PRP 2. IVR 0.5 mg on structured retreatment protocol	• Change in VA at 2 years • VA area under the curve, peripheral VF loss, rate of vitrectomy, DME development, retinal neovascularization	1. VA for IVR was not inferior to PRP at 2 years for treatment of PDR 2. VF loss, rate of vitrectomy, and DME development were worse in PDR arm	IVR per the Protocol S regimen may be considered for first-line PDR treatment

Continued

Protocol	Evaluation of	Study Group(s)	Outcome(s)	Results	Clinical Application
T	Phase III: IVA versus IVB versus IVR for DME	Using a strict retreatment protocol: 1. IVA 2.0 mg 2. IVB 1.25 mg 3. IVR 0.3 mg Focal/grid laser could be added at 6 months for persistent DME	• Changes in VA at 1 year • Study extended to 2 years • CST, adverse events, retreatment frequency	1. All 3 groups showed VA improvement in DME at 1 & 2 years 2. VA improvement was similar for eyes with better baseline VA 3. For eyes with worse baseline VA, IVA had better 2-year outcomes than IVB 4. Over 2 years, the cumulative number of injections was similar across all arms, with the number in year 2 being roughly half that in year 1	Offered data for choice of anti-VEGF agent
U	Phase II: IVR+IVDI versus IVR for persistent DME after anti-VEGF	1. IVR 0.3 mg + IVDI 2. IVR 0.3 mg + sham injection	• Change in VA at 24 weeks • CST	Ongoing	
V	Phase III: Treatment of DME in eyes with very good VA (20/25 or better)	1. Prompt focal/grid laser + deferred IVA 2. Prompt IVA 3. Observation + Deferred IVA	• % of eyes that have ≥5 letters of acuity at 2 years • VA, CST, change in DRSS, treatment crossovers	Ongoing	
W	Phase III: IVA for prevention of onset of PDR or CI-DME in high-risk eyes	1. Prompt sham (± deferred IVA or focal/grid laser) 2. Prompt IVA	• Efficacy of IVA on prevention of PDR/DME, VA between groups, • Should PDR/DME occur-> OCT, CST, DRSS, safety, costs	Ongoing	

Protocol	Evaluation of	Study Group(s)	Outcome(s)	Results	Clinical Application
AA	Detection of DR on UWF versus 7SF image on improvement of DR assessment and prediction of DR worsening	1. NPDR eyes will have protocol driven UWF imaging & ETDRS 7SF imaging 2. Risk of DRSS progression will be compared with the degree of far peripheral DR lesions seen in UWF but not in 7SF images	• Risk of DRSS progression over 4 years • Compare UWF to 7SF	Ongoing	
AB	Phase II/III: Prompt IVA versus prompt PPV/PRP for VH from PDR	1. Prompt IVA 2 mg 2. Prompt PPV/PRP	• VA area under curve • VA, rate of recurrent VH, CST	Ongoing	

7SF, 7 standard field; BMI, body mass index; BP, blood pressure; CI-DME, center-involved diabetic macular edema; CST, central subfield thickness on OCT; DM, diabetes mellitus; DME, diabetic macular edema; DR, diabetic retinopathy; DRSS, diabetic retinopathy severity score; ERM, epiretinal membrane; ETDRS, Early Treatment of Diabetic Retinopathy Study; HbA1c, hemoglobin A1c; ILM, internal limiting membrane; IVA, intravitreal aflibercept; IVB, intravitreal bevacizumab; IVDI, intravitreal dexamethasone implant; IVR, intravitreal ranibizumab; IVT, intravitreal triamcinolone acetonide; MMG, mild macular grid; NC-DME, non-center-involving DME; NPDR, nonproliferative diabetic retinopathy; OCT, optical coherence tomography; PC, photocoagulation; PDR, proliferative diabetic retinopathy; PPV, pars plana vitrectomy; PRP, panretinal laser photocoagulation; RCT, randomized controlled trial; SD, spectral domain; ST, subtenon injection; TA, triamcinolone acetonide; TD, time domain; UWF, ultrawide field; VA, visual acuity; VH, vitreous hemorrhage; VMT, vitreomacular traction.

APPENDIX B

Diabetic Terminology

APPENDIX: ABBREVIATIONS

The literature on diabetic retinopathy is full of abbreviations and acronyms that are continually being modified. The pertinent ones used in this book are the following.

ACE	angiotensin converting enzyme
ADA	American Diabetes Association
Anti-VEGF	Anti–vascular endothelial growth factor
ARB	angiotensin receptor blocker
BCVA	best corrected visual acuity
BMI	body mass index
BRB	blood-retinal barrier
CI-DME	center-involved diabetic macular edema
CS-DME	center-sparing diabetic macular edema
CMT	central macular thickness
CST	central subfield thickness on OCT
CSME	clinically significant diabetic macular edema
CTRRD	combined tractional rhegmatogenous retinal detachment
CVA	cerebrovascular accident
CVD	cardiovascular disease
DM	diabetes mellitus
DME	diabetic macular edema
DR	diabetic retinopathy
DRSS	diabetic retinopathy severity score
FA	fluorescein angiography
FDA	Food and Drug Administration of the United States
GWAS	genome-wide association studies
HE	hard exudate
HbA1c	hemoglobin A1c
HRC	high-risk characteristics
IDDM	insulin-dependent type 1 diabetes
ICG (A)	indocyanine green (angiography)
IL	interleukin
IOL	intraocular lens

IOP	intraocular pressure
IRMA	intraretinal microvascular abnormalities
IVA	intravitreal aflibercept (Eylea)
IVB	intravitreal bevacizumab (Avastin)
IVDI	intravitreal dexamethasone implant (Ozurdex)
IVR	intravitreal ranibizumab (Lucentis)
IVP	intravitreal pegaptanib (Macugen)
IVT	intravitreal triamcinolone acetonide
LCω3PUFA	long-chain polyunsaturated omega-3 fatty acid
LDL	low-density lipoprotein
LIO	laser indirect ophthalmoscopy
Ma	microaneurysm
MA	macroaneurysm
MVL	moderate visual loss, defined as doubling of the visual angle (i.e., 20/40 to 20/80) on two successive follow-up visits or loss of 15 or more ETDRS chart letters
MMG	mild macular grid laser
NC-DME	non-center-involving DME
NIDDM	non-insulin-dependent type 1 diabetes
NPDR	nonproliferative diabetic retinopathy
NV	neovascularization
NVD	neovascularization of the optic disc, or within 1 disc diameter from the disc margin
NVE	neovascularization elsewhere in the retina, located greater than 1 disc diameter from the optic disc margin
NVI	neovascularization of the iris
NVG	neovascular glaucoma
OCT	optical coherence tomography
OCTA	optical coherence tomography angiography
PC	photocoagulation
PDR	proliferative diabetic retinopathy
PKC	protein kinase C
PPV	pars plana vitrectomy

PRP	panretinal laser photocoagulation
RAS	renin-angiotensin system
RCT	randomized controlled trial
RPE	retinal pigment epithelium
SD-OCT	spectral domain optical coherence tomography
SNP	single nucleotide polymorphism
ST	Sub-Tenon injection
SVL	severe visual loss (defined as best corrected visual acuity of less than 5/200 on at least two consecutive 4-month follow-up visits
TA	triamcinolone acetonide
TD-OCT	time domain optical coherence tomography
TNFα	tumor necrosis factor alpha
TRD	tractional retinal detachment
UWF	ultrawide field
VA	visual acuity
VEGF	vascular endothelial growth factor
VH	vitreous hemorrhage
VMT	vitreomacular traction
WHR	waist to hip ratio
7SF	7 standard field

APPENDIX: ABBREVIATIONS FOR CLINICAL STUDIES RELATED TO DIABETES AND DIABETIC RETINOPATHY

ABCD	Appropriate Blood Pressure Control in Diabetes
ACCORD	Action to Control Cardiovascular Risk in Diabetes
BEVORDEX	Bevacizumab or Dexamethasone Implants for Diabetic Macular Edema
BOLT	Bevacizumab or Laser Therapy in the Management of Diabetic Macular Edema Study
DA VINCI	DME and VEGF Trap-Eye: Investigation of Clinical Impact study
DCCT	Diabetic Control and Complications Trial
DRCR.net	Diabetic Retinopathy Clinical Research Network
DRS	Diabetic Retinopathy Study
DRVS	Diabetic Retinopathy Vitrectomy Study

EDIC	Epidemiology of Diabetes Interventions and Complications
ETDRS	Early Treatment of Diabetic Retinopathy Study
FAME	Fluocinolone Acetonide in Diabetic Macular Edema
FIELD	Fenofibrate Intervention and Event Lowering in Diabetes
MEAD	Macular edema: Assessment of Implantable Dexamethasone in Diabetes
READ	Ranibizumab for Edema of the mAcula in Diabetes study
RESOLVE	Safety and Efficacy of Ranibizumab in Diabetic Macular Edema
RESTORE	Ranibizumab Monotherapy or Combined With Laser Versus Laser Monotherapy for Diabetic Macular Edema
REVEAL	Ranibizumab Monotherapy or Combined With Laser Versus Laser Monotherapy in Asian Patients with Diabetic Macular Edema
RISE & RIDE	Ranibizumab Injection in Subjects with Clinically Significant Macular Edema with Center-Involvement Secondary to Diabetes Mellitus
UKPDS	United Kingdom Prospective Diabetes Study
VIVID/VISTA	Intravitreal Administration of VEGF Trap-Eye (Aflibercept) in Patients with Diabetic Macular Edema
WESDR	Wisconsin Epidemiological Study of Diabetic Retinopathy

Index

A

ABCD trial. *See* Appropriate Blood Pressure Control in Diabetes trial (ABCD trial)
Absence of diabetic retinopathy, 15
ACE. *See* Angiotensin-1 converting enzyme (ACE)
Action to Control Cardiovascular Risk in Diabetes study (ACCORD study), 44–45
ADA. *See* American Diabetes Association (ADA)
Adaptive optics (AO), 33
Advanced glycation end products (AGEs), 38
Aflibercept, 54, 118, 124
Age-related macular degeneration (AMD), 53, 123
AGEs. *See* Advanced glycation end products (AGEs)
"Airlie House" classification, 15
AKB-9778 inhibitor, 127
Aldose reductase (ALR2), 37
ALG-1001, 128
ALR2. *See* Aldose reductase (ALR2)
AMD. *See* Age-related macular degeneration (AMD)
American Academy of Ophthalmology, 27
American Diabetes Association (ADA), 7, 44
Anesthesia, 92
Angelica gigas (*A. gigas*), 127
Angiopoietin 1 (Ang1), 127
Angiopoietin 2 (Ang2), 127
Angiopoietin pathway modulation, 127
Angiotensin receptor blockers (ARBs), 46
Angiotensin type I receptor (AT1 receptor), 37
Angiotensin-1 converting enzyme (ACE), 37
inhibitor, 45–46
Angiovue, 31–32
Anti-VEGF agents. *See* Anti–vascular endothelial growth factor agents (Anti-VEGF agents)
Anti-VEGF designed ankyrin repeat protein (DAPRin), 125–127
Antiangiogenesis therapies development, 53
Antibody fragment (Fab), 53

Antiplatelet agents, 102
Anti–vascular endothelial growth factor agents (Anti-VEGF agents), 4, 41, 101–102, 104, 111, 117–118, 124, 133
"crunch", 74
development of ocular, 75
in DME, 54–70, 56t–66t
aflibercept, 68–69, 69f
bevacizumab, 67–68
pegaptanib, 55
ranibizumab, 55–67
treatment, 133–140
drugs, 101
history and impact, 53
injections, 89, 103
and NVI/NVG, 56t–66t
in PDR, 56t–66t, 70–74, 70f–71f
combined anti-VEGF agents with PPV *vs.* PPV alone, 74
in eyes unresponsive to PRP, 73–74
plus PRP *vs.* PRP alone, 72–73
vs. PRP, 72
vs. sham or saline, 71–72
and non-center-involving DME, 142–145
and PPV, 56t–66t
for proliferative diabetic retinopathy, 96–97
role in treatment of NVI and NVG, 74–75
safety, 75
treatment, 124–125, 126t
AO. *See* Adaptive optics (AO)
AO-SLO, 33
Appropriate Blood Pressure Control in Diabetes trial (ABCD trial), 45–46
Arachidonic acid, 79–80
ARBs. *See* Angiotensin receptor blockers (ARBs)
Argon laser, 89
Arrhenius model, 89–90
Arteriothrombotic events (ATEs), 75
Aspirin therapy, 48
Asymmetric diabetic retinopathy, 140–142, 140f–141f
AT1 receptor. *See* Angiotensin type I receptor (AT1 receptor)
ATEs. *See* Arteriothrombotic events (ATEs)
Automated software, 27, 29–31
Avastin. *See* Bevacizumab

B

B-catenin, 54
B-scan ultrasonography, 103–104
Basement membrane thickening (BM thickening), 15–16
Best corrected visual acuity (BCVA), 9, 55
Bevacizumab, 53, 103, 124, 129, 133–134
injections, 74, 86
Bevacizumab or Laser Therapy (BOLT), 96, 134
BEVORDEX study, 85
Binocular indirect ophthalmoscopy, 10
Biomicroscopy, 13
Blood-retinal barrier (BRB), 79
Blot hemorrhages, 9–10
Blue spectrum range, 89
BM thickening. *See* Basement membrane thickening (BM thickening)
Body mass index (BMI), 47
BOLT. *See* Bevacizumab or Laser Therapy (BOLT)
Branch retinal vein occlusion, 123
BRB. *See* Blood-retinal barrier (BRB)
Broad-spectrum growth factor suppression, 127

C

Candidate Gene Association Resource (CARe), 38
Candidate genes, 37–38
ACE, 37
ALR2, 37
eNOS, 37–38
RAGE, 38
VEGF, 38
Capillary acellularity, 16–17
Capillary nonperfusion, 32
Cardiovascular disease (CVD), 44
CARe. *See* Candidate Gene Association Resource (CARe)
Carotid stenosis, 142
Cataract surgery, 110
Category C drug, 98
CDC. *See* Centers for Disease Control and Prevention (CDC)
Center-involving CSME, 19–20
Center-involving diabetic macular edema (CI-DME), 4, 31, 96, 110
treatment for, 96

Note: Page numbers followed by "f" indicate figures, "t" indicate tables.

Centers for Disease Control and Prevention (CDC), 7
Central macular thickness (CMT), 72, 80
Central retinal thickness (CRT), 55
Central subfield thickness (CST), 31
Cerebrovascular accident (CVA), 75
Chandelier illuminators, 109
Chandelier intraocular illumination, 101
Chromovitrectomy, 109–110
Chronic hyperglycemia, 41–43
CI-DME. *See* Center-involving diabetic macular edema (CI-DME)
Clinical diagnosis, 7
    asymmetric diabetic retinopathy with PDR and noncenter-involving DME, 140–142
    DME treatment with anti–VEGF injection and sustained-release steroid implant, 133–140
    examination features, 12t
    examination intervals and treatment options in diabetic eye disease, 8t
    history and examination, 8–13, 9t
    PDR and non-center-involving DME, treating with laser, 142–145
    rapidly progressive PDR to tractional retinal detachment in pregnancy, 145–148
    screening recommendations, 7–8
    timing of initial ophthalmic examination in diabetes, 8t
    wide-field fluorescein angiogram, 11f
Clinically significant macular edema (CSME), 4, 13, 15, 27, 73, 93
CMT. *See* Central macular thickness (CMT)
CNV process, 97
Collimation, 89
Combination therapy, 86–87
Combined tractional with rhegmatogenous retinal detachment (CTRRD), 101, 104, 108–109, 111
Complete diabetic eye examination, 8
Complete diabetic ocular examination, 9
Computer-guided scanning systems, 93–96
Concomitant cataract and vitreous pathologies, 101
Conventional diet control, 44
Corticosteroids, 79–80, 81t–82t, 89
    combination therapy, 86–87
    effect on progression, 86
    for treatment of diabetic macular edema, 80–86
Cotton wool spots (CWS), 15–16
CRT. *See* Central retinal thickness (CRT)
CSME. *See* Clinically significant macular edema (CSME)
CST. *See* Central subfield thickness (CST)

CTRRD. *See* Combined tractional with rhegmatogenous retinal detachment (CTRRD)
Cutting techniques, 104–105
CVA. *See* Cerebrovascular accident (CVA)
CVD. *See* Cardiovascular disease (CVD)
CWS. *See* Cotton wool spots (CWS)
Cyclooxygenase inhibitors, 129
Cyclopentolate, 116

D
DA VINCI studies, 68, 96
Danazol, 124
DAPRin. *See* Anti-VEGF designed ankyrin repeat protein (DAPRin)
DCCT. *See* Diabetes Control and Complications Trial (DCCT)
DCRC.net Protocol N, 97–98
Decursin, 127
DEGAS trial, 129
Delamination, 105–107
Dexamethasone implant, 118
DFE. *See* Dilated fundus examination (DFE)
Diabetes, 7, 101
    risk factors for diabetes progression, 115–116
    timing of initial ophthalmic examination in, 8t
Diabetes Control and Complications Trial (DCCT), 3, 43
Diabetes mellitus (DM), 1, 7, 79
    classification, pathogenesis, and epidemiology, 1–2
    economic burden, 2
    systemic manifestations, 2
Diabetic eye disease, anti–VEGF therapy for
    anti-VEGF agents, 53–54, 75
        development of ocular, 75
        in DME, 54–70
        in PDR, 70–74
        role in treatment of NVI and NVG, 74–75
    history and impact, 53
Diabetic eyes, 33, 102–103
Diabetic intraretinal hemorrhage, 9–10, 10f
Diabetic macular edema (DME), 2, 12–13, 19–20, 25, 29–31, 41, 54, 72, 79, 89, 101, 117–118, 123, 133
    anti-VEGF agents in, 54–70
    asymmetric diabetic retinopathy with PDR and noncenter-involving DME, 140–142
    corticosteroids for treatment, 80–86
        injection into suprachoroidal space, 86
        intravitreal injection, 83–84
        intravitreal injection of slow-release corticosteroid implants, 84–86

Diabetic macular edema (DME) *(Continued)*
        sub-tenon injection, 80–83
        topical administration of steroids, 80
    first-line treatment, 134
    management, 4
    modern DR and treatment, 123
    PDR in setting, 98
    prevalence, 3
    treatment, 117–118, 119f
        with anti–VEGF injection and sustained-release steroid implant, 133–140, 134f–135f, 137f, 139f
Diabetic retinopathy (DR), 1, 7, 25, 37, 79, 89, 101, 110, 123
    classification, 15
        absence, 15
        DME, 19–20
        NPDR, 15–19
        pathogenesis, 15
        proliferative, 20–21
    clinical studies of anti-VEGF agents, 56t–66t
    combination therapy, 86–87
    corticosteroids, 81t–82t
        effect on progression, 86
        for treatment of DME, 80–86
    diabetes mellitus, 1–2
    DME
        management, 4
        prevalence, 3
    epidemiology, 2–3
    inflammation role, 79–80
    laser for, 91–92
    natural history, 2
        in type I DM, 2–3
        in type II DM, 3
    NPDR and PDR management, 3–4
    treatments
        angiopoietin pathway modulation, 127
        anti-VEGF treatment, 124–125
        broad-spectrum growth factor suppression, 127
        diagnostic and treatment considerations during pregnancy, 116–117
        of DME, 117–118
        enzymatic vitreolysis, 128
        extended-release anti-VEGF technology, 125
        modern DR and DME treatment, 123
        nonsteroidal antiinflammatory therapy, 129–130
        novel anti-VEGF agents, 125–127
        novel large molecule therapy, 127–128
        of PDR, 117
        PKC β inhibition, 128–129
        in pregnancy, 115

Diabetic retinopathy (DR) *(Continued)*
   risk factors for diabetes
      progression during pregnancy,
      115–116
   screening guidelines for diabetic
      women, 116
   siRNA, 129
   somatostatin analogues, 124
   topical treatments, 128
Diabetic Retinopathy Candesartan
   Trials Protect 1 study (DIRECT
   Protect 1 study), 46
Diabetic Retinopathy Clinical Research
   Network (DRCR.net), 45, 83, 101–102
   protocols, 93, 96–97
      DRCR Protocol R, 129
      DRCR. net Protocol F, 92
      DRCR.net Protocol I, 96, 134
   studies, 83
Diabetic retinopathy severity score
   (DRSS), 25, 41
Diabetic Retinopathy Study (DRS), 92,
   101, 142–145
Diabetic Retinopathy Vitrectomy Study
   (DRVS), 101–102
Diabetic TRD, 11–12
Diabetic vitrectomy, complications of,
   110–111
Diabetic women, screening guidelines
   for, 116, 116t
Dietary intake of polyunsaturated fatty
   acids, 47
Diffuse DME, 19
Digital retinal imaging, 25
Dilated fundus examination (DFE), 7
Diode, 91–92
DIRECT Protect 1 study. *See* Diabetic
   Retinopathy Candesartan Trials Protect
   1 study (DIRECT Protect 1 study)
Distension of capillary wall, 16
DM. *See* Diabetes mellitus (DM)
DME. *See* Diabetic macular edema (DME)
DR. *See* Diabetic retinopathy (DR)
DRCR.net. *See* Diabetic Retinopathy
   Clinical Research Network (DRCR.net)
DRS. *See* Diabetic Retinopathy Study
   (DRS)
DRSS. *See* Diabetic retinopathy severity
   score (DRSS)
DRVS. *See* Diabetic Retinopathy
   Vitrectomy Study (DRVS)
Dye-based angiography, 27–29
   FA, 27–29

E

Early Anti-VEGF Response and Long-
   term efficacY (EARLY), 87
Early Treatment of Diabetic
   Retinopathy Study (ETDRS), 3–4,
   13, 15, 17t, 18f–20f, 21, 21t, 27, 48,
   54–55, 80–83, 92, 101, 129
   Protocol l, 96
   research group, 93

ECM. *See* Extracellular matrix (ECM)
EDIC study. *See* Epidemiology
   of Diabetes Interventions and
   Complications study (EDIC study)
Elevated blood glucose, 2
Enalapril, 45–46
Endothelial nitric oxide synthase
   (eNOS), 37–38
Enzymatic vitreolysis, 128
Epidemiology of Diabetes
   Interventions and Complications
   study (EDIC study), 3, 43
Epigenetics, 38–39
Epiretinal membrane (ERM), 104
ETDRS. *See* Early Treatment of Diabetic
   Retinopathy Study (ETDRS)
Extended-release anti-VEGF
   technology, 125
Extracellular matrix (ECM), 128
Eylea. *See* Aflibercept

F

FA. *See* Fluorescein angiography (FA)
Fab. *See* Antibody fragment (Fab)
Factor X, 53
FAF. *See* Fundus autofluorescence (FAF)
FAME. *See* Fluocinolone Acetonide in
   Diabetic Macular Edema (FAME)
Familial studies, 37
Family Investigation of Nephropathy
   and Diabetes Eye study (FIND Eye
   study), 37
Fasting plasma glucose (FPG), 44
FAZ. *See* Foveal avascular zone (FAZ)
FDA. *See* US Food and Drug
   Administration (FDA)
Fenofibrate Intervention and Event
   Lowering in Diabetes study (FIELD
   study), 47
Fibrovascular proliferation (FVP), 11–12
FIELD study. *See* Fenofibrate
   Intervention and Event Lowering in
   Diabetes study (FIELD study)
FIND Eye study. *See* Family
   Investigation of Nephropathy and
   Diabetes Eye study (FIND Eye study)
Fluocinolone acetonide, 85–86
Fluocinolone Acetonide in Diabetic
   Macular Edema (FAME), 85–86
Fluorescein angiography (FA), 10, 16,
   25, 27–29, 93, 116–117, 133
Focal DME, 19
Focal laser, 91
   effect, 90
   photocoagulation, 92–93, 94f, 95t, 96
Foveal avascular zone (FAZ), 16–17, 32
FPG. *See* Fasting plasma glucose (FPG)
Fundus autofluorescence (FAF), 25–27,
   33–34
Fundus photography, 25–27, 116–117
Funduscopic examination, 102–103
FVP. *See* Fibrovascular proliferation
   (FVP)

G

Genetics, 37
   candidate genes, 37–38
   epigenetics and diabetic retinopathy,
      38–39
   familial studies, 37
   linkage studies, 38
Genome-wide association studies
   (GWAS), 38
Gestational diabetes, 1–2
Glycemic control, 41–45
Gonioscopic evaluation, 102–103
Gonioscopy, 110
Green spectrum range, 89
Grid laser photocoagulation, 92–93,
   94f, 95t, 96
GWAS. *See* Genome-wide association
   studies (GWAS)

H

Hard exudates, 9–10, 10f, 16, 16f,
   29–31
HbA1C, 3
Hemoglobin, 91
Hemoglobin A1c (HgbA1c), 43
Hemorrhages, 9–10
HgbA1c. *See* Hemoglobin A1c
   (HgbA1c)
High-quality fundus photographs, 8
High-risk characteristics (HRC),
   141–142
High-risk PDR, 20
Hyaloid disruption, 103
3-Hydroxy-3-methylglutaryl coenzyme
   A, 46–47
Hyperglycemia, 79, 128–129
Hypertension, 45, 48, 115–116

I

ICG. *See* Indocyanine green (ICG)
IDDM. *See* Insulin-dependent diabetes
   mellitus (IDDM)
IL. *See* Interleukin (IL)
Illuminated lasers, 101
ILM. *See* Internal limiting membrane
   (ILM)
Iluvien. *See* Intravitreal fluocinolone
Imaging, 25
   AO, 33
   color standard and red-free
      photographs, 33f
   different modalities, 26f
   dye-based angiography, 27–29
   FAF, 33–34
   fundus photography, 25–27
   OCT, 29–31, 30f
   OCTA, 31–32
   telemedicine, 27
   ultrasound imaging, 34
In lifting techniques, 104–105
Indocyanine green (ICG),
   25–27, 29
Infectious endophthalmitis, 84

Inflammation role in diabetic
    retinopathy, 79–80
Infliximab, 129
Insulin-dependent diabetes mellitus
    (IDDM), 43, 70
Insulin-dependent type 1 diabetes. *See*
    Insulin-dependent diabetes mellitus
    (IDDM)
Integrin peptide therapy, 128
Intensive blood glucose control, 44
Interleukin (IL), 79, 127
    IL-6, 79
    IL-8, 79
Internal limiting membrane (ILM),
    109–110
International Clinical Diabetic
    Retinopathy Disease Severity Scale,
    15, 17–18, 18t
Intraocular corticosteroid
    development, 123
Intraocular lens (IOL), 103
Intraocular pressure (IOP), 71, 80,
    104, 110
Intraocular steroids, 98
Intraoperative considerations and
    complications, 111
Intraoperative OCT, 109–110
Intraretinal hemorrhage(s), 9–10, 16
Intraretinal microvascular
    abnormalities (IRMAs), 9–11,
    15–16
Intravenous TNF-α therapy, 129
Intravitreal aflibercept in DME, 69f
Intravitreal anti-VEGF
    injection, 96, 145–148
    medications, 98
Intravitreal bevacizumab (IVB), 67,
    68f, 104–105
Intravitreal corticosteroid, 103
Intravitreal dexamethasone,
    123, 133
Intravitreal fluocinolone, 123
Intravitreal injection, 83–84
    of slow-release corticosteroid
        implants, 84–86
Intravitreal pegaptanib (IVP), 53
Intravitreal ranibizumab (IVR), 53,
    71–72
Intravitreal steroids, 124
Intravitreal triamcinolone (IVT), 83,
    123
IOL. *See* Intraocular lens (IOL)
IOP. *See* Intraocular pressure (IOP)
IRMAs. *See* Intraretinal microvascular
    abnormalities (IRMAs)
Irregular vessel geometry, 31–32
Ischemia, 20
IVB. *See* Intravitreal bevacizumab
    (IVB)
IVP. *See* Intravitreal pegaptanib (IVP)
IVR. *See* Intravitreal ranibizumab (IVR)
IVT. *See* Intravitreal triamcinolone
    (IVT)

L
Large molecule therapy, 127–128
Laser indirect ophthalmoscope (LIO),
    90–91
Laser, 89, 96
    complications, 97
    parameters, 91
    PDR and non-center-involving DME,
        142–145
    photocoagulation, 89–90, 107
    PRP, 117
    radiation, 89
    therapy, 134
Laser treatment
    complications of laser, 97
    delivery systems, 90–91, 91t
    for diabetic retinopathy, 91–92
    focal/grid laser photocoagulation,
        92–93
    history of, 89
    laser parameters, 91
    laser *vs.* intravitreal anti-VEGF
        injection, 96
    laser-tissue interactions, 89–90
    navigated laser photocoagulation
        technique, 96
    noncompliant patient, 97
    pattern scanning, 93–96
    PDR
        in setting of DME, 98
        in setting of vitreous hemorrhage,
            97–98
    pregnancy, 98
    principles of, 89, 90f
    PRP, 92
        vs. anti-VEGF therapy for
            proliferative diabetic
            retinopathy, 96–97
    special considerations, 97
    subthreshold micropulse laser, 96
LCω3PUFAs. *See* Long-chain
    polyunsaturated omega-3 fatty acids
    (LCω3PUFAs)
LDL. *See* Low-density lipoprotein
    (LDL)
Lidocaine, 117
Linkage studies, 38
LIO. *See* Laser indirect
    ophthalmoscope (LIO)
Lipid exudation, 19
Long-chain polyunsaturated omega-3
    fatty acids (LCω3PUFAs), 47
Low-density lipoprotein (LDL), 46
Lucentis. *See* Ranibizumab

M
Macugen. *See* Pegaptanib
Macular interface pathologies, 109–110
Macular ischemia, 31
Mainster focal grid lenses, 90–91
Mainster PRP lenses, 90–91
Maturation of retinal neovascular
    complex, 11–12, 12f

MCP. *See* Monocyte chemotactic
    protein (MCP)
Melanin, 91–92
MI. *See* Myocardial infarction (MI)
Microaneurysms, 16, 16f, 32
Microcannulas, 111
Microincisional vitrectomy (MIVS),
    104, 109, 111
Microwave oscillator, 89
Mild macular grid laser technique
    (MMG laser technique), 93
Mild NPDR, 17
MIVS. *See* Microincisional vitrectomy
    (MIVS)
MMG laser technique. *See* Mild
    macular grid laser technique (MMG
    laser technique)
Moderate NPDR, 17
Modifiable risk factor effect, 41, 42t
    aspirin therapy, 48
    dietary intake of polyunsaturated
        fatty acids, 47
    evidence based assessment, 42t–43t
    evidence for, 41
    glycemic control, 41–45
    hypertension, 45
    inhibition of renin-angiotensin
        system, 45–46
    obesity, 48
    physical activity and sedentary
        behavior, 47
    serum lipid levels, 46–47
    smoking, 48
Modified Airlie House classification, 15
Monochromaticity, 89
Monocyte chemotactic protein (MCP),
    129
Multimodal imaging, 25
Myocardial infarction (MI), 41, 75

N
National Eye Institute (NEI), 7
Navigated laser photocoagulation
    technique, 96
NEI. *See* National Eye Institute (NEI)
Neodymium-doped yttrium aluminum
    garnet (Nd:YAG), 91–92
Neovascular glaucoma (NVG), 53, 101,
    110–111
    anti-VEGF agents role in treatment,
        74–75
Neovascularization (NVI), 20, 20f, 53
Neovascularization elsewhere (NVE),
    10–11, 20
Neovascularization of disc (NVD), 10,
    11f, 20, 140–141
Nephropathy, 1
Neuropathy, 1
NF-κB. *See* Nuclear factor kappalight-
    chain-enhancer of activated B cells
    (NF-κB)
Nisoldipine, 45–46
Nitric oxide (NO), 37–38

NO. *See* Nitric oxide (NO)
Non-center-involved DME (Non-CI-DME), 31, 110
asymmetric diabetic retinopathy with noncenter-involving DME, 140–142
treating with laser non-center-involving DME, 142–145
Noncompliant patient, 97
Noncontact condensing lens, 90–91
Noninferiority study, 96–97
Nonproliferative diabetic retinopathy (NPDR), 2, 7, 9–10, 15–19, 67–68, 115, 124, 133
management, 3–4
Nonsteroidal antiinflammatory drug (NSAID), 127
Nonsteroidal antiinflammatory therapy, 129–130
NPDR. *See* Nonproliferative diabetic retinopathy (NPDR)
NSAID. *See* Nonsteroidal antiinflammatory drug (NSAID)
Nuclear factor kappalight-chain-enhancer of activated B cells (NF-κB), 79
NVD. *See* Neovascularization of disc (NVD)
NVE. *See* Neovascularization elsewhere (NVE)
NVG. *See* Neovascular glaucoma (NVG)
NVI. *See* Neovascularization (NVI)

O
Obesity, 48
Occludin, 54
Ocriplasmin, 128
OCT. *See* Optical coherence tomography (OCT)
OCTA. *See* Optical coherence tomography angiography (OCTA)
Octreotide, 124
Ocular anti-VEGF agents development, 75
Ocular ischemic, 142
Ocular Therapeutix, 125
OHR-102. *See* Squalamine
Omega 3-fatty acids, 47
Ophthalmic ultrasound imaging, 34
Ophthalmology, anti-VEGF agents in, 53–54, 54t
Optical coherence tomography (OCT), 13, 16, 19–20, 25, 29–31, 30f, 55–67, 93, 102–104, 116–117, 133
Optical coherence tomography angiography (OCTA), 15, 25, 31–32, 102–103, 117
Optical light, 89
Optimal laser power, 91
Optina. *See* Danazol
Oxidative stress, 79
Ozurdex, 84, 85f, 123

P
PACORES study, 67
Panretinal laser photocoagulation (PRP), 70, 90–92, 96–97, 97t, 101, 117, 141–142
anti-VEGF agents plus PRP *vs.* PRP alone, 72–73
anti-VEGF agents *vs.*, 72
anti-VEGF in eyes unresponsive to, 73–74
Panretinal photocoagulation. *See* Panretinal laser photocoagulation (PRP)
Pars plana vitrectomy (PPV), 71–72, 101
combined anti-VEGF agents with PPV *vs.* PPV alone, 74
PASCAL. *See* Pattern scanning laser photocoagulator (PASCAL)
Pathogenesis of diabetic retinopathy, 15
Pattern scanning, 93–96
Pattern scanning laser photocoagulator (PASCAL), 93–96
Pazopanib, 128
PDR. *See* Proliferative diabetic retinopathy (PDR)
Pegaptanib, 53
PEGF. *See* Pigment-epithelium derived growth factor (PEGF)
Perfluoropropane (C_3F_8), 107
Peripheral diabetic pathology, 27–28
Persistent DME, 84
PF-655, 129
Phenylephrine, 116
Photochemical laser-tissue interactions, 89–90
Photomechanical laser-tissue interactions, 89–90
Photothermal effects, 89–90
Photothermal laser-tissue interactions, 89–90
Physical activity, 47
Pigment-epithelium derived growth factor (PEGF), 127
Pigmented dyes, 109–110
PKC β. *See* Protein kinase C β (PKC β)
PLACID study, 84
Platelet aggregation and disaggregation, 48
Polylactic-co-glycolic acid, 84
Polyol pathway, 37
Polyunsaturated fatty acids, dietary intake of, 47
Posterior segment neovascularization, 10–11
Posterior sub-Tenon Kenalog injection (PSTK injection), 118, 119f
Posterior vitreous detachment (PVD), 128
Postoperative anterior segment neovascularization, 111
PPV. *See* Pars plana vitrectomy (PPV)
Preeclampsia, 115–116

Pregnancy, 98
category C medications, 116
diabetic retinopathy treatment in, 115
hormonal changes, 1–2
rapidly progressive PDR to tractional retinal detachment in, 145–148
Preretinal hemorrhage, 11, 12f, 103–104
Progression of DR, 86
Progressive DME, 117–118
Progressive fibrovascular proliferation, 104
Proliferative diabetic retinopathy (PDR), 2, 7, 16–17, 20–21, 27–28, 41, 54, 89, 101, 115, 124, 140–141
anti-VEGF agents in, 70–74, 70f–71f
asymmetric diabetic retinopathy with, 140–142
management, 3–4
new treatments for, 101–102
rapidly progressive PDR to tractional retinal detachment in, 145–148, 146f–148f
in setting of DME, 98
in setting of vitreous hemorrhage, 97–98
treating with laser, 142–145, 143f–144f
treatment, 117
wide-field fluorescein angiogram in, 11f
Proparacaine, 92
Prospective interventional studies, 47
Prospective randomized studies, 98
Prostaglandin inhibitors, 129
Protein kinase C β (PKC β), 128–129
inhibition, 128–129
Protocol H of DRCR.net, 134
Protocol I, 98
Protocol S, 96–97
Protocol T of DRCR.net, 134
PRP. *See* Panretinal laser photocoagulation (PRP)
Pseudoendophthalmitis, 84
Pseudohypopyon, 84
Pseudophakic cystoid macular edema, 27
PSTK injection. *See* Posterior sub-Tenon Kenalog (PSTK injection)
PVD. *See* Posterior vitreous detachment (PVD)

Q
Quadraspheric lenses, 90–91

R
RAGE. *See* Receptor for advanced glycation end products (RAGE)
Randomized clinical control trials, 96
Ranibizumab, 53, 98, 101–102, 118, 124, 145–148

Ranibizumab Injection in Subjects with Clinically Significant Macular Edema with Center-Involvement Secondary to Diabetes Mellitus trials (RISE/RIDE trials), 44–45, 134

Ranibizumab Monotherapy, 134

Ranibizumab Monotherapy or Combined With Laser vs. Laser Monotherapy in Asian Patients with Diabetic Macular Edema study (REVEAL study), 67, 134

Ranibizumab monotherapy or combined with laser vs. laser monotherapy for diabetic macular edema study (RESTORE study), 67, 93, 96, 98

Rapamycin, 127

RAS. See Renin-angiotensin system (RAS)

READ-2 trials, 96, 98

Receptor for advanced glycation end products (RAGE), 37–38

Renin-angiotensin system (RAS), 37, 41
  inhibition of, 45–46

RESOLVE study, 98

RESTORE study. See Ranibizumab monotherapy or combined with laser vs. laser monotherapy for diabetic macular edema study (RESTORE study)

Retinal breaks, 11–12

Retinal capillary nonperfusion of neural retina, 16

Retinal imaging in diabetes, 25

Retinal ischemia, 104–105

Retinal neovascularization, 29–31

Retinal nerve fiber layer (RNFL), 25

Retinal pigment epithelium (RPE), 29–31, 90, 104

Retinal thinning, 92–93

Retinal vascular disease, 128

Retinal vein occlusion (RVO), 54

Retinopathy, 1
  progression, 44

REVEAL study. See Ranibizumab Monotherapy or Combined With Laser vs. Laser Monotherapy in Asian Patients with Diabetic Macular Edema study (REVEAL study)

RISE/RIDE trials. See Ranibizumab Injection in Subjects with Clinically Significant Macular Edema with Center-Involvement Secondary to Diabetes Mellitus trials (RISE/RIDE trials)

RNFL. See Retinal nerve fiber layer (RNFL)

Rod b-wave amplitude, 73

RPE. See Retinal pigment epithelium (RPE)

RTP801 gene, 129

Rubeosis iridis, 9, 123

Ruboxistaurin, 128–129

Ruby laser, 89

RVO. See Retinal vein occlusion (RVO)

S

Safety, anti-VEGF agents, 75

Saline, 71–72

Scanning laser ophthalmoscopy (SLO), 33

Scleral bucking surgery, 101

Screening recommendations, 7–8

SCS. See Suprachoroidal space (SCS)

Sedentary behavior, 47

Serum lipid levels, 46–47

Severe visual loss (SVL), 101

Sham injection, 71–72, 84–85

Sham subconjunctival saline injection, 83

Short-wave FAF, 33–34

Sight-threatening DME, 117–118

Silicone oil, 107, 117

Single nucleotide polymorphisms (SNPs), 38

siRNA. See Small interfering RNA (siRNA)

Slit lamp
  delivery systems, 90–91
  evaluation, 102–103

SLO. See Scanning laser ophthalmoscopy (SLO)

Slow-release corticosteroid implants, intravitreal injection of, 84–86

Small interfering RNA (siRNA), 129

Small-gauge instrumentation, 101

Small-gauge vitrectomy platforms, 101, 104–105

Smoking, 48

SNPs. See Single nucleotide polymorphisms (SNPs)

Somatostatin analogues, 124

Spatial coherence, 89

Squalamine, 128

Standard fundus photography, 25

Statins, 46–47

Stereoscopic imaging and viewing, 25

Sterile endophthalmitis, 84

Steroid(s), 123
  response, 80
  topical administration, 80

Stroke, 41

Sub-tenon injection, 80–83

Subthreshold micropulse laser, 96

SuperQuad lenses, 90–91

Suprachoroidal space (SCS), 123–124
  injection into, 86

Surgical treatment of diabetic retinopathy, 101
  cataract surgery, 110
  combined tractional with rhegmatogenous retinal detachment, 108–109
  complications of diabetic vitrectomy, 110–111

Surgical treatment of diabetic retinopathy (Continued)
  intraoperative considerations and complications, 111
  macular interface pathologies, 109–110
  new treatments for PDR, 101–102
  NVG, 110
  preoperative considerations, 102–103, 102f–103f
  TRD, 104–107
  vitreous hemorrhage and preretinal hemorrhages, 103–104

Sustained-release steroid implant, DME treatment with, 133–140

SVL. See Severe visual loss (SVL)

T

Telemedicine, 27

Tethadur, 125

Tetracaine, 92

TG10081 inhibitors, 128

3-D surgical viewing systems, 101

Tie-2 pathway, 127

TNFα. See Tumor necrosis factor α (TNFα)

Tobacco smoke, 48

Topical administration of steroids, 80

Topical anesthetic eye drop, 92

Traction retinal detachment (TRD), 10, 70, 101, 104–107, 105f–107f

Tractional pathology, 11–12

TRD. See Traction retinal detachment (TRD)

Triamcinolone
  intravitreal injection of, 83
  stain, 109–110
  sub-Tenon injection of, 83

Triesence, 118

Tropicamide, 116

Tumor necrosis factor α (TNFα), 79, 129

Type 1 diabetes, 1, 115
  natural history of diabetic retinopathy, 2–3

Type 2 diabetes, 1, 115, 133
  natural history of diabetic retinopathy, 3

Tyrosine kinase inhibitors, 128

Tyrosine phosphate β inhibitor, 127

U

UKPDS. See United Kingdom Prospective Diabetes Study (UKPDS)

UKPDS-HDS. See United Kingdom Prospective Diabetes Study-Hypertension in Diabetes Study (UKPDS-HDS)

Ultrafield lenses, 90–91

Ultrasound imaging, 34

Ultrawide field imaging (UWF imaging), 25–27, 28f

Ultrawide-angle photography, 108–109
Ultrawide-field photography, 102–103, 103f
United Kingdom Prospective Diabetes Study (UKPDS), 3, 43
United Kingdom Prospective Diabetes Study-Hypertension in Diabetes Study (UKPDS-HDS), 3
US Food and Drug Administration (FDA), 53, 83
UWF imaging. *See* Ultrawide field imaging (UWF imaging)

V

VA. *See* Visual acuity (VA)
Valsalva maneuvers, 11
Vascular endothelial growth factor (VEGF), 37–38, 53, 79
   VEGF-A, 54
   VEGF-trap and functions, 54
Vascular endothelial growth factor inhibitors (VEGF inhibitors). *See* Anti–vascular endothelial growth factor agents (Anti-VEGF agents)

Vascular leakage, 19
Vascular permeability factor, 53
VEGF. *See* Vascular endothelial growth factor (VEGF)
Venous beading, 9–10, 10f, 16
Viscoelastic dissection, 104–105, 106f
Vision-threatening retinopathy, 7
Visual acuity (VA), 80
Visual field loss, 97
Vitrectomy, 104–105, 109–110
Vitreomacular traction (VMT), 101
Vitreous hemorrhage, 11, 103–104
   PDR in setting of, 97–98
Vitreous traction, 11, 19
VIVID/VISTA studies, 134
VMT. *See* Vitreomacular traction (VMT)
Volk Area Centralis lenses, 90–91
Volk SuperQuad lens, 92

W

Waist-hip-ratio (WHR), 48
WDRS. *See* Wisconsin Diabetes Registry Study (WDRS)
Weight loss, 48

WESDR. *See* Wisconsin Epidemiologic Study of Diabetic Retinopathy (WESDR)
WHR. *See* Waist-hip-ratio (WHR)
Wide-angle viewing systems, 101, 104
Wide-field contact lenses, 90–91
Wisconsin Diabetes Registry Study (WDRS), 2–3
Wisconsin Epidemiologic Study of Diabetic Retinopathy (WESDR), 2–3, 15, 45

X

Xenon arc photocoagulator, 89

Z

Zonula occludens-1, 54

Printed in the United States
By Bookmasters